Psychedelic Experience

Revealing the Mind

AIDAN LYON

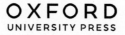

OXFORD
UNIVERSITY PRESS

Great Clarendon Street, Oxford, OX2 6DP,
United Kingdom

Oxford University Press is a department of the University of Oxford.
It furthers the University's objective of excellence in research, scholarship,
and education by publishing worldwide. Oxford is a registered trade mark of
Oxford University Press in the UK and in certain other countries

Published in the United States of America by Oxford University Press
198 Madison Avenue, New York, NY 10016, United States of America

British Library Cataloguing in Publication Data

Data available

Library of Congress Control Number: 2022948020

ISBN 978–0–19–884375–7

Printed and bound by
CPI Group (UK) Ltd, Croydon, CR0 4YY

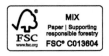

MIX
Paper | Supporting
responsible forestry
FSC
www.fsc.org   FSC® C013604

Contents

Preface

This book was born out of several psychedelic experiences I had in Amsterdam starting around 2014. There were four in particular that influenced its development.

The first experience kick-started the general philosophical project and, in a way, was the culmination of my initial series of experiences. Like so many people, I was deeply transformed by my psychedelic experiences. I found that they were helping me be more creative and insightful and generally live a better, healthier life. It was clear that these experiences were incredibly valuable. However, they were also curiously variegated in their qualities—each experience was so unlike all the others. At some point, I had the experience that launched this project: I realized that this variability posed a philosophical puzzle. While these experiences were extraordinarily different from one another, it was also clear they were unified in some important way. And so I started wondering what these experiences have in common and what sets them apart from other kinds of experience. In short, I realized there was an important philosophical question lying hidden in plain sight: what *are* psychedelic experiences? It seemed to me that it would be tremendously useful to have some kind of conceptual framework, even a rough one, for understanding these experiences from a subjective perspective. So, I started thinking about the question of what psychedelic experiences are, what they have in common, and how they relate to one another.

The second experience gave rise to an insight that set several major pieces of the puzzle in place and determined the general structure of the book. This insight was that whatever psychedelic experiences are, they constitute a category of experience that is much broader than how they are typically conceived. It is commonly thought that a psychedelic experience is an experience one has after consuming a psychedelic substance. (For example, the current Wikipedia page on 'psychedelic experience' defines the concept along these lines.) However, such an understanding ties the experience too tightly to its cause. You don't *need* to take a psychedelic to have a psychedelic experience. There are other ways. Indeed, part of the insight was that *meditation* (which I had been practising for a while) is another way of having a psychedelic experience. Thus, it became clear to me that our understanding of psychedelic *experiences* should be conceptually independent from psychedelic *substances*. This second experience also involved the realization that my most profound experiences were often attained by *combining* meditation and psychedelics. So, not only are there different ways of having psychedelic experiences, they can also be combined, with powerfully synergistic effects.

The third experience was a natural outcome of the second and my explorations with meditation and psychedelics (although I wasn't aware of this at the time). This experience made it clear that there are psychedelic experiences that are *radically* unlike the others—so much so that they seem to be yet another category of experience. In the literature, these experiences have come to be known as *mystical experiences*. While it can be difficult to describe psychedelic experiences, mystical experiences are a whole other ballgame. They are deeply *ineffable* and, as William James famously observed, they also have a *noetic* quality to them. Despite their ineffability, mystical experiences have been described as revelations of ultimate reality, glimpses of enlightenment, unions with the divine, and so on. Whereas "regular" psychedelic experiences appeared to be understandable within a naturalistic worldview, those that are mystical reveal that there is an entirely different way of looking at the world that should not be ignored. This inspired me to approach the topic with greater humility and opened up a new world of philosophical wonder—one in which naturalism and mysticism can be integrated as equals.

The fourth experience inverted my philosophical project. Up until that point, I was focused on using philosophy to make sense of psychedelic experiences. In this fourth experience, I had the insight that psychedelic experiences are themselves philosophical. It's difficult to describe what this means, exactly. Part of this insight was personal in nature: whatever it was that had originally drawn me to philosophy, as an academic, was the same thing drawing me into these experiences. However, it also seemed that this aspect of the experiences wasn't merely reflective of my own predispositions. As is well known, there is a plausible case to be made that many of the world's philosophical traditions find their origins in psychedelic experiences, whether they were induced with the help of substances such as *kykeon* in the Eleusinian Mysteries of ancient Greece, or *soma* of the *Rig Veda*, or the yogic and meditative practices of Hinduism and Buddhism. In short, it appears that these experiences can help us cultivate *wisdom*. They can help us become wiser in the sense of being better decision-makers and they can also help us pursue a deeper form of wisdom. This, I think, is the wisdom that Socrates and Plato were in love with, the wisdom of the Buddha's Noble Eightfold Path, the wisdom of the Dao, the wisdom of Suhrawardi's Illuminationism, and so on. Thus, I became fascinated with the idea that psychedelic experiences can help us do philosophy—in the sense of loving and pursuing wisdom.

Of course, there is nothing new under the sun: others before me have had similar experiences, insights, and thoughts, so I only mention them to help explain how this book came about. I was compelled to write it because I needed to reconcile all of these profound experiences, and their unusual forms of knowledge and wisdom, with the rest of my belief system. My background is primarily analytic and scientific: I grew up in an atheistic household and hold a Bachelors degree in mathematics and a PhD in analytic philosophy on the foundations of probability theory in statistical physics and mathematical biology. Because of my background and interests, I couldn't find anything written about psychedelic experiences that satisfied my philosophical curiosity. The scientific literature was helpful but often too focused on specific empirical details, and there was almost nothing in analytic philosophy (although that is now changing rapidly). And while there was plenty of important work on, and within, the mystical traditions, it tended to downplay, or just not even mention, psychedelics. I also found that many of the books about psychedelics were either lacking in rigour or didn't dive into the philosophical questions that I found to be important and was passionate about. So, I set out to write a book that I wish had existed when I first began having these experiences— something straightforward while still reasonably precise, and something philosophical but with a healthy respect for both naturalism and mysticism. As such, I think the book will be of value to others who are encountering these experiences for the first time (or are curious about them) or who share a similar background and mindset.

Given the importance and timeliness of the topic, I've also tried to make the book accessible to a wide audience. You don't need to be a philosopher or a scientist or a mystic to read it, but you may need to look a few things up here and there. Readers who are immersed in the field of psychedelic research may find that the book sometimes approaches things in a counterintuitive way—particularly my understanding of psychedelic experience as a kind of experience that can be had without consuming a psychedelic. However, based on feedback I've received, such readers tend to find that this counterintuitiveness eventually fades and, as one lets go of the tight association between psychedelic experiences and psychedelic substances, a more experiential and *a priori* perspective emerges that many find helpful. Other readers who are more immersed in the mystical traditions (or wisdom traditions, if you prefer) tend to have a different reaction. They find this perspective familiar and appealing but also that the book can sometimes emphasize the mind at the expense of the body, heart, and soul. This choice of emphasis mostly reflects one of the underlying goals of the book: to help show how an analytic and scientific mindset can accommodate a mystical one without compromising the scruples of either way of looking at the world. With that said, the emphasis is also somewhat illusory. 'Mind' can be understood here as broadly synonymous with *psychē*—historically interpreted as 'mind', 'soul', 'self', 'spirit', 'breath', etc.—and to include such things as somatic awareness, heartfulness, subtle energy, and so on. Thus, various somatic and energetic experiences—for example, those associated with *qìgōng*, *āsana*, *prānāyāma*, and *kundalinī* practices—can be understood as psychedelic (e.g. as spirit-revealing or as revealing of subtle energy).

There is one final aspect of the book that deserves prefatory comment, which is its overall positive and optimistic tone. This tone doesn't reflect a belief that psychedelics and meditation are panaceas or that the spiritual/self-development path is a smooth one (far from it!). In general, all interventions on the body and mind come with risks, and the consumption of psychedelics and the practice of meditation are no exception. Indeed, since risk and reward tend to go hand-in-hand, one may argue that these particular interventions can be especially risky. While there is something to that perspective, it also seems reasonably clear from the research literature that we can mitigate and manage those risks. That doesn't mean that psychedelics and meditation are for everyone, but it does mean that their risk-reward profiles can be suitable for certain kinds of people in the right sorts of circumstances. Thus, the positive and optimistic tone of the book reflects this assessment, along with a belief that a better philosophical understanding of psychedelic experiences can help us further refine the risk-reward profiles of these interventions. Indeed, this is one of my central motivations for writing the book: that we can benefit from a more philosophically precise understanding of these experiences.

I am indebted to many friends and colleagues who have helped and supported me through the process of researching and writing this book. First and foremost, I am extremely grateful to Anya Farennikova. Her insightfulness, creativity, critical feedback, and our many lengthy discussions about all things psychedelic and mystical, have made this book infinitely better than it would have been had I been left to my own devices. I'd also like to thank Joost Breeksema, Michiel van Elk, Branden Fitelson, Logan Fletcher, Alan Hájek, Ruben Laukkonen, Michael Morreau, Martijn Schirp, Ted Shear, Ida Stuij, and Karim Thebault for especially helpful feedback, discussions, and encouragement.

So many others have also helped in all sorts of ways—from general advice, to philosophical conversations, to help with making sense of the scientific literature, to detailed feedback on drafts of the manuscript. These people include (and my apologies to anyone I may have forgotten): Miri Albahari, Marshal Abrams, Marco Aqil, Matthijs Baas, Sam Baron, Cameron Beebe, Dekel Berenson, Huseyin Beykoylu, Jan-Willem Burgers, André van der Braak, Peter Brössel, Rachael Brown, Robin Carhart-Harris, David Chalmers, Matteo Colombo, Jack Cowan, Erik Curiel, Zoe Drayson, James Fadiman, Peter Fazekas, George Fejer, Fiona Fidler, Xaver Funk, Aaron Garret, Stephan Hartmann, Alan Houot, Silvia Jonas, Josef Kay, Daniel Kilov, Andrew Lee, David Lassiter, Jason Leddington, Stefan Leijnen, Chris Letheby, Jerry Levinson, Evan Lewis-Healey, Erick Llamas, Francesco Marchi, Kirsten McKimmie, Kelvin McQueen, Fiona Macpherson, Chris Morris, Daniel Moseley, Bence Nanay, Lois Nishizawa, Lensei Nishizawa, Catarina Dutilh Novaes, Patricia Palacios, Laurie Paul, Richard Pettigrew, Philip Pettit, Soroush Rafie Rad, Georges Rey, Bill Richards, Thijs Roes, Jan-Willem Romeijn, Siebe Rozendal, Jonathan Schaffer, Carlota Serrahima,

Susanna Siegel, Douglass Smith, Reuben Stern, Daniel Stoljar, Michael Strevens, Madelijn Strick, Mauricio Suarez, Enzo Tagliazuchi, Koji Tanaka, Mike Titelbaum, John Vervaeke, Joost Vervoort, and Cindy Woo. I'd also like to thank Peter Momtchiloff at Oxford University Press. Needless to say, I'm responsible for any remaining errors and omissions.

List of Figures

1
Introduction

Know thyself

—Delphic maxim

1.1 Psychedelic Philosophy

This book is about the philosophy of a special kind of experience known as *psychedelic experience*. The term 'psychedelic' derives from the ancient Greek words *psychē* (mind/soul) and *dēlos* (revealed/manifest) and means *mind-revealing*.[1] Accordingly, a psychedelic experience is a *mind-revealing experience*. It is an experience in which hidden parts or aspects of your mind are revealed and become manifest in your consciousness.

The concept of psychedelic experience is a profoundly important one, but it is also widely misunderstood. The main cause of this is the concept's historical connection with psychedelic *drugs* and the cultural baggage that comes along with them. Because of this connection, the term 'psychedelic' has become synonymous with "weird", "druggy", "mind-bending", "crazy", and so on. Understanding the term in this way is a mistake, but it is not just a mistake about the meaning of a word. This mistake obscures the true value of psychedelic experiences, and it prevents us from thinking clearly about them. This book aims to correct for this error.

Even when the error is corrected for, it is still easy to misunderstand the concept of psychedelic experience. This is because of how we relate to our minds. For example, some people seem to think that they have full access to their own minds, and so there is nothing about them to be revealed. One way to have this opinion is to think that all there is to the mind is *just* the conscious mind. This is a view that is often attributed to Descartes:

As to the fact that there can be nothing in the mind, in so far as it is a thinking thing, of which it is not aware, this seems to me to be self-evident. For there is nothing that we can understand to be in the mind, regarding this way, that is not

---

[1] The notion of mind will be understood broadly in this book so as to potentially include the soul, if such a thing exists, as well as other connotations or translations of *psychē* such as 'spirit' and 'self'.

a thought or dependent on a thought. If it were not a thought or dependent on a thought it would not belong to the mind *qua* thinking thing; and we cannot have any thought of which we are not aware at the very moment it is in us.

Descartes 1641[2]

From the perspective of this view, the idea of a mind-revealing experience can seem nonsensical: the mind is always fully present, and so it has no parts to be revealed. That's quite a strong view about the mind, and most people probably don't hold it. A view that is more reasonable, and which appears to be somewhat popular, is that there are, in fact, parts of our minds that exist outside of our awareness, but they are nonetheless accessible and can be made conscious at will. For example, right now you may not be consciously experiencing your love for chocolate, or your anxiety about finances, or your memory of eating breakfast today, but you can bring any of these into your awareness. From the perspective of this view, parts of the mind like these exist outside of awareness, but they are not *hidden* from awareness. And so the idea of a mind-revealing experience can still seem nonsensical: there is nothing inside our minds that is genuinely hidden.

Modern cognitive science shows that both of these views are false: it has given us overwhelming evidence that there are parts of our minds that are hidden from our awareness. For example, many of us have social biases that we are unaware of (Greenwald and Banaji 1995), we learn things implicitly without knowing we are doing so (Reber 1989), and there are factors that influence our decisions without us ever being conscious of them (Nisbett and Wilson 1977). One doesn't need cognitive science, though, to know that parts of our minds can be hidden from awareness. Anyone who has struggled on an exam is familiar with the fact that it can be frustratingly difficult to call up knowledge—that we *know* we have—into awareness. Similarly, anyone who has had a tip-of-the-tongue experience—where you can't remember a particular word, but you can *feel* that it's there, just beyond the reach of your awareness—is also familiar with this fact. And psychotherapists around the world witness this phenomenon on a daily basis: we are remarkably oblivious to the emotions, beliefs, desires, and mental habits that drive so much of our behaviour and decision-making. It can take a lot of work—sometimes years of therapy—to uncover those things.

So, there are definitely parts of the mind that are hidden from our awareness. However, some psychologists suggest that these parts are so hidden that we can *never* see them. For example:

[2] Cottingham 1985, p. 171. It should be noted that although this is a view often attributed to Descartes, it is not clear that it is exactly what he believed. For example, in *The Passions of the Soul*, Descartes remarks that a forgotten childhood experience can affect a person as an adult. See Simmons 2012 for a discussion of some of the possible nuances of Descartes' view of consciousness and the mind.

To understand better our own non-conscious personality dispositions, we cannot simply remove the veil obscuring our view, for there is no direct view. Instead, we are forced to make educated guesses about our non-conscious dispositions.

Wilson 2002, p. 90

According to this kind of view, there are chunks of our minds that we are forever locked out from accessing directly—much like how we are locked out from directly accessing *each other's* minds. So, the only way to come to know these aspects of ourselves is to do what we do when we try to understand someone else's mind: we have to observe our own behaviour, listen to what we tend to say, learn facts about human psychology, collect witness testimonies, and then draw *inferences* as to what is most likely going on in our hidden minds—as if we are strangers to ourselves.

A core thesis of this book is that in addition to these inferences, we can come to know our hidden minds through psychedelic experiences. That means there are parts of our minds that are not only *outside* of our awareness (contra Descartes) but also *hidden* from our awareness (contra popular opinion) and they can be revealed in conscious experience (contra Wilson). To put the point more vividly: I'll argue that we can have a kind of *x-ray vision* into our hidden minds, so that when one is having that x-ray vision, one is having a psychedelic experience.

The big question, then, is: how can we get this x-ray vision? Clearly, we don't always have it and yet many of us could greatly benefit from it, especially those who are struggling through years of expensive psychotherapy. Of course, this question about how we can get x-ray vision is really the question of how we can have a psychedelic experience. The answer that naturally suggests itself is that we can have a psychedelic experience by consuming a psychedelic substance. After all, that's why these substances are called 'psychedelics': they are thought to produce mind-revealing experiences. Although this is widely believed, it is nevertheless an empirical hypothesis that could easily be false—or perhaps not true in the way some people might expect. And so the hypothesis that psychedelics produce psychedelic experiences deserves careful examination. In the coming chapters, I'll evaluate the scientific evidence for this hypothesis. I'll also argue that such drug-induced experiences can be lacking in an important respect. In terms of our x-ray vision metaphor, these experiences are often not as clear as they could be and, therefore, can be misleading.

Naturally, that raises another big question: are there *other* ways of having psychedelic experiences? And are there ways to have psychedelic experiences that are clearer and less misleading than the drug-induced ones? I'll argue that there are. In particular, I will argue that *the practice of meditation* tends to induce psychedelic experiences that can complement the drug-induced ones.[3]

---

[3] As we will see, there are different meditative practices, which have measurably different effects on the mind, and they contribute to psychedelic experiences in different ways.

Although the acts of consuming a psychedelic and practising meditation can look quite different, many have noticed that they also have some strong similarities in their effects (e.g. Badiner et al. 2015, Millière et al. 2018). A general thesis of the book is that psychedelic experiences induced by psychedelic drugs tend to be fast, messy, and temporary, while those induced by meditation tend to be more gradual, less messy, and more enduring. However, it doesn't follow from this that meditation-induced psychedelic experiences give us *perfect* x-ray vision. Nor does it follow that practising meditation is uniformly superior to consuming psychedelics. Both methods have their advantages and disadvantages and both are valuable tools to have available in one's self-knowledge toolkit.

A third way of having a psychedelic experience that I haven't yet mentioned is to do nothing. That is, you can have a psychedelic experience during your normal, everyday life (at the office, say), without doing anything unusual like meditating or consuming strange substances. I call such experiences *spontaneous* psychedelic experiences. We are all familiar with them, even though we may not be familiar with them as such. For example, take a typical case of the tip-of-the-tongue phenomenon. An interesting feature of such cases is that the desired word often comes to you after you have stopped reaching for it. That's a spontaneous psychedelic experience: the word was hidden, and then it is suddenly revealed to you—without you doing anything weird. There are many other kinds of spontaneous psychedelic experiences, including epiphanies, creative insights, overcoming writer's block, when we laugh at some jokes, when we first have the insight of our own mortality—and when we become aware of it again in later years. There are many more examples. What they all have in common is that a previously hidden part or aspect of the mind suddenly appears in one's conscious experience.

The idea that we can have spontaneous psychedelic experiences will be counterintuitive to some readers. You could even frame this reaction in terms of an objection: if it is correct that we can have spontaneous psychedelic experiences, then why are psychedelic drugs such a big deal? Why do people report having such profound and life-changing experiences from them? My reply is that psychedelic drugs are a big deal because they tend to induce experiences that are *extremely* psychedelic and *far more* psychedelic than our spontaneous psychedelic experiences tend to be. In other words, the difference is a difference in *degree*, not a difference in *kind*. To be sure, the difference in degree is substantial—like the wealth difference between billionaires and regular people—but it is still just a difference in degree.

This reply requires a conceptualization of psychedelic experience that allows for experiences to vary in the *degree* to which they are psychedelic. It may be tempting to understand this idea in terms of experiences varying in how weird or mind-bending they are, but if we stick to our understanding of 'psychedelic' in terms of mind-revelation, then it must mean that experiences can vary in how mind-revealing they are. But what does *that* mean? What makes one experience more revealing of the mind than another? One of the objectives of this book is to answer this question and to unpack the idea of psychedelic experiences coming in degrees.

When we dig into that idea, it becomes clear that experiences can be more or less psychedelic in *different* ways. In other words, we'll see that psychedelic experiences are multidimensional with respect to how they may reveal the mind. There are different dimensions along which psychedelic experiences can vary, and the position of a psychedelic experience with respect to these dimensions determines the overall character and strength of the experience. I call the space entailed by these dimensions *psychedelic space*. As we will see, the conceptual framework of psychedelic space is extremely helpful for thinking clearly about the concept of psychedelic experience. For instance, it will help us analyse the similarities and differences that exist between the psychedelic experiences induced by psychedelics and those that are induced by meditation. And it will help us understand the phenomenon of psychedelic experience in general, no matter how it is brought about.

So far, we have been focusing on the ways one can have a psychedelic experience. However, we should also consider if, and how, one can have the *opposite* kind of experience. Such an experience would be one in which the mind is *concealed* rather than revealed. I will call such experiences *psychecryptic experiences*—derived from *psychē* (mind/soul) and *kryptos* (concealed/hidden). As in the case of psychedelic experiences, we regularly have psychecryptic experiences but often don't recognize them as such. A common example of such an experience is getting angry, which explains why one should avoid making decisions in such a state: you have temporarily lost access to the better parts of yourself. Another example is when a clever salesperson lures you into buying something you don't want: they know how to manipulate you so that you become disconnected from the parts of your mind that would prevent you from making the unwanted purchase. Various dissociative states—such as amnesia, fugues, derealization, and depersonalization—are also often psychecryptic in nature. Certain substances, such as alcohol and sedatives, may also have a tendency to cause psychecryptic experiences. Although we never use the terms 'psychecryptic' or 'mind-concealing' to describe these sorts of mental states, it's clear that we can recognize them as such. In some cases, we even label them in a way that reflects this idea. Take, for example, the experience of *brain fog*, which we all endure from time to time. We use the term 'fog' to indicate that we can't think clearly and that it's more difficult to see and move around in our minds the way we normally do—for example, by recalling memories in sufficient detail. Such an experience is clearly psychecryptic, and there are many more examples of psychecryptic experiences that we could find. Once you see a few of them, you start to see them everywhere—just like psychedelic experiences.

Although they are opposites, it is possible to have psychedelic and psychecryptic experiences at the same time. The metaphor of using a flashlight to find something in a dark and cluttered closet can help illustrate this idea. Turning on the flashlight is a psychedelic experience, making it brighter makes the experience more psychedelic, turning it off is psychecryptic, and moving it around is simultaneously psychedelic and psychecryptic: as you clamber through the closet, some parts of it are revealed and other parts are concealed (falling back into the darkness). In other words, in some of our experiences, some parts of the mind can be revealed while other parts are simultaneously concealed. Such experiences are both psychedelic and psychecryptic. Again, we're also familiar with these experiences, but we just may not be familiar with them as such. For example, part of the reason we tend to be bad at multitasking is because most tasks usually induce experiences that are both psychedelic and psychecryptic. As you pay attention to one thing, and thus bring it into awareness and hold it there, it becomes more difficult to pay attention to other things, and they consequently tend to fade from awareness and become hidden from it.[4]

This connection with attention is of fundamental importance in understanding how psychedelics and meditation can induce psychedelic experiences. The attentional system involves the allocation of attentional resources so as to bring things in and out of our awareness. There are two important facts to know about this resource: (i) it is limited, and (ii) we often don't use it as efficiently as we could. These two facts roughly correspond to the two ways that psychedelics and meditation can change our awareness, so that our experience becomes more psychedelic: psychedelics temporarily increase the amount of resource that can be allocated throughout the mind, and meditation increases our ability to use it more efficiently.[5] Although the primary effect on attention is different, the outcome can be the same: both psychedelics and meditation create an attentional surplus. This surplus of attentional resource can then be allocated to things in the mind that don't normally receive enough attention to appear in awareness.

The flashlight analogy is again useful here. The light of the flashlight is your attention, and what you can see is your awareness.[6] Roughly speaking, the effect of a psychedelic is to temporarily increase the amount of light shining from the flashlight.[7] Because of the increase in the amount of light, you can now see more of the closet than you otherwise would. However—continuing the analogy—most people are not very good at using a flashlight: it's difficult to hold it still or to move it

---

[4] There is a subtle issue here that will eventually need to be addressed. Normally, we speak of being aware of something in the external world (a penguin, for example) as though we are aware of *that thing* and not of our mental representation of it (our visual image of the penguin). Moving our attention around, then, might be better said to be *world*-revealing/concealing rather than mind-revealing/concealing. In Chapter 5, I'll discuss this issue in more detail. The upshot will be that if the experiences we are concerned with are world-revealing, then they are world-revealing by way of being mind-revealing.

[5] This is not to imply that these are the *only* effects of psychedelics and meditation.

[6] To be clear, this is just a metaphor for attention that can be useful in some situations and should not be understood as a general theory of attention.

[7] As we will see in Chapter 5, the truth is more complicated than this, but this metaphor is good enough for now.

around effectively and deliberately. Practising meditation develops your ability to use the flashlight more effectively. It also reduces the need for using the flashlight: you begin to be able to see things in the closet using less light.

It's important to note that this is only an analogy and the full situation is more complex. For example, increasing the brightness of the flashlight won't increase your ability to see in the closet if you shine the flashlight into your eyes or if you stumble around and create an even greater mess.[8] However, with that qualification kept in mind, the analogy is useful for getting a sense of how psychedelics and meditation can both reveal the mind in their different ways. They both bring more things into awareness by creating different attentional surpluses. This is the sense in which psychedelics and meditation are often said to "expand awareness" or "expand consciousness". While these concepts might appear unscientific (or sound outlandish), I'll argue that there is good evidence for them: by creating an attentional surplus, psychedelics and meditation can, in fact, expand awareness— and thus reveal the mind.

By now, I hope to have given a good sense of what this book is about. Given the title, you may have expected that it would primarily be about psychedelic *substances*. However, the book's central focus concerns psychedelic *experiences*. To some readers, it may seem that I am changing the definition of 'psychedelic experience'. However, as we'll see in Chapter 2, it is actually the *original* definition, and a core thesis of the book is that it's the best one for understanding the phenomenon of primary interest to many readers—that is, the experiences that are induced by psychedelics. Thus, the main goal of the book is to develop a precise philosophical and psychological understanding of psychedelic experiences, irrespective of how they are brought about.

Another goal of the book is to argue that appropriately engaging with psychedelic experiences can serve a higher purpose: that of cultivating wisdom. Seeking wisdom is the fundamental goal of philosophy (at least, historically speaking), and it is for achieving this goal that psychedelic experience finds its true philosophical significance. We'll see that by the lights of the major conceptions of wisdom that have been put forward by philosophers, psychedelic experiences can be valuable tools for cultivating wisdom. For example, according to Socrates, wisdom involves being aware of the limits of one's knowledge. Many of us fail to be wise in this respect, because we are often deeply unaware of our ignorance and because it can be inconvenient, and even painful, for us to acknowledge it. Indeed, what we do not know is often hidden from us by other things that we *also* cannot see. So, becoming wiser in this respect involves winning an internal struggle over that which obscures our ignorance. I will argue that psychedelic experiences

---

[8] The analogy also over-emphasizes the amplificatory aspect of attention. As is now well known, attention also has an inhibitory aspect to it.

can help us with that struggle and reveal the ignorance that lies hidden within our minds.

Being aware of one's ignorance is just one side to Socrates' conception of wisdom. The other side involves having knowledge about reality that is universal and timeless in nature. Arguably, this is the kind of knowledge that we associate with our best scientists, poets, writers, philosophers, musicians, spiritual leaders, artists, sages, mystics, and so on. Psychedelic experiences can help us become wise in this respect as well—for example, by helping us become more creative and insightful. In particular, psychedelic experiences can help us learn universal and timeless truths that may concern our minds (or souls). Many philosophers and mystics, for instance, have long thought that important philosophical and spiritual truths can be discovered through introspection, contemplation, and meditation. I won't take a stand on what those truths are, except that if those truths genuinely involve some hidden parts or aspects of the mind, then psychedelic experiences may help us come to know them.

Having knowledge of such truths and knowing the limits of one's knowledge are two important aspects of being wise. However, Aristotle thought that there must be more to wisdom than having these two kinds of knowledge. The essence of one of his arguments for this was that some philosophers of his time didn't appear wise in an important respect. What they lacked is what Aristotle called *phronesis*, which is commonly translated as 'practical wisdom'. To be wise in this practical sense is to know how to make good decisions—and to actually make them. I will argue that appropriately engaging with psychedelic experience can help us become wise in this sense as well.

At first glance, engaging with psychedelic experience might seem like the sort of thing that is antithetical to good decision-making. However, this impression is mostly because of the unfortunate connection between the concept of psychedelic experience and the world's turbulent history with psychedelic drugs. One way to begin to see through that cloud of confusion is to notice that we all recognize that the *opposite* is true: we know that *psychecryptic* experiences tend to be *bad* for decision-making. Recall: you don't want to make decisions when angry or drunk or when struggling with brain fog. So, if concealing the mind tends to be bad for decision-making, wouldn't it follow that revealing the mind tends to be good for it? I'll argue that the answer is yes, provided that we make some qualifications. Roughly speaking, my argument will be that appropriately engaging with psychedelic experiences can help us become more aware of the undue influences on our decisions and, consequently, help us manage or even alter them for the betterment of our decision-making.[9]

---

[9] To be clear, we should be mindful of the possibility that *psychedelic drugs* are not perfectly psychedelic. It might be that they are psychedelic in some respects, but psychecryptic in others, and so they may be both beneficial and harmful to decision-making.

Perhaps the ultimate notion of wisdom is that which is pointed to by the Delphic maxim, *know thyself*. Indeed, I think a case can be made that the Socratic and Aristotelian conceptions of wisdom are really just different aspects of—or perhaps threads that lead to—this ultimate form of wisdom. For example, knowing the limits of your knowledge must surely be part of knowing yourself. Similarly, knowing how to make good decisions must involve knowing what is good for oneself and being aware of one's decision-making dispositions (two strata of self-knowledge). However, the ultimate form of wisdom to which the Delphic maxim points arguably absorbs and transcends these conceptions of wisdom, taking on a mystical form that is divine and ineffable.

We also find a similar notion of wisdom in non-Western schools of thought. For example, in one translation of the *Dao De Ching*, we find: 'knowing others is intelligent; knowing yourself is enlightened' (Addiss and Lombardo 1993). Similarly, according to many Buddhist schools of thought, enlightenment involves the realization of one's true, and ineffable, self-nature.[10]

It would seem, therefore, that all roads of wisdom lead to—or through—the self. As we'll see, psychedelic experiences are not only beneficial in the pursuit of this ultimate form of wisdom, engaging with them is, arguably, the *only* way to attain it.

1.2 Book Outline

Now that we have a general understanding of the overall mission of the book, let's take a closer look at its structure. I'll start with an outline of the book and then review the plan for each chapter.

In Chapters 2–4, I lay out a philosophical framework that can help us think clearly about psychedelic experiences. This framework is needed because thinking clearly about psychedelic experiences is not an easy thing to do. There are at least three main reasons why. The first is that the general topic is emotionally charged and potentially has huge social and political implications. Such topics often invite passionate and nonrigorous thinking (on both sides of whatever debate). The second reason is that the method of inducing a psychedelic experience that most people are familiar with—namely, by consuming a psychedelic drug—has such a profound and disruptive effect on the mind that thinking clearly about *anything* can be challenging, let alone the disruption itself. The third reason is that the concept of psychedelic experience is both old and new—familiar and unfamiliar—and that can cause a lot of confusion. We don't yet really understand

---

[10] It should be noted, though, that it is a matter of debate as to what that true self-nature is, with many Buddhists believing that there is *no* self—a common interpretation of *anattā*. However, Buddhists are not universally agreed on this point. Some believe that *anattā* should not be treated as a metaphysical doctrine but instead engaged with as a practical method for discovering a hidden truth about the self (Albahari 2002).

these experiences, and the little bit of knowledge that we do have can fool us into thinking we know more than we actually do. For these reasons, we need to start slowly and carefully, and build up a philosophical framework—a conceptual architecture, if you like—that will help us avoid many obstacles down the road.

In Chapters 5–8, I will point this new philosophical machinery at the scientific literature, so that we can start to make sense of actual psychedelic experiences. I will focus primarily on three kinds of psychedelic experience: (i) those that occur spontaneously, (ii) those that are induced by the consumption of psychedelics, and (iii) those that are induced by meditation. By studying these three kinds of psychedelic experience, I believe we can get a good handle on the general phenomenon of psychedelic experience (abstracting away from how it is induced). One way to think about these four chapters is that they constitute an informal assessment of the likelihoods of various hypotheses that we may want to consider. For example, take the hypothesis that psychedelics tend to produce psychedelic experiences. How likely is that hypothesis given that we know that psychedelics produce hallucinations (which may seem like the opposite of the mind being revealed)? As another example, consider the hypothesis that meditation also induces psychedelic experiences. How likely is that hypothesis given that the experiences that typically result from psychedelics and meditation look so different? And so on. There are many other hypotheses and many other pieces of evidence that we can consider. As we'll see, some of these hypotheses can only be articulated once we have the philosophical framework in place.

In Chapters 9–11, I will come back to issues that are more philosophical in nature. In particular, I will discuss how psychedelic experience relates to two philosophically substantial issues: (i) that of mystical experience and (ii) that of wisdom and enlightenment. Necessarily, these issues will be less grounded in the scientific literature. However, they will be analysed within the confines of the philosophical framework that will—if the previous four chapters are successful—have received indirect support from the empirical research. So, although the issues of these three chapters may seem unusual or perhaps unscientific, the plan is to discuss them in a manner that meets the usual standards of analytic philosophy and scientific inquiry. Indeed, one of the exciting aspects of the latest research into psychedelics and meditation is that we can begin to scientifically investigate these issues, which have long been thought to lie outside the domain of science.

With that overview of the book's structure in place, let's now look at the goals of the particular chapters.

In Chapter 2, I introduce the central question of the book: what is psychedelic experience? A core objective of this chapter is to argue that this question is best understood as a *conceptual* question rather than an *empirical* question about the effects of psychedelic drugs (as might be expected by some readers). Approaching our topic in this way allows us to cleanly separate the concept of psychedelic *experience* from the baggage that often comes with the topic of psychedelic *drugs*.

This, in turn, makes it easier for us to think about things like psychedelic drugs in a baggage-free way. For example, we can ask whether so-called psychedelic drugs are actually psychedelic. That is, do psychedelics actually produce mind-revealing experiences?[11] Perhaps they don't—perhaps they only produce mind-*scrambling* experiences. Or perhaps they do, but perhaps they only reveal the mind in particular ways. If so, then are there methods for revealing the mind in *other* ways? And so on. By establishing this clear separation of conceptual and empirical matters, it will be easier to address each appropriately and find answers to our questions.

In Chapter 3, having established the central question as a conceptual one, I will then develop an answer to it. We already have the hint of an answer: a psychedelic experience is a mind-revealing experience. That must mean that it is an experience in which the mind is revealed in some way. But in what way? As we will see, we need to be careful here. If we are not, then all sorts of experiences will count as being psychedelic—for example, when you discover facts about your mind by reading a psychology textbook. As we dig into this issue, we'll see that it is essential to stipulate that psychedelic experiences *come in degrees*. That is, experiences can be *more or less psychedelic* than other experiences. This raises the question of what it means for one experience to be more (or less) psychedelic than another experience. My answer is that an experience is more psychedelic than another if it is more revealing of the mind. And, as we'll see, there are four main ways an experience can be more revealing of the mind: (i) *scope*: it can uncover larger parts of the mind; (ii) *clarity*: it can uncover parts of the mind more clearly; (iii) *novelty*: it can uncover more novel (or more deeply hidden) parts of the mind; and (iv) *duration*: it can uncover parts of the mind for longer periods of time. These four ways of being more mind-revealing constitute the four dimensions of what I call *psychedelic space*. All possible psychedelic experiences have a location within this conceptual space, and the overall phenomenological character of a psychedelic experience is determined by its position with respect to these four dimensions. In general, the further out along these dimensions an experience is, the more psychedelic it is.

In Chapter 4, I use the conceptual framework of psychedelic space to begin developing some empirical hypotheses about psychedelic experience that we may want to consider. This is necessary because it will help us avoid many pitfalls later on. For example, a common objection to the hypothesis that psychedelics produce psychedelic experiences is that many of the hallucinatory experiences that psychedelics are known to cause seem to be anything but mind-revealing. The point that psychedelic experiences can vary in terms of their clarity is important

[11] Although it often isn't clear in the scientific literature, it is a *hypothesis* (or at least an empirical claim) that so-called psychedelic drugs produce psychedelic experiences. One notable exception to this lack of clarity is Carhart-Harris 2018, p. 170, who clearly recognizes this point and also the fact that it often isn't recognized.

to consider when we think about this objection. It may be that psychedelics do produce mind-revealing experiences, but they tend to produce them with *low clarity*. That's a hypothesis that is more specific than the one that just says that psychedelics produce mind-revealing experiences. According to this more specific hypothesis, hallucinations may be like the imperfections in the lens of an old telescope: despite these imperfections, the telescope can still reveal things to us— the craters of the moon, for example. Similarly, another pitfall we can avoid concerns the question of whether meditation produces psychedelic experiences. This question is often asked in a lopsided way, where 'psychedelic experience' is used to refer to the kind of experience typically produced by psychedelic *drugs*. This causes unnecessary confusion, and we can do better by reframing the question as asking whether meditation produces psychedelic experiences understood as mind-revealing experiences. Understanding the question in this way makes it clear that meditation may tend to produce psychedelic experiences that are different from those that tend to be produced by psychedelic substances. For example, one salient hypothesis in this regard is that meditation-induced psychedelic experiences tend to be *higher in clarity* than those induced by psychedelics. As we'll see, we need to be careful in how we articulate these hypotheses, and there are many complicating factors that need to be considered.

With these conceptual issues sorted out, we are then ready to begin examining the empirical evidence concerning psychedelic experiences. The first step in this direction is Chapter 5, in which I put forward a unifying theory of the psychedelic experiences induced by psychedelics and meditation in terms of their effects on *attention*. Psychedelics and meditation are often said to *expand awareness*, and awareness and attention have an intimate relationship with each other. Some philosophers even think they are *identical*, but the consensus appears to be that attention and awareness are separable but intimately related (Lopez 2022). Either way, given this close connection between awareness and attention, it stands to reason that psychedelics and meditation must have an important effect on attention. In fact, we'll see that some meditative practices are, by definition, the repeated and deliberate manipulation of attentional resources. We can see, then, one way in which meditation expands awareness and thus reveals the mind: it helps one allocate attentional resources to things in the mind that don't normally receive those resources, making it more likely that they appear in awareness. Whereas meditation improves the control over the allocation of one's attentional resources, I'll suggest that the effect of psychedelics is to free up one's attentional resources. These additional resources then have to go somewhere—that is, they end up being reallocated throughout the mind. When this happens, the effect is similar to that of meditation: the parts or aspects of the mind that receive extra attentional resources are more likely to appear in awareness—or to appear in awareness more vividly. I'll argue that this hypothesis helps us understand the various psychological and phenomenological effects of psychedelics.

It will also help us explain the overlapping and synergistic effects of psychedelics and meditation. The result of this chapter will be a unified theory of how psychedelics and meditation can reveal the mind: they do so by changing how attentional resources are allocated.

In Chapter 6, we will then consider what is, arguably, the simplest kind of psychedelic experience: when a long-lost memory suddenly floods one's consciousness. We are all familiar with such experiences since they can be triggered by the most mundane events, such as when we happen to come across a scent that we haven't smelled since childhood. Although we don't normally think of them in this way, these sorts of memory flashbacks are *spontaneous* psychedelic experiences—they can happen without unusual interventions such as the consumption of psychedelics or the practice of meditation. Because these experiences are so familiar to us, they provide us with a convenient starting point for studying psychedelic experience as an empirical phenomenon.

Another reason why it is useful to focus on memory in this context is that there is an important relationship between memory and meditative practices that cultivate *mindfulness*. In various Western/modern contexts, the concept of mindfulness is often defined as paying attention to the present moment in a particular way. However, this sort of definition is mistaken—or at least, it is incomplete.[12] We will see that mindfulness has a subtle but crucial connection to memory that needs to be accounted for in order for us to have a complete understanding of mindfulness. This better understanding of mindfulness will result in two major consequences. The first is that we will establish an elegant connection between psychedelic experience and mindfulness. Roughly speaking, a psychedelic experience is like suddenly finding your keys after having lost them, and mindfulness is like not having lost them in the first place. This connection between psychedelic experience and mindfulness will be especially useful later on, when we begin to consider the relationship between psychedelic experience and wisdom (Chapter 11). It will also help make sense of a somewhat surprising body of evidence: that *psychedelics* can induce long-lasting improvements in mindfulness. The second major consequence of this better understanding of mindfulness is that it implies that the practice of meditation should have an observable and beneficial impact on one's recollective abilities. Indeed, there is a growing body of scientific research that supports this prediction, and so we will take a look at that literature.

Finally, in this same chapter, we will consider the evidence that psychedelics bring about experiences that involve the recollection of long-lost memories. Based on the fact that such experiences are psychedelic when they happen spontaneously, it seems reasonable to expect that if so-called psychedelics are genuinely deserving of their name, then they should result in these kinds of experiences. With that in

---

[12] The definition is perhaps better understood as a definition of a mindfulness *practice* rather than mindfulness itself.

mind, we will consider what the evidence says about this prediction. We will see that while the evidence is positive overall, it is only suggestive. One of the major weaknesses of the current body of evidence in this regard is that we lack controlled and well-designed studies that demonstrate that the supposed memories recovered during psychedelic trips are *genuine* and not merely fantasies that are constructed on the fly.

In Chapter 7, I turn to the common objection that I mentioned earlier: how can the visual hallucinations that psychedelics are renowned for producing possibly count as mind-revealing? As I mentioned, some of the hallucinations may simply be imperfections, and so although they themselves may not be mind-revealing, there may nonetheless be some aspect of the larger experience that is. However, I will argue that at least some hallucinations are, in fact, instances of mind-revelation. My argument for this will involve making a distinction between two kinds of visual hallucinations: (i) simple hallucinations and (ii) complex hallucinations. Simple hallucinations tend to be the colourful geometric patterns that psychedelics are famous for causing. Complex hallucinations tend to involve more meaningful experiences, such as the apparent perception of a person who isn't real, or walking through an alien city, or talking to a dragon about your life. I'll argue that both kinds of hallucinations may be mind-revealing, but the simpler ones appear to be the clearest case of hallucinations that are revealing of the mind.

In Chapter 8, I examine how mind-revelation may be responsible for the supposed increases in *creativity* that psychedelics have a reputation for causing. Indeed, if psychedelics increase creativity, then this may form the basis for an objection to a view such as mine: far from being mind-revealing, it would seem that psychedelics are mind-*creating* (Shanon 2002). My reply is that a lot of our creativity exists hidden from our awareness and that psychedelics can increase our effective creativity by bringing more of it into our conscious experience. I also argue that meditation has a similar effect and consider the evidence that meditation increases our creativity by revealing the mind. Although it may seem unintuitive at first—that is, that we have hidden creativity that can be revealed—I argue that this view about creativity is well supported by contemporary cognitive science.

In Chapter 9, the next issue we will tackle concerns the extent to which the *psychotherapeutic benefits* of psychedelics and meditation can be explained in terms of their tendency to produce mind-revealing experiences. This is an important issue to consider because it is the therapeutic value of these interventions that is the primary driver for most of the current research, especially in the case of psychedelics. We don't yet know how to explain these effects, but some plausible hypotheses have been put forward. One natural hypothesis to consider is that by inducing psychedelic experiences, psychedelics facilitate *psychological insights*, which either have immediate therapeutic value in themselves or enable substantial and long-term improvements in behaviour and thinking.

A similar explanation could be put forward for meditation: various meditative practices are known to reliably afford psychological insights. I think there is some truth to these explanations, but they are also somewhat incomplete. I will argue that there is a more comprehensive explanation available: with the appropriate qualifications in place, both psychedelics and meditation tend to result in increases in *mindfulness*, which is what is ultimately responsible for the therapeutic benefits we observe (or at least, a substantial portion of them). My argument will rely on the connection between psychedelic experience and mindfulness that is established in Chapter 6. Considering this explanation in terms of mindfulness can help us appreciate how psychedelics and meditation may benefit our well-being in general, which will help pave the way for some of the arguments in Chapter 11 concerning how psychedelics and meditation may enhance our wisdom.

In Chapter 10, I turn to the topic of *mystical experience*. This is necessary because both psychedelics and meditation are widely reported to lead to mystical experiences, which are often thought of as *peak* or *maximally psychedelic* experiences. Since the conceptual framework of psychedelic space is designed to account for experiences being more or less psychedelic, mystical experience presents us with an important test case. A natural question to consider is whether mystical experience can be located within psychedelic space as a maximally psychedelic experience—that is, an experience that maximizes the four dimensions of scope, clarity, novelty, and duration. I'll argue that there is a sense in which we can't answer this question. This is because mystical experiences are deeply *ineffable* and, as a result, they form a kind of *singularity* for analytic philosophy (and any downstream field of investigation). The best we can do is to reason *around* the experience, which the framework of psychedelic space allows us to do. So, although we can't speak directly to the question of whether mystical experiences are maximally psychedelic—or even if they are psychedelic to *any* degree—we will be able to develop an understanding of them that is still valuable.

In Chapter 11, I argue that psychedelic experience, when appropriately engaged with, is conducive to *wisdom*. It is important to be clear upfront that this is not the same as the statement that consuming psychedelics is conducive to wisdom. Indeed, if psychedelics tend to produce psychedelic experiences that are very low in clarity, then they may do more harm than good when it comes to wisdom. Moreover, whereas many of the effects of psychedelics are clearly temporary, the effects of meditation appear to be more enduring. In so far as we think that being wise is a stable, long-term attribute of a person, then it could be that meditation may be more conducive to wisdom than psychedelics are. At any rate, we needn't take a stand on such issues here—psychedelics and meditation may provide different and complementary methods for cultivating wisdom. In this chapter, I will unpack in more detail how psychedelic experience, regardless of how it is brought about, can help us become wiser. This gives rise to a different way of doing philosophy, which I will refer to as *psychedelic philosophy*.

Finally, in Chapter 12, I will bring everything together with some concluding remarks.

We've already covered a lot of territory in this introductory chapter. We'll now go back over it more carefully. In the next chapter, we will start with our central question: what is psychedelic experience? That will help us get a better idea of what that question is asking, why we should ask it, and how we can go about in trying to answer it.

2

What Is Psychedelic Experience?

2.1 Introduction

Every year in the former USSR, children across the region drowned an untold number of guinea pigs. What on Earth did these children have against these poor animals, you may wonder?

Well, it turns out that the Russian name for guinea pig is *morskaya svinka*, which literally means 'sea pig'. Because of this name, some of the children thought that guinea pigs live in the sea. Naturally, some of these well-intentioned children ended up finding a home for their guinea pigs in containers filled with water, and the inevitable happened. What the children didn't realize is that the name *morskaya svinka* is likely an abbreviation of *zamorskaya svinka*, which means 'overseas pig', indicating that the animals come from overseas. If the children understood the real meaning of the name of their pets, they wouldn't conceive of them as animals that live in water, and they would be less likely to drown them.[1]

Psychedelic experiences are like guinea pigs in the former USSR. Some of us have the wrong idea about what they are, and because of this, we make some serious mistakes in how we think about them. The goal of this chapter is to take a first step in correcting our misconceptions about psychedelic experiences by returning to the original sense of psychedelic experience as a *mind-revealing experience*. I'll argue that this is not only the original meaning of 'psychedelic experience', but that this meaning is also *better* than other contemporary understandings of the term.

We will begin, in Section 2.2, by reflecting on how the term 'psychedelic experience' was first introduced. This will give us a better understanding of the question and an initial sketch of what a psychedelic experience is. In Section 2.3, I will discuss some crucial methodological points about how we should proceed in answering the question and in developing the definition of psychedelic experience. This will set up the basic rules for the rest of the book and thus determine how the entire project ought to be evaluated.

---

[1] Fortunately, awareness of this mistake is growing, and it is becoming increasingly rare.

2.2 The Question

What is psychedelic experience? At first glance, it might seem as though we don't need to spend much time on grappling with the meaning of this question. After all, it appears to be clear enough since it seems to simply ask about the kind of experience that people typically have after consuming a psychedelic drug. Can't we go straight to explaining what people experience when they are in such a state? Similarly, can't we just start answering other related questions, such as whether meditation also produces psychedelic experiences?

Unfortunately, we can't. The problem is that the concept of psychedelic experience is not as clear-cut as it may initially seem. In part, this is because the meaning of 'psychedelic' has evolved over time and come to take on all sorts of meanings. As Brian Wells noted, the term 'psychedelic' underwent a semantic shift in the 1960s and early 1970s, and soon came to mean 'anything in youth culture which is colourful, or unusual, or fashionable' (Wells 1974, pp. 19–20). The term also often—but not always—functions as a *name* for a class of substances with some family resemblance to the so-called "classic" psychedelics, such as LSD, psilocybin, and mescaline (Nichols 1986, p. 306). However, the original meaning of the term is also still in use. For example, in the foreword to the edited collection *Manifesting Minds*, Rick Doblin and Brad Burge write:

> [...] above all else, psychedelic describes what happens when the contents of the mind and body are made more visible or more clear—in other words, when the mind is manifested. This process by which hidden memories and experiences are revealed is both feared and revered in our society.
>
> Doblin and Burge 2014, p. x

Later on, we will unpack this meaning in more detail and see another notable example of it being used in the scientific literature. The essential point for now is that different people mean different things by 'psychedelic', and so it isn't immediately clear what we are asking when we ask what a psychedelic experience is. It follows, then, that we need to define our concept of psychedelic experience.

To do this, there are two main strategies available to us. The first is to identify some version of the concept that is currently in use and then say explicitly what that concept is. For example, one common conception in use today (especially in informal contexts) would be that of a "weird" or "mind-bending" or "trippy" experience. So we could try to unpack this idea and give it a more precise definition. Alternatively, another conception in use today is that a psychedelic experience is an experience induced by certain drugs, such as mescaline, psilocybin, LSD, and so on.[2] We could then, similarly, choose to unpack this idea and give it a precise

---

[2] For example, the Wikipedia entry on *psychedelic experience* currently defines it as: 'a temporary altered state of consciousness induced by the consumption of a psychedelic substance (most commonly LSD, mescaline, psilocybin mushrooms, or DMT)'.

definition. Those are two examples of how we can pursue the first strategy available to us. The second strategy is to return to the *original* concept of psychedelic experience, understood as a mind-revealing experience, and then see if we can define it more precisely. It is this second strategy that I will pursue in this book.

The main reason for pursuing this second strategy is that it ultimately provides us with a definition of psychedelic experience that is more useful for scientific and philosophical purposes. This stems, in part, from the fact that the term's original meaning was carefully designed to capture a core insight concerning the nature of the experiences produced by the substances in question. It is also because this approach gives us a broader conceptualization of psychedelic experience that allows us to connect it with other important notions we have. Ultimately, whichever strategy we choose should be judged by the fruit it bears. Can it be used to give good explanations of known phenomena? Does it help us avoid unnecessary confusion? Does it give us a precise concept that is linked to other well-defined concepts that we already have? Does it give us the conceptual flexibility to identify and evaluate new hypotheses and theories? And so on. These are standard criteria for any successful definition of a concept, but they are critical in this context since the topic of psychedelic experience can be a conceptual minefield. A goal of this book is to demonstrate that the second strategy for defining the concept of psychedelic experience pays off best in terms of meeting these criteria.

The term 'psychedelic' was first introduced by the psychiatrist Humphry Osmond in 1957 as he thought it to be the most appropriate name for the class of drugs in question, which at the time had captured the attention of psychiatrists and psychologists (as well as the wider public). Before Osmond, these drugs received a variety of other names. One popular name for them was 'hallucinogen', signifying that these drugs produce hallucinations. Another common term in use was 'psychotomimetic', indicating that these drugs produce psychological states that resemble psychosis. Osmond argued that these names were inappropriate because they failed to capture the core characteristic of the experiences that the drugs tend to produce. He believed that the term 'psychedelic' did a much better job in this respect, and we will see why in a moment.

An important point that is often overlooked is that each of these names implies a different *hypothesis* about the effects of the drugs. For example, by calling a drug a 'psychotomimetic', one implies that the production of psychosis-like states is a central characteristic of the drug. Similarly, by calling a drug a 'hallucinogen', one implies that the production of hallucinations is a central characteristic of the drug. These are empirical hypotheses that may be true or false. So, by suggesting that we call these drugs 'psychedelic', Osmond intended to introduce a new hypothesis about their central characteristic—namely, that they produce psychedelic experiences. It then follows that in order to sensibly advance such a hypothesis, Osmond must have had some independent conception of what a psychedelic experience is. Otherwise, his hypothesis would be circular and meaningless.

This point becomes clear when we consider how the other hypotheses work in this regard. For example, consider the 'hallucinogenic' hypothesis. A common definition of 'hallucination' is that it is an apparent perception of an object that is not actually present.[3] Clearly, this definition does not refer to drugs in any way. The terms involved in the definition only refer to *other* things—apparent perception, an object, and actual presence. This is important because if we did not have some independent grasp of the concept of hallucination, then we would not know what it would mean for the drugs to be hallucinogens. Consequently, we wouldn't know what would count as evidence for or against that hypothesis. Therefore, when Osmond argued that the drugs in question are neither psychotomimetics nor hallucinogens, and put forward the alternative claim that they are *psychedelics*, he must have had some independent understanding of that concept.

It is clear, then, that there must be some way to understand the concept of psychedelic experience independently of the drugs in question. However, this observation introduces a complication: whereas the concept of hallucination was familiar to most people in 1957, the concept of psychedelic experience was not. This is because Osmond introduced 'psychedelic' as a new term of art. He intended it to be a technical term that expressed a new idea—or, at least, one that hadn't yet been clearly recognized in connection with the drugs in question. Because of this, Osmond needed to explain the new idea, either by defining it carefully or at least by providing some sketch of its meaning. Without doing so, he could have just as well given the drugs some completely meaningless name, like *fumble-wumbles*. Therefore, Osmond not only had to have a concept that could be understood independently of the drugs in question, but he also had to explain its meaning—at least, in rough outline.

Indeed, this is exactly what Osmond did. His sketch of the concept was contained in the term's etymology and in his consideration of alternatives:

> I have tried to find an appropriate name for the agents under discussion: a name that will include the concepts of enriching the mind and enlarging the vision. Some possibilities are: *psychephoric*, mind-moving; *psychehormic*, mind-rousing; and *psycheplastic*, mind-molding. *Psychezymic*, mind-fermenting, is indeed appropriate. *Psycherhexic*, mind bursting forth, though difficult, is memorable. *Psychelytic*, mind-releasing, is satisfactory. My choice, because it is clear, euphonious, and uncontaminated by other associations, is *psychedelic*, mind-manifesting.
>
> Osmond 1957, p. 429

As we can see, Osmond's idea was that the drugs in question produce experiences that involve the mind manifesting or revealing itself.[4] If correct, this was a major

---

[3] Cases of veridical hallucination may be possible (Lewis 1980), but these subtleties won't concern us here.

[4] The term 'psychedelic', when used in the sense of mind-manifestation, has become synonymous with the term 'mind-revelation'. I will follow suit and treat this as a purely terminological choice.

insight with potentially paradigm-changing implications. In this single paragraph, Osmond was simultaneously performing two significant tasks: (i) introducing the *concept* of a psychedelic experience and (ii) proposing the *hypothesis* that the drugs in question produce psychedelic experiences. However, this was a lot to happen all at once. Such a major insight ought to be unpacked carefully so that the concept and the hypothesis are disentangled from each other. That will be the primary task for the following two chapters, with Chapter 3 defining the concept more precisely and Chapter 4 exploring the range of hypotheses involving the concept that we may consider evaluating.

To better understand why Osmond identified these drugs by this name, it will help to retrace his thought process. Prior to coining his new term, he and Aldous Huxley had already been discussing this issue for a few years. In their exchanges, we see that they were looking for a name that would capture the mind-revealing aspect of the experiences that they thought the drugs induced. In a letter to Huxley, we see Osmond exploring the issue:

> It is absurd [...] to label them as psychotomimetics. I make several suggestions, have you any other ones? [...] The name should have a clear meaning, be reasonably easy to spell and pronounce and not be too like some other name. Psychophrenics had to be abandoned and so did psychoplastics. Psychorhexics and psychohormics are doubtful. So far psychodelics-mind manifestors seems the most promising, psycholytics-mind releasers is doubtful because lysis in medicine is now associated with dissolution rather than release. Euleutheropsychics, though accurate and euphonious is too much of a mouthful. Psychodelics seems unambiguous, not loaded with old associations and clear.
>
> Osmond, 25 March 1956[5]

And then Huxley replies:

> About a name for these drugs—what a problem! I have looked into Liddell and Scott and find that there is a verb *phaneroein*, 'to make visible or manifest,' and an adjective *phaneros*, meaning 'manifest, open to sight, evident'. The word is used in botany—phanerogam as opposed to cryptogam. Psychodetic is something I don't quite get the hang of.[6] Is it an analogue of geodetic, geodesy? If so, it would mean mind-dividing, as geodesy means earth-dividing, from *ge* and *daiein*. Could you call these drugs psychophans? Or phaneropsychic drugs? Or what about phanerothymes? *Thumos* means soul, in its primary usage, and is the equivalent of Latin *animus*. The word is euphonious and easy to pronounce; besides it has

---

[5] Bisbee et al. 2018, p. 261.
[6] It appears that Huxley misread Osmond's suggestion of 'psychodelic' as 'psychodetic', which would explain why he was initially confused by Osmond's proposal.

relatives in the jargon of psychology—e.g. cyclothyme. On the whole I think this is better than psychophan or phaneropsychic.

Huxley, 30 March 1956[7]

Following up on that letter, Huxley continues:

Psychodetic seems to me wrong, as it would mean mind-dividing (on the analogy of geodetic) rather than mind revealing. Revealing would be phaneros, phaneroein. So you get either phaneropsychic, or psychophan or (as I feel, much better) phanerothyme as a substantive and phanerothymic as the adjective. *Thumos* is the Greek equivalent of Latin animus and, in its primary sense, signifies soul. (*Phaneros* means evident, manifest, open to sight. *Phaneroein* means to make manifest, make visible.)

Huxley, April 1956[8]

A passage from one of Osmond's letters a year later also makes it clear that he was not necessarily concerned with the drugs themselves, but with the experiences they produce:

I can't see any point in considering an experience of the other derived from epilepsy, schizophrenia, starvation, flagellation, vitamin deficiency, the reduced environment, dervish dancing, yogistic practices, more or less valuable than one derived from hashish, soma, peyote, cohoba, ololiuqui, harmola, ayahuesca, cohoba, amanita muscaria, Wasson's new ones [psilocybin mushrooms], or for that matter mescaline, LSD-25, TAM, LSM, adrenochrome, adrenolutin, Alles' compounds [amphetamines], or Szára's DMT and T-9 which are derivatives of the amino acid tryptophan. *It is all one to me. The whole point is whether the experience justifies the risk, discomfort or time involved and whether its fruits are good or evil.*

Osmond, June 1957 (emphasis added)[9]

Clearly, then, the concept of psychedelic experience can be understood independently of the drugs in question. This is because we have an independent grasp of the component concepts: we have some idea of what the mind is, what it means to reveal something, and what it means to have an experience. Although we do not yet know precisely what a mind-revealing experience is, we can nevertheless see how it can be understood without any reference to drugs: it has something to

---

[7] Bisbee et al. 2018, pp. 265–6.   [8] Bisbee et al. 2018, pp. 266–7.
[9] Bisbee et al. 2018, pp. 333–4. It is worth noting that Osmond also appears to be echoing William James' famous pragmatic principle of focusing on the fruits and not the roots of mystical/spiritual/religious experiences (James 1902).

do with the mind being hidden or obscured in some way and then being revealed or made visible. Clearly, more needs to be said about what this idea amounts to, which is one of this book's main tasks. However, the important takeaway here is that we can understand the concept of psychedelic experience independently of any drug that may cause such an experience. Consequently, the phenomenon of psychedelic experience is more general than that of an experience induced by the consumption of a so-called psychedelic drug.

To some readers, it may seem that I am belabouring this point. However, the reason I am unpacking it in such a painstaking manner is because this important point is so easily misunderstood. As I noted earlier, the term 'psychedelic' has evolved over the decades since to take on several meanings, and this can cloud discussions with unnecessary confusion. For instance, because the meaning of the term 'psychedelic' is sometimes heavily anchored on the drugs in question (and on popular conceptions of their effects), it is difficult to ask if anything else is psychedelic. If someone were to ask, for example, whether meditation also produces psychedelic experiences, then that question would be understood—in this drug-oriented way—as asking whether meditation produces experiences that are the same as those that psychedelics produce. One might then reasonably reply that the answer is no simply because the drug-induced experiences can be so unlike the meditative ones.

In contrast, if we understand the question as asking whether meditation also produces *mind-revealing experiences*, then we can see that the answer could easily be yes, even though the experiences induced by psychedelics and meditation have substantial differences. The point can be illustrated using an analogy with restaurant experiences: even though one's experience of a sushi restaurant in Tokyo may differ substantially from one's experience of a Mughlai restaurant in Srinagar, they are both recognizable as restaurant experiences. Accordingly, both meditation and psychedelics may be methods for producing psychedelic experiences—understood as mind-revealing experiences—and it may be that they produce mind-revealing experiences of different *kinds*. It is difficult to achieve this kind of flexibility and clarity in our thinking if we discard Osmond's original conception of a psychedelic experience.

Among psychedelics enthusiasts (and especially the evangelists), merely considering the possibility that psychedelic drugs are not actually psychedelic might be seen as a form of blasphemy. However, if our desire to understand these experiences is genuine, then we need to be open to the possibility that psychedelics are not actually psychedelic. Alternatively, perhaps they are psychedelic, but not *as* psychedelic as the enthusiasts like to think. Or, still further, maybe they are considerably psychedelic, but only in a particular way, implying that there are other ways of being psychedelic.

In this regard, it is worth noting that Robin Carhart-Harris, one of the world's leading psychedelic researchers, makes a similar observation:

Thankfully, the true origin and meaning of [the] neologism 'psychedelic' is becoming increasingly well recognized and understood. It dates back to the mid-1950s and an exchange between two Brits (one, the famous author, Aldous Huxley) in which they sought to find a more appropriate term for these compounds (Huxley et al. 1977). The objective was to devise a word that would better capture their core psychological properties than the relatively shallow and arguably misleading alternative 'hallucinogen'. It was Huxley's interlocutor, the psychiatrist and psychedelic research pioneer Humphrey Osmond who would coin the term 'psychedelic'—combining two ancient Greek words for 'mind' or 'soul' (*psyche*) and 'to reveal' or make manifest' or 'visible' (*delein*)—to lay principal emphasis on these compounds' mind-revealing effects. The notion that a principal property of psychedelics is their ability to reveal aspects of the mind that are normally not fully visible, was (Cohen 1964, Grof 1975, Sandison et al. 1954), and remains (Carhart-Harris and Friston 2010, Kraehenmann et al. 2017, Kraehenmann et al. 2017, Richards 2015), widely accepted among those most familiar with their effects, if through direct personal experience, or second or third-hand observation. *Remarkably however, that psychedelics do this, remains a mere assumption/hypothesis that has never been systematically measured and tested, and therefore given an opportunity to be verified or falsified.*

It seems reasonable to begin by acknowledging that this relatively major oversight may be explainable—if not excusable—by the unreasonable difficulty of conducting human research with psychedelics (Nutt et al. 2013), *let alone testing such an abstract and paradigm-challenging idea.*

Carhart-Harris 2018, p. 170 (emphasis added)

Carhart-Harris then goes on to operationalize the idea of mind-revelation in a specific way, namely, by defining *emotional insight* as a kind of mind-revelation. He then considers whether psychedelic drugs may facilitate or enhance subjects' abilities to have emotional insights (Carbonaro et al. 2017). Carhart-Harris' strategy exemplifies how we should proceed: we first clarify what it means to have a mind-revealing experience and *then* consider the evidence that something—say, a particular drug—tends to produce such experiences. Emotional insight is one way the mind may be revealed; however, as we will see in the next chapter, there are many others as well.

Separating the concept and hypothesis in this way gives us a cleaner way of approaching our topic. Once we have unpacked the idea of a psychedelic experience, we can consider which of our experiences are psychedelic. Perhaps the experiences that people have after consuming a drug such as psilocybin are psychedelic, but perhaps other experiences are psychedelic as well. It may even be that some people have psychedelic experiences in response to substances that are not typically considered psychedelic. For example, in Chapter 8, we will see that Henri Poincaré had a psychedelic experience after drinking *coffee*.[10] Moreover, if, in unpacking the idea of a psychedelic experience, we find that there are *different kinds* of psychedelic experiences, then even more possibilities arise. It may be that psychedelics tend to induce psychedelic experiences of a particular kind, while meditation may tend to induce psychedelic experiences of another kind. We may also consider the possibility that different kinds of psychedelics reliably produce different kinds of psychedelic experiences. And so on. The possibilities are endless, and they come more clearly into our view when we clean up our concepts.[11]

With this perspective in place, there is one terminological issue that needs to be sorted out: we need some convenient way of referring to the series of experiences that one typically has after consuming a psychedelic drug. For convenience, I will stick to what has become convention and refer to these as *psychedelic trips* or *psychedelic sessions*. Thus, a psychedelic trip is a series of experiences one has after consuming a psychedelic drug, but those experiences may or may not be psychedelic (i.e. mind-revealing)—and some may be psychedelic, while others are not. This terminological setup is not ideal, but it is a reasonable compromise between how these terms are now commonly used and the mission of staying true to the original meaning of 'psychedelic'.

To summarize, our question is about the concept of psychedelic experience. So far, we only have a rather rough understanding of this concept: we know it has something to do with revealing the mind in some way. In order for us to answer the question—and thus develop a more precise understanding of psychedelic experience—we first need to sort out our methodology for doing so.

2.3 Methodology

Now that we have clarified the question, let's consider how we should go about answering it.

Since our central question is a conceptual one, the most suitable way of answering it is by using some method of conceptual analysis (broadly construed). Moreover, since the concept in question is relatively new, largely undefined, and intended for scientific and philosophical discourse, the most appropriate kind of method would be one of *conceptual explication*.

---

[10] For what it's worth, several friends have also reported experiencing similar effects from coffee.

[11] Concepts are like mental lenses. By cleaning them up and choosing them carefully, we can put our experiences more sharply into focus. As we will see in the coming chapters, the practice of meditation can also be extremely useful in this process. It can help us notice when our concepts are distorting our experiences and help us become more flexible in adapting our conceptual schemes to whatever is present.

A conceptual explication is an analysis of a vague or relatively undefined concept that provides a transformative definition, making the concept more suitable for scientific and philosophical use. For example, consider the concept of the hardness of a material. Before the early nineteenth century, this concept was relatively undefined, despite its increasing use in scientific and engineering applications. It was clear that some materials were harder than others, but there was no systematic way of defining the hardness of a given material. The situation improved dramatically when Mohs and Haidinger (1825) introduced the Mohs scale of mineral hardness, which defined the hardness of a material in terms of its resistance to being scratched by other materials. The introduction of this definition is a classic example of explication: the Mohs scale gave us a definition of hardness that is more precise than our intuitive, pre-theoretical notion of hardness, and this increase in precision allowed for novel theoretical and practical applications (including even better explications that were subsequently developed).

The goal here is to do the same sort of thing for the concept of psychedelic experience. As things stand, we only have a rough idea of what psychedelic experiences are—they have something to do with the mind being revealed. We also have the idea that emotional insights are one kind of psychedelic experience. Presumably, though, there are other kinds of psychedelic experiences. It also seems clear that some experiences are more psychedelic than others and that psychedelic experiences can vary in their qualities in theoretically and therapeutically important ways. However, we currently lack any way of making these ideas precise. Indeed, the present situation regarding the concept of psychedelic experience is somewhat similar to that of the concept of hardness prior to the early nineteenth century. So, one goal of this book is to help bring about some conceptual clarity by introducing an explication of the concept of psychedelic experience.

Different philosophical theories of explication have advanced different criteria for a successful explication. I won't take a stand on these issues because settling them would take us too far afield, and they would have little impact on the success of the particular explication that I will offer. To keep things simple, I will follow a broadly Carnapian view of explication (Carnap 1951). According to this view, an explication is successful to the extent that it is: (i) *simple*, (ii) *precise*, (iii) *faithful* to the original concept, and (iv) theoretically *fruitful*. Let us take a moment to discuss how these criteria work to define a successful explication. This will give us some concrete tools we can use to evaluate the explication of psychedelic experience that we will develop in the next chapter.

First, let's consider simplicity. This criterion is relatively straightforward, and there are two reasons for including it. The first is that our ultimate goal is to improve our understanding of psychedelic experience. In general, complexity tends to be detrimental to our understanding of anything. So, we should aim to keep things as simple as possible, all else being equal. The second reason is that keeping things simple helps protect us from the problem of overfitting. A complex explication of a concept will have many moving parts, and so hypotheses that involve its application will tend to have many degrees of freedom, making it difficult for us to test the hypotheses empirically. So, whatever explication of psychedelic experience we give, it should be as simple as possible. The more complicated an explication is, the more sceptical we should be of it, all other things being equal.

Second, let's consider precision. A primary motivation for giving an explication is to make an imprecise concept more precise. Therefore, it makes sense that when we judge how successful an explication is, one dimension of evaluation should be its precision. One way to develop a more precise formulation of a concept is to unpack it in terms of other concepts that are already more precise. For example, instead of focusing on mind-revealing experiences, we could unpack *emotion-revealing* experiences. Similarly, another concept that is more precise is *memory*, and in this regard, one specific kind of psychedelic experience would be a *memory-revealing* experience. And so on.[12] By unpacking the concept according to these more specific formulations, we can get a better grasp of the more general term. From these different formulations, we can start to develop testable hypotheses involving their application. For example, if psychedelic drugs produce various mind-revealing experiences, it seems reasonable to expect that they may produce memory-revealing experiences. The question would then be: do we have any evidence that psychedelics tend to cause people to have experiences in which their memories are revealed? (We will consider this question in Chapter 6.)

Another way to formulate the concept in more precise terms would be to quantify it. The analogy with hardness is helpful here. In everyday language, we speak of materials as being hard or soft as though this is a binary matter. However, we also recognize that some materials are *harder* than others. The Mohs scale of hardness gives us a precise way of saying what it means for one material to be harder than the other: the former can scratch the latter but not vice versa. This principle gives us an *ordinal ranking* of materials in terms of their hardness.[13] The same idea may hold for psychedelic experiences: just as one material may be harder than another, one experience may be more psychedelic than another. In this way, we can develop a more precise conception of psychedelic experience by defining what it means for experiences to be more or less psychedelic. We may not arrive at a numerical measure of how psychedelic any given experience is, but developing an understanding of how one experience may be more psychedelic than another would count as an increase in precision.

[12] For example, we could also consider the revelation of different forms of memory—episodic, semantic, procedural, etc.
[13] Subsequent explications of hardness have given us even more quantitative, and thus even more precise, definitions of hardness (Walley 2012).

Yet another way to define a concept more precisely is to highlight its contrasts. For example, we are interested in the concept of psychedelic *experience*, as opposed to, say, psychedelic *inference*. While some philosophers have debated the distinction between experiences and inferences, our pre-theoretical grasp of these notions is that they correspond to two ways of acquiring knowledge. For example, I may learn some facts about Tibet by experiencing them first-hand or by reading about them in a book and inferring that they are true (assuming I think the book is reliable). In our case, a psychedelic experience is one in which a person may learn certain facts about one's mind by experiencing them directly. In contrast, a psychedelic experience is not an experience in which facts about one's mind are learned, say, by reading a psychology textbook. Highlighting this contrast increases our capacity to formulate a more precise concept of psychedelic experience.

It also opens the door to additional ways of increasing precision. For example, we could be more precise about the distinction between experience and inference by considering to what degree knowledge acquired by experience involves some form of inference. Furthermore, philosophers of mind may ask how debates around direct realism and representationalism relate to the idea of psychedelic experience. For example, are experiences of the mind direct, or are they always mediated by cognitive models or representations? We may also wonder how psychedelic experiences relate to other kinds of experiences, such as *aesthetic experiences*. These are important and fascinating questions that should eventually be addressed, and I touch on them briefly in the coming chapters. However, my goal in this book is only to develop the explication with enough precision that is sufficient for us to evaluate the merit of this general approach.

Third, let's consider the criterion of faithfulness. According to this criterion, an explication's definition must not be *too* transformative. That is, the end result must bear some resemblance to the original concept (and the more the better, all else being equal). Otherwise, if this criterion is not satisfied, the new definition might end up counting as the introduction of a new concept rather than the explication of an already existing one. Of course, that would not necessarily be a bad outcome, since we sometimes need to introduce new concepts and discard old ones. Nevertheless, since the goal here is to define psychedelic experience, understood as the kind of experience that Osmond thought psychedelics tend to induce, the explication should be at least recognizably similar to that original concept.

With that said, it should be acknowledged that there are some subtleties in identifying the original concept. Although the term 'psychedelic' is due to Osmond and Huxley, it is not as though they were the first humans to think of the idea of mind-revelation. As we will see in the next chapter, the idea (or at least a version of it) can be traced back, for example, to William James in 1882 and even de Quincey's 1821 *Confessions of an Opium Eater*. Moreover, depending on how we think about the mind—and how open we are to the interpretation of *psyche* as 'soul' or 'spirit' (or 'breath')—the idea can arguably be traced back to ancient Greek philosophy and various Buddhist and Hindu schools of thought. Since it is clear that Osmond and Huxley were influenced by this history of philosophical thinking, it makes sense for us to use this rich history as a source of data that can ground the original concept.[14]

Fourth, and finally: fruitfulness. The criterion of fruitfulness says that the explication should be theoretically fruitful. This means we should get some kind of scientific or philosophical payoff from the explication—and the bigger the payoff, the better. This criterion of fruitfulness therefore places substantial scientific and philosophical constraints on the explication. For example, in order for the explication to have any chance of being useful in our scientific theorizing, it can't presuppose something that is not in line with our current scientific theories. If our best science says, for instance, that there is no such thing as the Oedipus complex, then the explication better not rely on such complexes as the sorts of things that could be revealed in experience. It should only say that the sorts of things that can be revealed are the sorts of things that science says exist and might possibly be revealed—things such as memories, desires, emotions, knowledge, ideas, and so on. The criterion of fruitfulness therefore prevents the explication from doing anything unscientific.

However, the criterion does much more than that. Not being unscientific is only a *minimal* standard that an explication must meet in order for it to be fruitful. Ideally, it should do much more. In particular, it should help us make scientific and philosophical *progress*. For example, if it makes it easier for us to articulate testable hypotheses and disentangle them from one another, then the explication scores some fruitfulness points. Importantly, these hypotheses need not be true in order for them to advance our understanding. In science, knowing what is false can be just as important as knowing what is true. As I mentioned, it may turn out that psychedelics are not actually psychedelic, or not psychedelic in the ways we may initially expect. Being able to articulate these possibilities, and knowing what would count as evidence for or against them, is a form of fruitfulness.

However, if *all* of the hypotheses turn out to be false, this would be bad news for the explication. Such an outcome would indicate that the explicated concept of psychedelic experience fails to refer to anything real. An analogy may help clarify this point. Suppose I introduced a new concept: the Emperor of Australia. With that new concept, we can articulate new hypotheses. For example: the Emperor of Australia will go to the beach today. If we searched the beaches and found no

[14] One could argue that these various traditions do not share a unified concept of a mind-revealing experience. That may be true, but it is beside the point. The key assumption is that Osmond and Huxley had a single concept of psychedelic experience in mind and that the inspiration for their understanding of this concept is traceable back to these traditions, which may have had different (but perhaps somewhat similar) concepts in use.

sign of Australian emperors, this would serve as evidence against the hypothesis. However, it would also be evidence against the more general hypothesis presumed by the concept, namely, that there is an Emperor of Australia in the first place. As we articulate other hypotheses—for example, the Emperor of Australia sells sausage rolls on Flinders Lane—only to continually find evidence against them, it would become increasingly clear that the new concept is useless. Therefore, although not all of the hypotheses involving the concept need to be true, at least *some* of them should be.[15]

The explication also scores more fruitfulness points to the extent that *diverse* hypotheses involving its application are true. This is because useful concepts help us give unifying explanations of seemingly disparate phenomena. The classic example of this is Newton's theory of gravity (often known as the 'first great unification'), which explained such disparate phenomena as the orbits of celestial bodies and the behaviour of objects on Earth. The unifications proposed in this book are much more modest in scope, but the same fundamental idea applies: to the extent that the concept of psychedelic experience can unify seemingly disparate phenomena, it counts as being fruitful. For example, although the typical experiences induced by meditation and psychedelics may appear quite different from each other, I will argue that they are, in fact, essentially the same kind of experience. Similarly, I will argue that a disparate array of phenomena—from binocular rivalry to certain kinds of memory flashbacks, hallucinations, creative insights, and improvements in well-being—can all be usefully united by the concept of psychedelic experience. The point of making the case of these unifications is twofold: (i) they can advance our understanding of the phenomena in question, and (ii) they help demonstrate the explication's fruitfulness.

One final comment about fruitfulness is worth making. Although the criterion of fruitfulness is often understood in terms of scientific fruitfulness, I will use a broader conception that also includes *philosophical* fruitfulness. In part, this is based on the view that good philosophy and science are continuous with each other. However, there is also another reason. As I mentioned in the previous chapter, I will argue that my explication of the concept of psychedelic experience is also useful for specifically *philosophical* purposes (where philosophy is understood as the pursuit of *wisdom*). In Chapter 11, I will argue that the explication can help us see how we can use the phenomenon of psychedelic experience to do better philosophy. To the extent that this is true, the explication scores additional fruitfulness points.

In total, an explication should be judged by the degree to which it is simple, precise, faithful, and fruitful. Of course, there can be some trade-offs between these

---

[15] To be sure, theoretical context and pragmatic factors play a crucial role in determining the space of hypotheses to be quantified over. This is because we can always find trivial hypotheses that are true.

criteria. For example, we might decide that sacrificing some degree of faithfulness is worthwhile if it means acquiring a greater degree of fruitfulness. Generally speaking, however, a good explication should score high on all of these criteria simultaneously. Similarly, any *alternative* explication should score at least as high on all of the criteria (though, again, some trade-offs may be permitted).

This discussion of conceptual explication gives us the basic rules of the game. These are the rules that any conceptual explication project should follow (generally speaking). However, there are some additional rules that are more specific to the topic of psychedelic experience, which we should also review.

The first such rule concerns the role played by first-person experience in a project such as this one. If someone—let's call her Mary—decided to pursue this kind of philosophical research, would she need to have had a psychedelic experience? It seems that the answer to this question ought to be yes. Otherwise, it would be like trying to conduct a philosophical analysis of colour without having experienced a single one. Moreover, given that there appears to be a considerable variation in the qualities of psychedelic experiences, wouldn't Mary need to have *several* such experiences? Otherwise, this would be like trying to understand colour while only having ever experienced one colour—a particular shade of red, say. If you are trying to understand colour, then it seems you need to experience more than one of them. However, we also don't want to say that one must experience *every* colour. It seems reasonable to expect that experiencing some sufficiently rich set of colours may suffice. For example, perhaps it would be sufficient to experience the primary, secondary, and tertiary colours, and then the mind can use that set of experiences as a basis for imagining or conceiving all others. If this is true of colour, then something similar may also be true of psychedelic experience.

That would help address the concern that it would be a bad outcome if the philosophical investigation of psychedelic experience required its investigators to sample every kind of psychedelic experience. However, we don't yet know what the equivalent of primary, secondary, and tertiary psychedelic experiences would even be. Without knowing what would constitute a minimally sufficient set of base experiences, researchers could fall into the trap of having to sample every kind of psychedelic experience that could ever be generated. For every strange substance that's considered potentially psychedelic—from a mushroom, to toad venom, to nitrous oxide, to a new synthetic compound produced in a mobile laboratory in Florida—Mary and her fellow researchers would have to be well versed in the experiences it induces. Moreover, they would need to be familiar with the experiences produced by *combinations* of these substances (and how they combine with other, non-psychedelic substances). Perhaps worst of all, there would potentially be a competition in terms of dosages. For instance, it is not uncommon for self-professed *psychonauts* to take "heroic" doses of psychedelics, all in the name of exploring the great unknown that is the human mind.

This is a serious problem because of the obvious health risks it poses, but also because of the epistemological instability that ensues. How can we build any serious theory without having some idea of the full gamut of psychedelic experience? The issue does not just arise for drugs, by the way. Pick anything that has the slightest reputation of causing psychedelic experiences—meditation, sensory deprivation, fasting, yoga, etc.—and a similar issue arises. If Mary hasn't experienced the effects of smoking toad venom while doing hot yoga after having fasted for seven days at high altitude, how can we be sure she really knows what she's talking about? There seems to be no limit to such challenges.

I'm not aware of a completely satisfactory solution to this problem. It seems that the best we can do is basically the same as what we do for colour. In the case of colour, we build an initial model that we think might define the space of all possible colours. For example, according to the CMYK model, each colour is defined as a linear combination of the primary colours of cyan, magenta, yellow, and black. Using this model, we can then map each colour in CMYK space, where each dimension of the space corresponds to a primary colour. For example, suppose that someone finds a new pigment that can only be created from some rare Amazonian plant. Furthermore, let's suppose that when we look at this pigment, we experience a colour that is new to us. Nevertheless, even though this colour experience is new for us, if we believe the CMYK model is complete, then we will expect that the colour is located within the model's colour space. There would, thus, be a reasonable expectation that the new pigment would not require a new model of colour. The thought is, then, that perhaps we can accomplish something similar for psychedelic experiences.

Unfortunately, we can't be certain that the CMYK model is complete (indeed, colour theory is much more complex than this simple model). We can bolster our confidence in the completeness of the model by studying the neurophysiology of human perceptual system—how our light cones respond to different stimuli, etc. However, we won't be able to rule out the possibility that there are colours that can be experienced that are not captured by the model. For example, for all we know, it may be possible to *imagine* a colour that is not perceptible via stimulation of our light cones. Indeed, bringing things closer to home, Klüver 1928 noted that people often report that mescaline induces experiences of mental imagery with entirely new colours that they have never seen before. As far as I can tell, there is no way to rule out such possibilities with certainty. The worry, then, is just as we can't be confident that the CMYK model of colour space is complete, we also wouldn't know that any model of psychedelic space that we come up with is complete. The best we can do, I think, is to start with a fairly comprehensive space, ground it in human neurophysiology as much as possible, and then treat potential counterexamples with open-minded scepticism.

With that in mind, let's come back to the original question about the role of first-person experience in a project such as this. Does Mary need to have had some minimal set of psychedelic experiences? The answer is yes—or, at least, it certainly help if she does. However, it's important to be clear that it doesn't follow from this that Mary needs to have had any *drug*-induced experiences. It's entirely possible that a minimal set of psychedelic experiences can consist of experiences induced by other means (by meditation, for example). Ultimately, this will depend on the space of possible experiences and how our eventual theories allow us to make extrapolations across it.

One final methodological issue needs to be addressed before we can proceed. This final issue concerns the question of what epistemic attitude we should have towards mystical traditions such as Buddhism, Daoism, Hinduism, and so on. This book draws upon many of the ideas of these traditions. In particular, there will be much discussion of meditation and mindfulness, which are predominantly Hindu and Buddhist notions. This raises an important difficulty when it comes to interpreting these ideas. For example, as is well known, Buddhism is a plurality of belief systems, and there can be disagreement between Buddhists (and Buddhist scholars) about all sorts of issues.[16] For instance, there is disagreement as to whether the doctrine of non-self (*anattā*) should be interpreted as the metaphysical claim that there is no self or as a methodological technique for attaining self-knowledge (Albahari 2002). This creates a problem. On the one hand, it would be desirable to avoid getting caught up in these intricate debates since they can take us far afield (and have been going on for centuries). On the other hand, the existence of these debates reflects the subtleties of the corresponding issues, and so it would be irresponsible to ignore them.

My solution is to strike a middle ground between these two extremes by embedding the discussion of these issues within the project's larger methodological framework. We will occasionally engage with the discussion surrounding these issues, but the objective is not to settle any debates within the traditions. Instead, the goal is to use these discussions to better inform our own thinking about the relevant concepts. For example, in the case of mindfulness, it makes sense for us to have a definition that doesn't depart radically from traditional definitions and belief systems. However, we also want to have a definition that can be understood in terms of other concepts that are familiar to us—such as attention, memory, unconscious processing, etc. This will help ensure that the concept can be sensibly deployed in experimental settings, so that we can test hypotheses involving mindfulness. It will also help ensure that we can develop explanations of observed phenomena with theoretically grounded concepts. In other words, we want a definition that is simple, precise, fruitful, and which also stays as faithful as possible to tradition. As before, some trade-offs between these criteria are to be expected. Whereas debates within and between these traditions

---

[16] For transparency, my personal orientation is generally ecumenical but I find the most resonance with Advaita Vedanta, Daoism, Rāja and Tantric yoga, and the Soto school of Zen.

(or their scholarship) may place more emphasis on the criterion of faithfulness, in this project we will put more weight on the other criteria. In short, the approach is to use the richness of these traditions to inform our thinking without being beholden to their internal debates.

With that said, it should be noted that what it means to be faithful to these traditions is not as straightforward as might be expected. This is because many of these traditions teach the importance of not clinging to their teachings. For example, various schools of Buddhism emphasize the importance of orthopraxy (correct practice) over orthodoxy (correct belief), resulting in a form of spiritual pragmatism (Braak 2011, p. xii). As Seung Sahn put it in the case of Zen:

> There are many misconceptions about the nature of Zen teaching and practice. Zen teaching simply means not attaching to language. If you want to attain the Buddha's way, then don't attach to speech and words.
>
> Sahn 2012, p. 254

And, in Verse 18 of the *Amritabindu Upanishad*, we find:

> Having studied books, the wise man, solely devoted to knowledge and wisdom, should give up the books entirely, like the man who, seeking for rice, gives up the husk.[17]

From this perspective, staying faithful to the mystical traditions isn't a matter of maintaining propositional verisimilitude. However, it's difficult to say what it does amount to—not surprisingly.[18] My take is that it involves conducting one's philosophy in this area with kindness, flexibility, and an authenticity that is ineffable but nonetheless recognizable (you know it when you see it). To the extent that this can be articulated in the language of analytic philosophy, staying faithful to these traditions involves, somewhat paradoxically, a reflexive relaxing of the faithfulness condition (understood propositionally) for the benefit of greater simplicity, precision, and fruitfulness.

2.4 Conclusion

The point of this chapter was to set up a particular way of approaching our topic and to make sure that we are clear about what question we are asking and

---

[17] Sastri 1921, p. 74.
[18] The Buddhist concept of *upaya* (skilful or expedient means) is relevant here, but it requires a lengthy discussion that would take us too far afield. In part, this is because this concept has received multiple interpretations, including consequentialist ones that can lead to predictably undesirable outcomes.

how we should go about answering it. Because of how the term 'psychedelic' is generally used in society, it is tempting to think of our question as primarily being one about drugs. I have argued that we should resist that temptation. There is a theoretical advantage to understanding the concept of psychedelic experience as the concept of *mind-revealing* experience rather than, say, some kind of *drug-induced* experience.

We now have a sound methodological framework for tackling this fascinating topic. In the next chapter, I will give an explication of the concept of psychedelic experience. This will answer our question of what psychedelic experience is and then allow us to consider hypotheses involving the application of that concept.

3

Psychedelic Space

3.1 Introduction

In the previous chapter, we established that our central question is a conceptual one. It is the question of what it means for an experience to be psychedelic. I then provided a rough answer: an experience is psychedelic if it is a *mind-revealing* experience. However, we don't really know what a mind-revealing experience is yet. This chapter aims to unpack this idea in more detail.

To get started, in Section 3.2, we will explore the history of the idea of a psychedelic experience. Although the *term* 'psychedelic' is due to Humphrey Osmond, we will see that the *idea* of a psychedelic experience dates back to well before his time. Appreciating the history of the idea will help us develop a more contextual understanding of the concept of psychedelic experience. As I mentioned in the previous chapter, having this contextual understanding is important because a precise explication of the idea should be *faithful* to the original concept (however vague or undefined it may be). So, we need to understand what the original concept is.

With that understanding in place, we will then turn to the main task of unpacking the concept in more precise and familiar terms. Section 3.3 will provide the first step in this direction. In this section, we will examine the three component concepts of psychedelic experience—(i) the mind, (ii) revelation, and (iii) experience—and how they combine to form the aggregate concept. This will help us determine a set of conditions that may usefully be regarded as being necessary and sufficient for an experience to be psychedelic. As part of this discussion, I will give some concrete examples of experiences that satisfy these conditions and of others that do not. In order to help delineate the concept of psychedelic experience, we will also consider its conceptual opposite: *psychecryptic experience*.

The main result of Section 3.3 will be an explication of the concept of psychedelic experience. However, it will be a relatively rough-and-ready explication. This is because the explication will treat the concept only in categorical terms: it will say that an experience will count as psychedelic if it meets the necessary and sufficient conditions. Although there is value in having such an explication, it needs to be refined to account for the fact that psychedelic experiences come in *degrees*. This will be the task of Section 3.4, where we will explore what it means for one experience to be *more psychedelic* than another. This exploration will lead us to a multi-dimensional conceptual space of experiences that I call *psychedelic space*. The final explication of the concept of psychedelic experience will be in terms of this space. Roughly speaking, it will say that the deeper an experience is in psychedelic space, the more psychedelic it is. This framework will form the philosophical backbone of the rest of the book.

3.2 History

As we saw in the previous chapter, the *term* 'psychedelic' was coined by Humphrey Osmond, with the help of Aldous Huxley (Bisbee et al. 2018). However, the *concept* had already been around for quite some time. For example, one can see a version of the idea in Williams James' reflections on his experiences with nitrous oxide:

> I myself made some observations on [...] nitrous oxide intoxication, and reported them in print. One conclusion was forced upon my mind at that time, and my impression of its truth has ever since remained unshaken. It is that our normal waking consciousness, rational consciousness as we call it, is but one special type of consciousness, whilst all about it, parted from it by the filmiest of screens, there lie potential forms of consciousness entirely different. We may go through life without suspecting their existence; but apply the requisite stimulus, and at a touch they are there in all their completeness, definite types of mentality which probably somewhere have their field of application and adaptation.
>
> James 1902, pp. 300–1[1]

James' metaphor of the filmiest of screens evokes the idea of something being hidden and which could be revealed—in this case, by nitrous oxide, but also potentially by some other stimulus. Note that the implication is not that nitrous oxide *creates* the alternative forms of consciousness, nor that it *transforms* the normal form into a new one. Rather, the nitrous oxide *reveals* what was always there.[2]

Although James is typically associated with this insight about the effects of nitrous oxide, he was clearly inspired by Benjamin Paul Blood, who described the general idea in an 1874 article entitled *The Anaesthetic Revelation and the Gist of Philosophy*:

> By the Anaesthetic Revelation I mean a certain survived condition, (or uncondition,) in which is the satisfaction of philosophy an appreciation of the genius of being, which appreciation cannot be brought out of that condition into the

---

[1] James made his original comments on the effects of nitrous oxide in James 1882.

[2] To be clear: nitrous oxide isn't typically considered a psychedelic substance. The point is simply that James' *experience* was psychedelic. Nevertheless, it is interesting to note that recent evidence indicates that nitrous oxide may have an important similarity to classic psychedelics in that it might be effective in treating major depression (Nagele et al. 2021).

normal sanity of sense—cannot be formally remembered, but remains informal, forgotten until we return to it.

'As here we find in trances, men
Forget the dream that happens then,
Until they fall in trance again'

Of this condition, although it may have been attained otherwise, I know only by the use of anaesthetic agents. After experiments ranging over nearly fourteen years I affirm—what any man may prove at will—that there is an invariable and reliable condition (or uncondition) ensuring about the instant of recall from anaesthetic stupor to sensible observation or 'coming to,' in which the genius of being is revealed; but because it cannot be remembered in the normal condition it is lost altogether through the infrequency of anaesthetic treatment in any individual's case ordinarily, and buried, amid the hum of returning common sense, under that epitaph of all illumination: 'this is a queer world'. Yet I have warned others to expect this wonder on entering the anaesthetic slumber, and none so cautioned has failed to report of it in terms which assured me of its realization.

Blood 1874, pp. 33–4

The rest of Blood's article indicates that the experience he is describing is likely a *mystical experience*. We will address such experiences in Chapter 10. For now, it is enough to observe that Blood had the idea that there can be a condition that is lost, or forgotten, but which can be revealed in experience by anaesthetic agents—and potentially by other means.

About half a century earlier, we find the idea of a psychedelic experience in Thomas de Quincey's *Confessions of an English Opium-Eater*:

The minutest incidents of childhood, or forgotten scenes of later years, were often revived: I could not be said to recollect them; for if I had been told of them when waking, I should not have been able to acknowledge them as parts of my past experience. But placed as they were before me, in dreams like intuitions, and clothed in all their evanescent circumstances and accompanying feelings, I *recognized* them instantaneously. [...] Of this at least I feel assured, that there is no such thing as *forgetting* possible to the mind; a thousand accidents may and will interpose a veil between our present consciousness and the secret inscriptions on the mind; accidents of the same sort will also rend away this veil; but alike, whether veiled or unveiled, the inscription remains forever, just as stars seem to withdraw before the common light of day, whereas in fact we all know that it is the light which is drawn over them as a veil, and that they are waiting to be revealed when the obscuring daylight shall have withdrawn.

Quincey 1821, p. 581

Whereas James focused on forms of consciousness being separated by the filmiest of screens, de Quincey expresses the idea in terms of *memories* being obscured by a veil. Indeed, Blood also expressed his idea in terms of memory but, in his case, it was the memory of a condition (or uncondition)—one that 'cannot be formally remembered, but remains informal, forgotten until we return to it'. The fundamental idea among these different authors is clearly the same: some parts or aspects of the mind are hidden from conscious experience during everyday life, and the consumption of a psychoactive substance can reveal them. They also share another important insight: James describes the screen as filmy and removable by a requisite stimulus, de Quincey says that accidents may rend away the veil, and Blood supposes that his anaesthetic revelation could be attained by other means. All three converge on the thought that, although consuming a psychoactive substance brought about the novel experience, it may be that the experience can be brought about by other means.

It is more difficult to find explicit traces of the idea of psychedelic experience before 1821, at least in Western texts. Much of what the Christian mystics wrote is very suggestive, but they were primarily focused on searching for God, so it is not clear that they conceptualized their experiences in terms of the mind being revealed. The Neoplatonists come closer, especially Plotinus. For example:

> What is our course and what is our means of flight? We should not rely on our feet to get us there, for our feet just take us everywhere on earth, one place after another. Nor should you saddle up a horse or prepare some sea-going vessel. You should put aside all such things and stop looking; just shut your eyes, and change your way of looking, and wake up. Everyone has this ability, but few use it.
>
> Plotinus, *Ennead I*, 6.8.25[3]

> So if there is going to be apprehension of things present in this way, then that which is to apprehend must revert inward, and focus its attention there. Just as if someone were waiting to hear a voice that he wanted to hear, and, distancing himself from other voices, were to prick up his ears to hear the best of sounds, waiting for the time when it will come—so, too, in this case one must let go of sensible sounds, except insofar as they are necessary, and guard the soul's pure power of apprehension and be ready to listen to the sounds from above.
>
> Plotinus, *Ennead V*, 1.2.15[4]

In these passages, we see Plotinus expressing the idea that there is something hidden within that can be revealed and that this can be achieved by disengaging from the external world and concentrating one's attention inwards. As we will see in Chapter 5, this is a form of meditation. Similar ideas are also found in gnostic writings, such as the Gospel of Thomas:

---

[3] Boys-Stones et al. 2018, p. 101.   [4] Ibid. p. 547.

When you bring forth *that* within you,
then *that* will save you.
If you do not,
then *that* will kill you.

Gospel of Thomas, Logion 70[5]

How to interpret the mysterious 'that' is open to debate, with Love, Being, Oneness, or some form of ineffable knowledge as plausible candidates.

Going back even earlier, we can see traces of the idea in ancient Greek philosophy but, as with the Christian mystics, it is not easy to disentangle their beliefs about the divine from their beliefs about the mind. In this regard, it is worth highlighting that the term *psychē* has been interpreted with several meanings, including "mind", "soul", and "breath"—understood as spirit, subtle energy, or animating life force. A psychedelic experience could, therefore, also be understood as a *soul*-revealing experience. Indeed, psychedelic substances are sometimes called *entheogens*, derived from *entheos* and *genesthai*, to signify that they fill one with spirit or make one divinely inspired. Our focus for now, however, is primarily the concept of a mind-revealing experience (while leaving open the possibility that the soul, spirit, or divinity can also be revealed).

Coming back now to the point about the ancient Greek philosophers, much of what Socrates said—or, rather, what Plato wrote—stands out as particularly psychedelic. For example, in *Phaedrus*, we see:

[...] not every soul is easily reminded of the reality there [the place beyond heaven[6]] by what it finds here [mortal life]—not souls that got only a brief glance at the reality there, not souls who had such bad luck when they fell down here that they were twisted by bad company into lives of injustice so that they forgot the sacred objects they had seen before. Only a few remain whose memory is good enough; and they are startled when they see an image of what they saw up there. Then they are beside themselves, and their experience is beyond their comprehension because they cannot fully grasp what it is that they are seeing.

[...] the senses are so murky that only a few people are able to make out, with difficulty, the original of the likenesses they encounter here. But beauty was radiant to see at that time when the souls [...] saw that blessed and spectacular vision and were ushered into the mystery that we may rightly call the most blessed of all. And we who celebrated it were wholly perfect and free of all the troubles that awaited us in time to come, and we gazed in rapture at sacred revealed objects that were perfect, and simple, and unshakeable and blissful. That was the

---

[5] Leloup and Rowe 2005, p. 41.

[6] Interestingly, Socrates' description of the place beyond heaven has striking similarities to some reports of particularly extreme psychedelic trips: 'What is in this place is without color and without shape and without solidity, a being that really is what it is, the subject of all true knowledge, visible only to intelligence, the soul's steersman'.

ultimate vision, and we saw it in pure light because we were pure ourselves, not buried in this thing we are carrying around now, which we call a body, locked in it like an oyster in its shell.

Socrates in Phaedrus, 250a–250c[7]

Although this passage involves reference to souls and 'a place beyond heaven', it is clear that what Plato is referring to here is a psychedelic experience (indeed, one that has mystical qualities). For Plato, especially in *Phaedrus* and *Symposium*, instances of worldly beauty can awaken the soul by reminding one of Beauty in its perfect and ultimate form.

In *Phaedo*, Socrates' argument for the permanence of the soul involves a reflection that could easily be a praise of meditation:

> Surely the soul can best reflect when it is free of all distractions such as hearing or sight or pain or pleasure of any kind—that is, when it ignores the body and becomes as far as possible independent (of it), avoiding all physical contacts and associations as much as it can, in its search for reality [...] cutting himself off as much as possible from his eyes and ears and virtually all the rest of his body, as an impediment which by its presence prevents the soul from attaining to truth.

Socrates, in Phaedo, 65b[8]

And, quite famously, he likened his method of *elenchos* (now commonly known as the Socratic method) to the practice of midwifery:

> Now my art of midwifery is just like theirs in most respects. The difference is that I attend men and not women,[9] and that I watch over the labor of their souls, not of their bodies. And the most important thing about my art is the ability to apply all possible tests to the offspring, to determine whether the young mind is being delivered of a phantom, that is, an error, or a fertile truth. [...] At first some of them may give the impression of being ignorant and stupid; but as time goes on and our association continues, all whom God permits are seen to make a progress which is amazing both to other people and to themselves. And yet it is clear that this is not due to anything they have learned from me; it is that they discover within themselves a multitude of beautiful things, which they bring forth into the light. But it is I, with God's help, who deliver them of this offspring.

Socrates, Theaetetus, 150b–c[10]

It's also worth noting that Socrates' method of *elenchos* was part of Plato's theory of *anamnēsis*, according to which philosophical learning is actually the *remembering*

---

[7] Reeve 2012.   [8] Hamilton and Cairns 1980.
[9] Unfortunately, such sexism was common at the time.
[10] Cooper and Hutchinson 1997.

of knowledge that was acquired by the soul before one's birth but has since been forgotten (as described in the above passage from *Phaedrus*). Finally, we know that a central point of focus for Socrates' philosophizing was to *know thyself*, with the implication being that knowing oneself is not a trivial matter.[11]

Finally, it seems likely that many of the Athenian philosophers took part in the Eleusinian Mysteries, which have been argued to have involved the consumption of a psychedelic substance known as *kykeon* (Hillman 2008, Clark 2017, Muraresku 2020). Plato's *Symposium* appears to be especially oriented towards these mystery rites, and the Socrates-Diotima speech on *eros* (love) is divided into two parts that are modelled on the lesser and greater Mysteries. After having established the connection between love and procreation (of body and soul), Diotima says:

> These are aspects of the mystery of love that perhaps you too, Socrates, might be initiated into. But for the final initiation and revelation, to which all this has been merely preliminary for someone on the right track, I am not sure if you have the capability. However I will do my utmost to explain to you, and you must try to follow if you can.
>
> Diotima in *Symposium*, 209e–210b[12]

She then goes on to explain how someone who is appropriately guided by a love for beauty will eventually perceive its ultimate form. The qualities of this experience give it a striking resemblance to those experiences that we now call mystical:

> Anyone who has been guided to this point in the study of love [. . .] will suddenly perceive [. . .] a beauty that is marvellous in its nature—the very thing, Socrates, for the sake of which all the earlier labours were undertaken. What he sees is, in the first place, eternal; [. . .] Secondly, [. . .] it exists on its own, single in substance and everlasting. [. . .] What, then, do we suppose it would be like for someone actually to see the beautiful itself, separate, clear and pure, unsullied by the flesh or by colour or by the rest of our mortal dross, but to perceive the beautiful itself, single in substance and divine? Do you think that a person who directs his gaze to that object and contemplates it with that faculty by which it has to be viewed, and stays close to it, has a poor life? Do you not reflect that it is there alone, when he sees the beautiful with that by which it has to be viewed, that he will give birth to true virtue? He will give birth not to mere images of virtue but to true virtue, because it is not an image that he is grasping but the truth. When he has given birth to and nurtured true virtue it is possible for him to be loved by the gods and to become, if any human can, immortal himself.
>
> Diotima in *Symposium*, 210e–212a[13]

---

[11] Incidentally, the maxim was inscribed above the entrance to the temple of Delphi, and there is evidence that the temple was regularly filled with light hydrocarbon gases from bituminous limestone, known to have effects similar to those of classic psychedelics (Boer et al. 2001).

[12] Howatson and Sheffield 2008.   [13] Ibid.

Plato is clearly drawing a connection between the wisdom that philosophers seek and the revelation of the greater Mysteries.[14] Because of the secrecy surrounding Eleusinian Mysteries, which may have been due to the ineffability of the final revelation, we know very little about them. However, we have second-hand knowledge from Aristotle that the initiates did not *learn* anything but instead experienced the revelations and were brought to an appropriate state of mind (Burkert 1985, p. 286).

Going back further, we also know that Pythagoras travelled frequently to learn the practices of the Egyptian mystics, which also involved the ritualistic consumption of unknown pharmacological concoctions (Hillman 2008). So, it is plausible that the golden age of Athenian philosophy was grounded in regular substance-induced psychedelic experiences. However, whether substances were involved is not our concern here. At the moment, we are only considering whether the Athenian philosophers were familiar with psychedelic *experiences*, irrespective of how they were brought about.

Another plausible way of tracing the history of the concept of psychedelic experience comes from Ellenberger's 1966 discussion of what he calls the *pathogenic secret*. Ellenberger argued that many indigenous and shamanic populations have, for many centuries (if not millennia), understood illness and disease as involving pathogenic secrets, defined as parts or aspects of the mind (broadly construed) that are hidden from the person suffering from poor health and the cause of their condition. For example, many shamanic traditions have understood disease to occur when the soul accidentally leaves the body—perhaps because it is somehow stolen or becomes lost. This would seem to correspond to the opposite of psychedelic experience, namely, a *psychecryptic experience*: a mind- or soul-*concealing* experience. According to such traditions, solving this problem involves finding and returning the soul to the individual through some kind of intervention, which would then presumably result in a psychedelic experience. The intervention could involve anything from a "spell" being cast by a shaman (perhaps as a form of hypnosis), to a dance being performed by the community, to the individual consuming a psychedelic substance.

To be clear, we needn't believe these ideas in order to recognize that the same *concept* is in play: namely, that a part or aspect of the mind (understood broadly) can be hidden and then revealed via some intervention. With that said, it should be

---

[14] In *Phaedo*, we also see a connection drawn between philosophy and the mystic rites:

> It is likely that those who established the mystic rites for us were not inferior persons but were speaking in riddles long ago when they said that whoever arrives in the underworld uninitiated and unsanctified will wallow in the mire, whereas he who arrives there purified and initiated will dwell with the gods. There are indeed, as those concerned with the mysteries say, many who carry the thyrsus but the Bacchants are few. These latter are, in my opinion, no other than those who have practiced philosophy in the right way. I have in my life left nothing undone in order to be counted among these as far as possible, as I have been eager to be in every way.
>
> Socrates in *Phaedo*, 69c–d (Grube and Cooper 2002, p. 106)

noted that Ellenberger 1970 argues that although such interventions and theories may seem misguided to us, they have a lot in common with early Western theories of the unconscious and even modern theories of psychological conditions, such as depression and anxiety. We also have growing scientific evidence that psychedelics are particularly effective in treating such conditions (Nutt and Carhart-Harris 2020). So, it is not implausible that there is more psychological knowledge in these traditions than has been previously recognized, especially in connection to psychedelics (Schultes et al. 2001).

If we turn our attention to the Eastern traditions, we again find the same idea, but with a strong focus on meditation as the method for inducing psychedelic experiences. For example, the concept of *ekō henshō* captures the idea of turning one's attention from the external world and directing it inward, into the mind, in order to experience a hidden truth:

> Calm yourself, quiet your senses. Look right into the source of mind, always keeping it shining bright, clear and pure.
>
> Daman Hongren 601–74[15]

> When you do not think of good and do not think of bad, what is your original face? (At these words, Huiming was greatly enlightened) What I have told you is no secret. If you reflect inwardly, the secret is in you.
>
> Dajian Huineng 617–713[16]

> The thinker is the mind and the thought-of is the environment. Therein are mountains, rivers [. . .] and so forth; reverse your thought to think of the thinking mind—are there so many things there? You people should all turn back your light and reflect; do not memorize my words. Since beginning-less eons you have turned your backs on the light and plunged into darkness; the roots of your false conceptions are deep.
>
> Yangshan Huiji 807–83[17]

> As a beginner, knowing there is something fundamental in oneself when one turns the light around (shifts attention from sense experience to the essence of mind), one ejects form, sound, smell, flavor, touch, and phenomena, and attains tranquility. Then, after fully accomplishing this, one does not grasp the sense data but descends among them without being blinded, letting them be, without interference.
>
> Sōzan Honjaku 840–901[18]

> The most important thing is for people of great faculties and sharp wisdom to turn the light of mind around and shine back and clearly awaken to this mind before a single thought is born [. . .].
>
> Yuanwu Keqin 1063–1135[19]

---

[15] Cleary 1995, p. 9. [16] Cleary 1998, p. 13. [17] Cleary 1998, p. 140.
[18] Cleary 1986, p. 9. [19] Cleary and Cleary 1994, p. 66.

Everyone without exception holds on to the jewel that glows in the night. [...]
Unless we turn the light within to illuminate the self, how can we hold close the
jewel when we are lost in the outlying countryside?

Eihei Dogen 1200–53[20]

These passages highlight four key points. First, they express the idea that meditation is fundamental to attaining the revelatory experience. Second, they give
us a sense of what a meditation practice would involve: turning our *attention*
('the light') inward and letting the regular activity of the mind settle down, so
that one achieves a *clarity* of mind that makes it easier to *see* something hidden
in the mind ('the secret is in you', 'the jewel that glows in the night'). Third, we
see that meditation is not only about relaxation or stress reduction, but involves
having 'great faculties' and 'sharp wisdom', and achieving something substantial
and rare ('[s]ince beginning-less eons you have turned your backs on the light and
plunged into darkness'). Fourth, and finally, the passages also resonate with the
Western examples we have already seen—for example, the Delphic maxim to *know
thyself*, Socrates' notion of the soul contemplating without sensory distractions,
and Plotinus' idea of directing the faculty of sensation inwards. As before, we do
not have to agree with the statements contained in these passages to recognize that
they involve the concept of a psychedelic experience. The point, rather, is that the
authors clearly had the idea that something about (or in) the mind can, in some
sense, be hidden from us, and can be revealed in experience via the appropriate
intervention—in this case, *ekō henshō*.

Many Eastern schools of thought tend to refrain from using substances as
part of their practices and instead place a strong emphasis on meditation and
contemplation (of koans, for example).[21] The Vedic traditions also tend to have a
somewhat similar orientation, but in some cases, they are open to the consumption
of psychoactive substances. Quite famously, the *Rig Veda* describes the practice of
drinking a substance known as *soma*:

We have drunk the soma; we have become immortal; we have gone to the light;
we have found the gods.

Rigveda Mandala 8.48.3[22]

Although the exact pharmacological makeup of soma is unknown, many
have argued that it was a psychedelic substance.[23] In particular, some recent

---

[20] Leighton and Okumura 2010, pp. 268–9.
[21] One exception is the use of tea, which is sometimes used to sustain alertness during long
periods of meditation. Another notable exception is Vajrayana Buddhism, which sometimes permits
small amounts of alcohol and potentially other substances, including psychedelics (Crowley and
Shulgin 2019).
[22] Jamison and Brereton 2014, p. 1129.
[23] In a letter to Huxley, Osmond wrote: 'Soma might be the herb which would restore vision of the
inner and so would justly be considered king of the herbs. This would put psychedelics among the
earliest pieces of pharmacological equipment and mean that medicine has been deeply concerned with
them from its inception'. Osmond, February 1958 (Bisbee et al. 2018, p. 370).

archaeological evidence suggests that it was made out of psilocybin mushrooms (Polosmak 2010), but there is also evidence that it was made out of *Amanita muscaria* mushrooms (Maillart-Garg and Winkelman 2019), and others yet have argued that it was a plant-based analogue of ayahuasca (Clark 2017, 2019).

Putting aside the question of whether soma was a psychedelic substance, it seems reasonably clear that the Vedics were familiar with the possibility of psychedelic experiences. For example, in the *Katha Upanishad*, we find reference to a hidden self that can be seen by certain kinds of people:

> Hidden in all the beings,
> this self is not visibly displayed.
> Yet, people of keen vision see him,
> with eminent and sharp minds.
>
> *Katha Upanishad*, Section 3, Verse 12[24]

And, in the *Amritabindu Upanishad*, we're told how this self can be revealed (through a form of meditation):

> Quite concealed in all beings dwells *Vijñāna* [pure consciousness/Self] as butter in milk; ever churn [meditate], O aspirant! with *manas* [mind] as the churning stick.
>
> *Amritabindu Upanishad*, Verse 20[25]

It should be noted, however, that we need to be careful with these translations (which are subject to debate) and remember that the conceptualization of a hidden self (Atman) in the Vedas may differ from that of other traditions. Like the Greek philosophers and Christian mystics, the conceptualization is not easily separable from the hidden divinity or ultimate truth that is supposedly revealed. Nevertheless, it seems reasonably clear that the concept of a psychedelic experience appears to be deployed in the Vedas: something important (e.g. a certain kind of knowledge) is hidden within the mind (broadly construed) that can be revealed via an appropriate intervention (meditation/contemplation). At the very least, this *interpretation* of the Vedas appears to have been a strong influence on Osmond and Huxley's thinking when they were coining the term 'psychedelic'.

That's a brief (and incomplete) summary of the history of the concept of psychedelic experience.[26] It is important to remember that it has *not* been a brief

---

[24] Olivelle 1998, p. 391.   [25] Sastri 1921, p. 76.

[26] It should be emphasized that this summary is not intended to be complete. For example, the above includes no discussion of the related ideas that appear in other Abrahamic religions and mystical traditions. A detailed discussion of the varieties of shamanism and indigenous belief systems (such as 'the Dreaming' of the Aboriginal peoples of Australia) would also be warranted as part of a complete discussion. The goal here was simply to give some of the historical context behind the concept that Osmond and Huxley were using to account for the effects of psychedelic substances.

history of psychedelic *drugs*, nor has it been the etymological history of the *term* 'psychedelic'. It's the history of an *idea*: the idea that there are parts or aspects of the mind that are normally hidden from us and which can be unveiled through an experience. Let's now see if we can make this idea more precise.

3.3 Psychedelic Experience

Let's think more carefully about what it means for the mind to be revealed in experience—that is, for an experience to be psychedelic. We can begin by thinking about the component concepts—mind, revelation, and experience—and how they combine to form the aggregate concept.

Let's consider revelation. What does it mean to reveal something? It means that the entity in question was in some way obscured from someone and then something happens to change that. A poker player may reveal their cards by turning them over. A child playing a game of hide-and-seek may choose to step out from their hiding place and reveal themselves. An artist may reveal their latest painting to the critics at an exhibition by removing the cloth that was covering it. Your partner may reveal their new tattoo to you by pulling up their sleeve. And so on.

The concept of revelation is relatively straightforward, but one of its subtleties comes to light when we combine it with the concept of *experience*. This subtlety arises because of a distinction between revealing something via *inference* or via *experience*.[27] Using the tattoo example, there are two different things that your partner could reveal to you: (i) the fact that they have a tattoo or (ii) the tattoo itself. They may reveal the fact that they have a tattoo simply by telling you that they have a tattoo. However, if they are to reveal the tattoo itself, you have to actually *see* it. In this second case, we may say that you had a tattoo-revealing experience and that in the first case, you did not. In the first case, you *inferred* the fact from what your partner said—you have to trust that, for instance, they were not lying to you and that you heard them correctly. It is the second kind of case that we are interested in here: we can have tattoo-revealing experiences, painting-revealing experiences, and so on.[28]

We have combined the concepts of revelation and experience to form the aggregate concept of a revelatory experience. Let's now add the concept of the mind by replacing the general idea of a revelatory experience with the more specific

---

[27] Some philosophers and psychologists think that experiences are just certain kinds of unconscious inferences—or the outputs thereof. I will discuss this issue later on. For now, we can make do with our everyday, pre-theoretical understanding of the difference between inference and experience.

[28] This distinction between revelation via inference and revelation via experience is similar to Bertrand Russell's distinction between knowledge by description and knowledge by acquaintance (Russell 1912, ch. 5, Russell 1910a). However, one difference is that whereas knowledge by acquaintance is non-judgemental and non-conceptual, revelation via experience doesn't have to be, and thus can be fallible. For the sake of keeping the discussion as simple as possible, I'm going to avoid discussing such nuances except when they are absolutely necessary.

idea of an experience that is revelatory of the mind. For that more specific idea to make sense, there must be some way in which the mind is hidden and some way in which it can become unhidden via experience. Moreover, it is also clear that the experience in question must be self-referential: it is the mind being revealed *to itself*. But how can the mind be hidden from itself in the first place?

We can see St. Augustine grappling with this issue in his reflections on the nature of memory:

> Great is this power of memory, exceedingly great, O my God—a large and boundless inner hall! Who has plumbed the depths of it? Yet it is a power of my mind, and it belongs to my nature. But I do not myself grasp all that I am. Thus the mind is far too narrow to contain itself. But where can that part of it be which it does not contain? Is it outside and not in itself? How can it be, then, that the mind cannot grasp itself?
>
> St. Augustine ca. 400 CE, *Confessions*, 10.8.15[29]

A natural solution to this puzzle would be to treat the mind as divided into parts, where some parts are hidden from others. Perhaps the simplest way to implement this solution would be to make use of the conscious/unconscious distinction. Thus, we may understand a mind-revealing experience to be one in which some part or aspect of the unconscious mind is revealed to the conscious mind. Or, to put it in terms that are more familiar to cognitive science: unconscious contents or processes normally not easily accessible suddenly appear in conscious experience.

Although this is a natural solution to the puzzle—and one that, I think, does justice to the phenomenology of psychedelic experiences—we should be aware that it entails making a substantial assumption about the structure of the mind. Moreover, it isn't the only available option. For example, Block 1995 has argued we should divide consciousness up into what he calls *access* consciousness and *phenomenal* consciousness. Using this division, we could say, for instance, that a psychedelic experience is an experience in which content that is normally only available to phenomenal consciousness appears in access consciousness. Alternatively, we could say that it is an experience in which any content that is not ordinarily available to access consciousness, whether it is in phenomenal consciousness or in the unconscious, appears in access consciousness. It's not clear that the evidence supports Block's division of consciousness (Kouider et al. 2010, Kentridge 2013, Thibault et al. 2016), but if it does, these two options could be alternative ways of making sense of the mind being revealed to itself (or of distinguishing different kinds of psychedelic experience). Similarly, some have argued that conscious experience is actually much richer than it is often conceived and contains content or has aspects to it that we are not aware of (Schwitzgebel 2002) or cannot easily report with language (O'Brien and Jureidini 2002a, 2002b).

---

[29] Outler 2006, p. 210.

These views give us alternative ways of understanding the idea of the mind being revealed to itself by relying on subdivisions within the *conscious* mind. There is also the possibility that the *unconscious* mind could be subdivided to allow for additional ways of making sense of how the mind can be revealed to itself. For example, if we adopted a modularity theory of the mind (Fodor 1983), then we might say that a psychedelic experience can occur when content that is normally encapsulated in one module is suddenly transferred to another. Such an experience may not involve any unconscious content appearing in consciousness, but the transfer of content between modules may nevertheless result in substantial alterations to the phenomenological character of conscious experience. For instance, psychedelic-induced synaesthesia may be an example of this phenomenon.

So we see that there are various ways to make sense of the mind being revealed to itself. These are all reasonable options, especially since they may fit well with some of the phenomenological data (e.g. synaesthesia) and neuroimaging evidence (e.g. increased global connectivity, Daws et al. 2022). Perhaps we should say, then, that a psychedelic experience occurs when *any* part of the mind that is normally hidden from another part of the mind appears (or is represented) in that other part of the mind. However, to simplify matters, from now on I will focus on the idea that a psychedelic experience is one in which a part or aspect of the unconscious mind is revealed in consciousness. We can think of this as a useful idealization—a modelling choice—that we can revise later.

Although the idea of an unconscious mind still occasionally triggers some unfortunate Freudian associations, it is nevertheless a well-accepted concept in cognitive science. Indeed, as Fodor once put it, 'practically all psychologically interesting cognitive states are unconscious' (Fodor 1983, p. 86). Moreover, as I mentioned in Chapter 1, some parts of the mind appear to be not only unconscious but *stubbornly* so; that is, it is *difficult* for some parts of the mind to appear in conscious experience. We need this to be the case in order to get the concept of psychedelic experience off the ground.

We also require the possibility for these parts to be *revealed*. Some psychologists appear to take a particularly strong stance on the unconscious, arguing that many, if not all, parts of the unconscious mind can *never* be made available to the conscious mind (Wilson 2002, Wilson 2009, Wilson and Dunn 2004). According to this kind of view, our access to these parts of our minds is much like our access to other people's minds. All we can do is observe what we can see in our behaviour and conscious experience and then make educated guesses as to what is going on in the hidden parts of our minds. This is quite a strong position. Although it is probably true for some parts of the unconscious mind, it is unlikely true for *all* of them.[30] Indeed, from the simple fact that we know that some of our memories can

---

[30] It is not entirely clear how general Wilson's view is. Especially in more recent work (for example, Hofmann and Wilson 2010), Wilson develops a view in which the outputs of some unconscious processes can appear as phenomenal cues, which he categorizes as experiential and preconscious.

temporarily be difficult to remember, we know that access to certain parts of our mind can be blocked and then later permitted.

The question, then, is how much of the unconscious mind can be revealed. One of the exciting features of the experiences induced by psychedelics is that they appear to reveal a lot more than we might otherwise expect. To quote a famous passage by Stanislav Grof:

> It does not seem to be an exaggeration to say that psychedelics, used responsibly and with proper caution, would be for psychiatry what the microscope is for biology and medicine or the telescope is for astronomy. These tools make it possible to study important processes that under normal circumstances are not available for direct observation.
>
> Grof 1980, p. 12

And again in a later work:

> In one of my early books I suggested that the potential significance of LSD and other psychedelics for psychiatry and psychology was comparable to the value the microscope has for biology or the telescope has for astronomy. My later experience with psychedelics only confirmed this initial impression. These substances function as unspecific amplifiers that increase the cathexis (energetic charge) associated with the deep unconscious contents of the psyche and make them available for conscious processing. This unique property of psychedelics makes it possible to study psychological undercurrents that govern our experiences and behaviours to a depth that cannot be matched by any other method and tool available in modern mainstream psychiatry and psychology.
>
> Grof 2009, p. xxv

To be clear, the claim that psychedelics actually reveal hidden parts of the unconscious mind is a *hypothesis* that we have not yet evaluated. The point for now is simply that it must be *possible* for psychedelics to do this. This possibility is necessary for our explication of psychedelic experience to have a chance of being successful. With that said, one of the main reasons why this hypothesis is interesting is because of the intriguing idea that psychedelics may reveal hidden parts or aspects of the mind in unprecedented ways.

We now have a clearer idea of the concept of psychedelic experience: an experience is psychedelic if it is an experience of a hidden part or aspect of the unconscious mind being revealed to the conscious mind. Nevertheless, the concept may still feel rather abstract to some readers. So, let's consider some concrete examples.

1. Emotional insights: We briefly came across this kind of example in the previous chapter. There are different kinds of emotional insights, but one example that many people will be familiar with is that of suddenly realizing that they have been attracted to someone for a long time. It's important to note that this realization doesn't have to come by way of an inference. For example, it is not as if you suddenly notice that you have been behaving differently around the person in question and then start to contemplate the possibility that you are attracted to them (although this can certainly happen). Instead, the realization may come to you in an experience. For example, it may come to you as an epiphany when you are by yourself: perhaps your mind becomes quiet enough for you to notice the attraction. Or perhaps one day, when you encounter the person, the attraction is amplified to the point that you cannot fail to notice it. Whatever the details of the experience are, the crucial point is that the attraction has been there for a while, entirely (or mostly) unbeknownst to you, and is then made manifest in your conscious awareness.

2. **Episodic memories:** Another kind of example, which we have already come across, is that of a long-lost memory appearing in one's conscious experience. We saw this in de Quincey's description of his opium dream, in which he was confronted by memories of his childhood he would otherwise not be able to recollect. We find similar examples from the literature on psychedelic-assisted psychotherapy, where patients suddenly recollect forgotten traumas, triggering a cathartic release, or providing material for further analysis (Grof 2009). Experiences in which we become aware of a lost memory can also be induced by substances that are not typically thought of as psychedelic. Almost everyone has had the experience of an aroma triggering a long-forgotten memory. The classic example of this type of experience is Proust's sudden recollection of eating a tea-soaked madeleine as a child (we will come back to this example in Chapter 6). For these examples to count as psychedelic, the memories should be real and not fantasies made up on the fly. If they are momentary constructions, then they are not revealing something hidden and therefore won't be psychedelic in our sense of the term.

3. **Tip-of-the-tongue experiences:** This kind of example also involves memory, but of a different kind: semantic rather than episodic. Pretty much everyone has had a tip-of-the-tongue experience: it happens when you are unable to recall a familiar word. Indeed, it isn't just that you are unable to recall the word. You also feel that you are *almost* able to recall it. Hence the name for these experiences: it can feel like the word is right on the tip of your tongue. These experiences themselves are not psychedelic, but they are followed by a psychedelic experience—when you finally recall the word. That moment in which the word pops into your awareness is a mind-revealing experience: for a while, the word was hidden from you, despite your best efforts to recall it, and then it is suddenly revealed.

4. **Creative insights:** This example is another case of something suddenly popping into your mind: this time in the form of *a new idea*. Many of our creative ideas often seem like they come from nowhere: they seem to just magically appear in

our minds. However, our creative ideas are most likely generated via unconscious processes, and some of these ideas eventually appear in the conscious mind for evaluation or execution. As we'll see in Chapter 9, it is also likely that many of these ideas *remain* in the unconscious mind—even some of the good ones—because they do not pass an initial unconscious phase of evaluation for relevance and quality. This filter keeps many of our ideas hidden from the conscious mind. However, sometimes, some of these hidden ideas do make it through the filter. There could be all sorts of reasons: the filter is not perfect and occasionally makes errors, or it is temporarily relaxed somehow, or the criteria for relevance and quality have changed. Whatever the reason, some ideas manage to make it through, and when one of these hidden ideas pops into your awareness, you have a psychedelic experience.

5. Visual processes: A completely different class of examples involves our visual system. The popular view of vision is that it starts by light reflecting off objects and hitting our eyes, which then convert that light into a neural signal, which then is processed by the brain, resulting in the visual experience of the objects before us. However, cognitive science paints a rather different picture: roughly speaking, the mind proactively creates visual scenes it thinks are likely to be real (or useful) and then checks to see if this matches the incoming signals from the eyes.[31] We typically don't notice this process because the visual system works smoothly and does an adequate job of showing the world in front of us. However, we can get glimpses of the process by putting it in unusual situations that evolution didn't optimize for—such as closing one's eyes in a pitch-black room for an extended period of time. For many people, intricate geometric patterns of colour eventually emerge from the initially dark visual scene. In Chapter 7, I'll argue that these patterns are the result of the visual system actively trying to find low-level visual features, such as edges, colours, contours, motion, and so on. In such cases, we get a glimpse of the processes that create our everyday visual scenes. These glimpses are psychedelic experiences.

Other situations for which the visual system is not well tuned, and which give rise to psychedelic experiences, are some cases of visual illusion. As we will see later, not all visual illusions are psychedelic experiences, but some are. One example is that of illusory motion, as shown in Figure 3.1. Although the image is static, most people perceive it as moving. When you look at the image, you have a psychedelic experience; however, this isn't because the image looks "psychedelic" (in the colloquial sense of the word). Instead, your experience is psychedelic because you are getting a glimpse of a visual process (or of its intermediary outputs) that is normally hidden from your awareness. Note that the relevant

[31] This view is often associated with predictive processing (Friston 2002, Hohwy 2013), but it is also compatible with other Bayesian (Griffiths et al. 2008) and non-Bayesian (Bowers and Davis 2012) theories of perception.

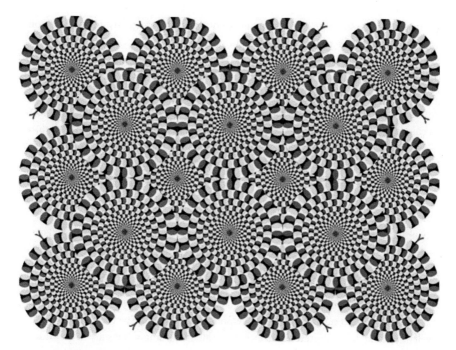

Figure 3.1 Illusory motion.

point here is not that you learn that your mind is proactively constructing your visual experience when you look at the image. Nor is it the point that you learn something about how your mind constructs your visual experience. The illusory motion experience is psychedelic even if you are entirely oblivious to such facts about your visual system. The experience is psychedelic because you experience a part of the visual process (or of its intermediary outputs) that is normally hidden from your consciousness.[32]

6. Perspectives: Another kind of example involves perspectives being revealed to us in experience. For example, anyone who flies regularly likely knows the perspective that arises from looking down at your home city and realizing that the vast majority of your problems are immaterial. From this perspective, you begin to have insights about how to live better—you should relax more, spend more time with loved ones, quit your dead-end job, etc.[33] This change in perspective can be a psychedelic experience since it is often accompanied by the realization that one had *forgotten* the better perspective.[34] Also, many of the insights that arise through

[32] Metzinger 2003 makes a similar point about low-level geometric hallucinations induced by psychedelics (p. 171), and we will come back to this in more detail in Chapter 7.

[33] The *overview effect* that astronauts frequently report having while in space (Yaden et al. 2016) is an extreme form of this kind of experience.

[34] Forgotten in the sense that the better perspective was available but had merely become inaccessible.

this revealed perspective are not *new*—they tend to be old insights, or lessons learned, that are *remembered*.

7. **Mystical experiences:** We will come back to mystical experiences in Chapter 10, so for now I just want to flag the example and warm us up to thinking about whether they are psychedelic. If the nitrous oxide experiences of James and Blood were genuinely mind-revealing, then what was it about the mind that was being revealed? Perhaps the experience simply revealed to them a set of latent religious beliefs they were unknowingly committed to? Or perhaps they accessed another kind of hidden perspective that is available to us all? On this point, it is worth noting James' own hypothesis about mystical experiences:

> My hypothesis is that [it will] bring a mass of subconscious memories, conceptions, emotional feelings, and perceptions of relation, etc., into view all at once; and that if this enlargement of the nimbus that surrounds the sensational present is vast enough, while no one of the items it contains attracts our attention singly, we shall have the conditions fulfilled for a kind of consciousness in all essential respects like that termed mystical. [...] Its form will be intuitive or perceptual, not conceptual, for the remembered or conceived objects in the enlarged field are supposed not to attract the attention singly, but only to give the sense of a tremendous muchness suddenly revealed. If they attracted attention separately, we should have the ordinary steep-waved consciousness, and the mystical character would depart.
>
> James 1910, p. 87

According to James, a mystical experience involves revealing ordinary elements of the mind—memories, emotions, etc.—but on the condition that these elements do not attract one's attention singly. If they were to do so, that would minimize the degree to which the experience is psychedelic and, consequently, end the possibility of it being mystical. (In addition to the idea of revelation, the distribution of *attention* is clearly an important aspect of James' hypothesis. This will be important to keep in mind as we consider the role of attention in psychedelic experience in Chapter 5 and in mystical experience in Chapter 10.)

This list of examples is by no means exhaustive. There are plenty more examples of mind-revealing experiences. The human mind is incredibly rich and complex, and there is a great variety of ways in which parts of it can be revealed. It is also important to remember that we are using the notion of mind rather broadly here so as to include, without being committed to, other notions such as the soul and spirit (or *prāna*). The above examples are also not intended to be definitive, and there may be good reasons to reject some of them. For example, the theory of creativity I used may turn out to be false (if, for instance, creative ideas are never hidden and are always easily accessible). If all the examples end up overturned, and no new ones replace them, then this would be a problem for the fruitfulness of the explication of psychedelic experience. However, the above examples seem plausible, and as we'll see, they involve phenomena that are modulated or induced by the consumption of psychedelics and the practice of meditation.

One important kind of example that some readers may notice is missing from the above list is that of *dreams*. This is because dreams are somewhat tricky to classify. On the one hand, there are some compelling reasons to think of dream experiences as psychedelic. Famously, psychoanalysts have long thought that dreams provide access to the unconscious; however, the scientific evidence for this hypothesis is rather scant. This could be due to the particular way that the psychoanalysts have conceptualized the unconscious. If instead we work with a conceptualization of the unconscious that is more aligned with contemporary cognitive science, then the evidence for the view that dreams are psychedelic starts to look more promising. For example, there is evidence that dreaming and, in particular, lucid dreaming, enhances memory and creative problem-solving.[35] These results suggest that dream experiences may involve a novel kind of access to hidden parts or aspects of the mind (similar to the above examples of hidden perspectives and insights). If this is correct, then dreams would count as psychedelic experiences, in that they reveal the unconscious parts of our minds to us. There is also growing evidence that psychedelic trips have many similarities to dreams, especially lucid ones.[36] So, there is some intuitive support for the *faithfulness* of this classification (recall from Chapter 2 that faithfulness is one of the criteria for a successful explication).

On the other hand, a major difference between dreams and clear-cut psychedelic experiences is that of *wakefulness*. This difference provides some intuitive support in the opposite direction. Also, importantly, dreams do not seem to have the same kind of psychotherapeutic benefits as psychedelic trips or meditative practices (Chapter 9).[37] This suggests that classifying dream experiences as psychedelic may, in fact, undermine the faithfulness of our explication. Therefore, it might make sense to amend the explication to rule out dream experiences as being psychedelic. For example, we might want to say that a psychedelic experience is an experience in which a hidden part or aspect of the unconscious is revealed to the *wakeful* conscious mind. It's not obvious how to best resolve this issue, so for now, let's leave our explication unamended and stay open to the possibility that some (though perhaps not all) dream experiences are psychedelic.

Now that we have reviewed some concrete examples, it is worth considering an objection that some readers may have in mind: if experiences such as having

---

[35] For example, see Barrett 1993, Barrett 2001, Barrett 2017, Cai et al. 2009, Stumbrys and Daniels 2010, Wamsley et al. 2010, Lewis et al. 2018, and Wamsley and Stickgold 2019.

[36] For example, see Kraehenmann 2017, Kraehenmann et al. 2017, Sanz et al. 2018, and Fox et al. 2018.

[37] However, this is not to say that dreaming is entirely disconnected from well-being—see, for example, Lara-Carrasco et al. 2009 and Scarpelli et al. 2019.

new ideas and remembering past events count as psychedelic experiences, then surely this is a misuse, and trivialization, of the term 'psychedelic'. The primary motivation behind this kind of objection is that such experiences look very little like the experiences that are typically induced by psychedelic substances. There are three points that we can make in response to this. First, there isn't as much dissimilarity between these experiences as one might think. For example, many people report feeling more creative after having consumed psychedelics (Chapter 8), and some psychotherapists claim to have used psychedelics to help their patients uncover deeply buried memories (Chapters 6 and 9). Second, we have yet to say anything about what makes an experience *more psychedelic* than another. Once we have defined that criterion, we will be able to consider the possibility that psychedelics induce experiences that are much more psychedelic than naturally occurring psychedelic experiences. That will help dispel some of the counterintuitiveness of this way of using the term 'psychedelic'. Third, we must remain open to the empirical possibility that some of the paradigmatic effects produced by psychedelic drugs are not actually psychedelic, and so it may be that some of the experiential qualities we have come to think of as "psychedelic" may not be an appropriate basis of evaluation.

Let's recap. We now have a definition of psychedelic experience that gives us necessary and sufficient conditions for an experience to count as psychedelic: it is an experience in which a part or aspect of the mind that is normally hidden in the unconscious is revealed in conscious experience. We also have a diverse list of concrete examples that plausibly meet these conditions. And we have the promise of a more sophisticated definition (coming in the next section) that will tell us how an experience can be more or less psychedelic and thus help us to handle the trivialization objection.

However, before we get to that, it will help to see some examples of experiences that might seem like they are psychedelic but actually are not. This will give us a better sense of the boundaries defined by the necessary and sufficient conditions.

1. Reading a psychology textbook: Suppose you read a psychology textbook and learn a new fact about the human mind, and consequently, a new fact about your own mind. For example, you might learn that most people cannot hold their attention on a fixed, unchanging object for more than a few seconds. In learning this new fact, did you have a psychedelic experience? It's unlikely. If anything, you made a psychedelic *inference*: a fact about your mind was in some sense revealed to you, but you learned it by way of inference. (In Chapter 5, we will see how this fact can also be learned experientially.)

2. Visual illusions: Earlier, I presented a visual illusion as one kind of example of a psychedelic experience. However, not all visual illusions are psychedelic in this way. For example, consider the Müller-Lyer illusion, depicted in Figure 3.2. Although it may not look like it, the two horizontal lines are equal in length. To discover this, however, you have to perform some kind of inference. For example,

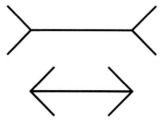

Figure 3.2 The Müller-Lyer illusion.

if someone tells you that the lines are of the same length, you need to trust their testimony and then compare it with the evidence from your visual experience. Alternatively, if you measure the lines yourself, you need to be confident that you measured them accurately and hold the difference in measurements against your visual experience. There is nothing about your experience of the lines that is in itself mind-revealing: all the new insights are acquired via inferences.

Note that the distinction between inference and experience in this context is not entirely clear-cut, and some philosophers consider experiences to be simply fast, unconscious inferences—or the outputs thereof. For example, Carruthers 2011 adopts such a view and argues that much of the mind can only be known via inference. On the face of it, this would rule out the possibility of psychedelic experience: we would only have inferences about the mind. However, from the perspective of this kind of view, the relevant distinction for our purposes would be the one between fast, unconscious inferences (corresponding to what we normally call 'experiences') and slower, conscious inferences. To detect that the mind is behaving strangely with the Müller-Lyer illusion, you need to conduct a slow, conscious inference (for instance, checking the lengths of the lines). In contrast, in the case of illusory motion, a fast, unconscious inference (which you have no control over) causes you to become aware of a novel aspect of the mind.

3. Regular memories: Suppose that right now you call to mind your memory of eating breakfast today. Is that a psychedelic experience? It's unlikely. Although this example is experiential (in contrast to the previous two examples), it doesn't involve a part of the mind that is *hidden* from awareness. This is because this memory would be easy to recall. In contrast, it is much more difficult for you to remember eating breakfast one week ago. This older memory is hidden to some degree (assuming it has been retained), and so if it were to appear in awareness suddenly, you would have an experience that is somewhat psychedelic. This example highlights the central point of the next section: experiences can vary in the degree to which they are psychedelic. Suddenly remembering eating breakfast one week ago is somewhat psychedelic, but suddenly reliving your first day of school would be much more psychedelic. As we will see in the coming chapters, a plausible hypothesis is that a distinctive feature of psychedelic substances is that they induce experiences that are *very* psychedelic. If correct, this hypothesis would explain why people tend to relive early childhood memories during psychedelic trips. At any rate, the point for now is just that not any memory recollection counts as a psychedelic experience—the memory in question has to be *hidden* from awareness.

4. New sensations: Suppose you suddenly experience some kind of pain. If the pain is new—say, because you kicked your toe—then the experience won't be psychedelic. In contrast, if the pain is an old one, then the experience might be psychedelic. For example, suppose you suffer from chronic pain which fades in and out of awareness. If the chronic pain is hidden (e.g. because of suppression or being crowded out by sensations), then when it fades into awareness, this will count as a psychedelic experience. However, if the pain is new or is not hidden, then the experience won't be psychedelic. It is important to note that there is some debate as to whether pain can be unconscious (Hill 2006, Gligorov 2008, Byrne 2012). If pain can't ever be unconscious, then it also can't be hidden from awareness, and so the experience of a pain will never be psychedelic.

Another class of non-psychedelic experiences are those experiences that are *psychecryptic*. In Chapter 1, I introduced the term 'psychecryptic' as deriving from the ancient Greek words *psychē* (mind/soul) and *kruptos* (to conceal/hide). Psychecryptic experiences are, thus, mind-*concealing* experiences. Alongside the notion of a psychecryptic *experience*, it is also helpful for us to have the concept of a psychecryptic *state*. In a psychecryptic state, some parts or aspects of the mind are hidden from awareness. The difference between these concepts is analogous to that of a ship sailing into the fog and a ship already being in the fog. In other words, a psychecryptic experience is the process of something becoming concealed, and a psychecryptic state is a state in which something is already concealed. The more your mind is hidden from your awareness, the more psychecryptic your mental state is. It follows that if you can have a psychedelic experience, then your mental state is, by default, psychecryptic to some degree. Below are some examples of psychecryptic experiences and states.

1. Tip-of-the-tongue experiences (again): Earlier, I used the example of this phenomenon as involving a psychedelic experience. However, recall that the psychedelic experience occurs when the needed word finally pops into your awareness. Until that happens, you are in a psychecryptic *state*, and one noteworthy feature of this example is that you can recognize that this is the case: you are aware that you know the word and that you temporarily lack access to it. At that moment, something is preventing the word from appearing in your consciousness. Occasionally, this phenomenon can also involve psychecryptic *experiences*. For example, you may feel that you are getting close to remembering the word, but then it slips away. That feeling of the word slipping away is a psychecryptic experience (the ship sailing into the fog). The state of not being able to recall the word is a psychecryptic state.

2. Brain fog: This is an example that I mentioned briefly in Chapter 1. The fact that we use the term 'fog' to describe this state is quite telling: under these circumstances, we can tell that we are unable to see as much of our mind as we normally do—or that we can't see it *as well* as we normally do. For whatever reason—poor diet, lack of sleep, stress, etc.—something prevents us from accessing parts or aspects of our mind that we can normally access. Brain fog tends to creep up on us, and so we fail to notice the process of it concealing our mind. However, there are some exceptions. For example, if you eat a heavy meal after a period of fasting, the transition may be pronounced enough to be noticeable, and you can feel access to your mind slipping away. Such an experience is a psychecryptic experience.

3. Inattentional blindness: A classic example of inattentional blindness involves subjects being given the task of counting how many times some basketball players have passed the ball to each other (Simons and Chabris 1999). When observers focus on this task, they tend to perform it well, but they also tend to fail to notice something odd about the situation: a person in a gorilla suit strolls into the scene, does a little dance, and then walks away. The explanation for why observers fail to notice this is that the task of counting requires so much attention that little is left over to notice the unexpected event. Several other studies have shown that this effect, first reported by Neisser and Becklen 1975, holds across a wide range of conditions and stimuli. Importantly, studies have also shown that although subjects fail to be aware of the unexpected stimulus, the stimulus may nevertheless undergo substantial unconscious processing (Moore and Egeth 1997, Mack and Rock 1998, Wood and Simons 2019, Kreitz et al. 2020, Nobre et al. 2020). So there is a sense in which a perception of the stimulus (the dancing gorilla) is in the mind, even though it may not appear in one's awareness. Moreover, and importantly, the perception appears to be *hidden* to some degree from one's awareness due to the focusing of limited attentional resources on the counting task. On this interpretation, cases of inattentional blindness may be viewed as different ways in which we temporarily instantiate psychecryptic states.

4. Binocular rivalry: This example involves an experience that is psychedelic and psychecryptic *at the same time*. Binocular rivalry occurs when each eye is presented with a different image simultaneously. Instead of seeing some blurry fusion of the two images, as you might expect, you end up seeing one image for a few seconds, then the other image for a few seconds, then the first again, and so on. In other words, your experience oscillates between the two images. When one image appears and the other disappears, you are having a psychedelic experience and a psychecryptic experience all at once: in one moment, one image is revealed and the other is concealed. Of course, the phenomenon of binocular rivalry is not normally explicated in these terms but, as we'll see in Chapter 5, understanding it this way will help make sense of how it can be modulated by psychedelics and meditation.[38]

---

[38] For a review of neuroimaging studies of cortical competition and suppression of the percepts during binocular rivalry, see Zhang et al. 2017.

5. Selective attention: These last two examples are somewhat artificial cases involving the general phenomenon of *selective attention*. An everyday example of selective attention occurs when you are in a conversation at a party and suddenly hear someone in another conversation say your name: your attention is drawn away from your current conversation and towards the other one. In this situation, it can become difficult, or even impossible, to hear what the person in front of you is saying and to *not* hear what the person in the other conversation is saying about you. One explanation for this is that your mind has been unconsciously tracking both conversations, dampening the other conversation and amplifying your present one—until you hear your name. However, although it dampens the other conversation, it remains alert to signals that are potentially important—such as someone saying something about you. When it detects such a signal, the mind automatically flips around its dampening and amplifying processes, and you start hearing the other conversation more clearly. If this explanation is correct, then there is a sense in which the other conversation is hidden from your awareness— that is, before you hear your name. The sudden incoming signal of your name being spoken changes that priority assessment, and the other conversation then appears more clearly in your conscious experience. And, as a result, the conversation you are meant to be participating in becomes partially hidden from your awareness— as evidenced by the fact that it can be difficult to re-engage with the person you are talking to.

6. Dissociative states: While dissociation is a complex phenomenon, various dissociative states can be understood as psychecryptic in nature. Cases of amnesia are perhaps the clearest cases involving psychecryptic states (assuming that the memories in question can be recovered). Similarly, fugue states that involve the forgetting of an identity that is later recovered (with perhaps no recollection of the intervening identity) are psychecryptic. In cases of depersonalization, awareness of one's identity can remain but in a detached form, whereby the person's sense of selfhood feels hindered or suppressed. Individuals can feel divorced from their usual sense of self, emotions, empathy, bodily sensations, etc. Relatedly, experience of derealization can involve a disconnection from one's usual perceptual perspective of the world, with the external world feeling distant, distorted, unreal, as though it is being veiled by a sensory fog. Experiences involving dissociation are not necessarily psychecryptic *simpliciter* since a dissociation from one thing may allow the revelation of another. Indeed, ketamine is often recognized as having intertwining effects that are psychedelic and dissociative (psychecryptic) in nature (Mashour 2022). Similarly, MDMA can cause experiences of dissociation (Puxty et al. 2017), and classic psychedelics such as psilocybin can induce experiences with dissociative-like effects (Studerus et al. 2010).

With all the examples and distinctions in place, the concept of psychedelic experience should be clearer. According to our definition, an experience is psychedelic if and only if it reveals a part or aspect of the mind that is normally hidden from conscious awareness. It is important to remember that this is only an initial sketch. In particular, it assumes that the hiding and revealing can happen only between the unconscious and conscious parts of the mind. We've started with this assumption because it is reasonably well grounded in cognitive science and fits the common conception of the effects of psychedelics. However, we should be open to the possibility that there are other ways of revealing the mind. Another reason why this is only an initial definition is that it treats the issue of an experience being psychedelic as a binary, all-or-nothing matter. In order to account for the fact that experiences can be *more or less* psychedelic, we need to refine the definition. That will be the task of the next section.

3.4 Psychedelic Space

We need to refine our initial explication of psychedelic experience to account for the fact that experiences can be more or less psychedelic. To do this, it is helpful to think of our initial explication as an equation:

Psychedelic experience = Mind-revealing experience.

If we want the term on the left-hand side to come in degrees, then we need at least one of the terms on the right-hand side to come in degrees. There are three salient options here:

1. There are degrees to which something is a part or aspect of the *mind*.
2. There are degrees to which something can be an *experience*.
3. There are degrees to which something can be *revealed*.

For each of the three component concepts, if there is a sense in which it comes in degrees, then that may give us an insight into how the aggregate concept may come in degrees. So let's consider each of these in turn.

Exploring the first option, we could say that there are degrees to which something is a part of the mind. For instance, one could argue that our proprioceptive and kinaesthetic sensations are less mental and more bodily than our emotions and desires are. To take a specific example, some people who sit slouched over their laptops all day may not know how to contract their rhomboid muscles (the two muscles on the upper back that attach the shoulder blades to the spine). They have the ability to contract these muscles, but this ability is obscured from them. Suddenly seeing how to contract these muscles—say, during physical therapy—can take the form of a psychedelic experience, since it involves becoming aware of the kinaesthetic sensation of contracting these muscles.[39] In general, this phenomenon is known as *sensory motor amnesia*. Nevertheless, perhaps we should say that such an experience is less mind-revealing than, say, attaining an emotional insight, because the kinaesthetic sensation is less mental.[40] If that kind of analysis makes sense, then we could say, all else being equal, that an experience is psychedelic to the extent that the thing being revealed is part of the mind.

Exploring the second option, we could consider exploiting the distinction between experience and inference and say that processes of knowledge acquisition can be more or less experiential (and, correspondingly, more or less inferential). We could then say that an experience is psychedelic, all else being equal, to the extent that it is experiential. For example, to know that you are experiencing an illusion with the Müller-Lyer lines, you need to carry out a fair amount of inferential reasoning. In contrast, the case of illusory motion seems to be much more experiential in nature. However, one could argue that the case of illusory motion is also partly inferential. For example, there seems to be a difference between seeing the image on a computer screen, which may conceivably be moving, and seeing it printed on a piece of paper, which is surely not moving. If you look at the image on the computer screen, you may need to perform some kind of inferential check to convince yourself that the image is not actually moving. If so, then one might say that the example is less psychedelic than it otherwise would be.

Both of these two options are conceptually plausible, but the third option is more intuitive and appears to be a more fruitful line of investigation. This is because *revelation* clearly comes in degrees. For example, during a poker game, you may only see *some* of the cards in someone's hand, which would thus be a *partial* revelation of their hand. Similarly, your partner may choose to only reveal part of their new tattoo to you. The thought, then, is that we can say that an experience is psychedelic to the extent that it is revealing of the mind.

To start unpacking this idea, let's first think about how revelation can come in degrees. To help fix our concepts, let's consider a concrete example: there is a new

---

[39] The distinction between revealing abilities one already has and developing new abilities is not always clear-cut. To use the well-known example from Lewis 1976: compared to an ape, I have the ability to speak Finnish, but don't take me to Helsinki as your interpreter—I can't speak a word of Finnish. Thus, for someone who has never known a word of Finnish, we wouldn't expect that having a psychedelic experience would result in them suddenly speaking the language. In contrast, if they once knew how to speak Finnish but have long forgotten it, then a psychedelic experience may uncover that ability. One can find anecdotal reports that also speak to this point. For example, Paul Stamets reports that a single psilocybin-induced psychedelic trip cured his congenital stuttering. Does this amount to a revelation of an ability to speak fluently or its creation? Perhaps the ability was created because the condition was congenital? Another related example is that of a single ayahuasca session curing acquired aphantasia (Santos et al. 2018). This example seems to be the revelation of an ability. In contrast, Luke 2018 reports a case of apparently congenital aphantasia remaining unaffected by over a thousand psychedelic trips (induced by inhaled DMT).

[40] If one is inclined to think that kinaesthetic sensations are just as mental as emotional insights (as I do), then replace the example with something else—say, of muscle memory or of monosynaptic "knee-jerk" reflexes.

painting in an art gallery that is covered by a cloth, and it will soon be revealed to a group of art critics. What are the different ways in which this revelation can come in degrees?

Perhaps the most obvious way is that only a portion of the painting is uncovered. For example, if the critics only get to see half of the painting, then, all else being equal, this would be less revelatory than if the critics saw the full painting. Let's call this the *scope* of the revelation. All else being equal, increasing the scope of a revelatory experience makes it more revelatory.

There is another way in which the revelation of the painting may come in degrees. Suppose that the painting is fully uncovered but the room is filled with smoke. Although the critics will be able to see the painting in full, they won't be able to see it *clearly*. Similarly, suppose that the painting was not completely dry when it was covered, and so when the cloth is removed, some of the paint becomes smeared. Or, as another example, suppose that brightly coloured lights are shone on the painting, altering its apparent colours. In all of these cases, the critics can see the full scope of the painting, but they do not see the painting as it is—in its true, original state. In all these cases, the *clarity* of the revelation is imperfect. All else being equal, increasing the clarity of a revelatory experience makes it more revelatory.

A third way that a revelation can come in degrees is by varying in its *duration*. Let's suppose that the painting is uncovered entirely and the critics' view of it is not corrupted in any way. That is, let's suppose that the scope and clarity of the revelation are perfect. Nevertheless, the critics would be right to complain if the painting were only uncovered for a fraction of a second. They might be able to get a vague sense of the colour palette used in the painting and the kind of painting it is (say, a portrait), but apart from that, they wouldn't get enough time to really take it in. Thus, their experience of the painting would be more revelatory if they could examine it for a greater amount of time. This, of course, only holds up until a certain point. After a certain amount of time has passed, the critics can stop looking at the painting and be satisfied with their experience of it. The amount of time will depend, in part, on the painting itself. Small and simple paintings don't need much time, whereas large and complex paintings require more. Also, some critics will need less time than others. Therefore, the way in which the duration of the experience affects the degree to which it is revelatory depends on (i) the nature of the thing being revealed and (ii) the mind to which it is being revealed. With these qualifications in place, we can say that increasing the duration of a revelatory experience makes it more revelatory, all else being equal.

A fourth factor that affects the degree to which an experience is revelatory is the *novelty* of the thing being revealed. Suppose that the painting being revealed is an exact copy of the one revealed last week, which itself was a copy of the one from the previous week, and so on. Suppose, further, that the art critics know this and fully expect to see the same painting being uncovered yet again.

It would be reasonable for the critics to complain that they have already seen the painting. Therefore, in this scenario, there is little sense in which uncovering the painting counts as *revealing* it to the critics—revelation generally involves making something known that is surprising or was previously secret.[41] And this wasn't true in our case. In contrast, if the artist has a reputation for being highly creative, or if the painting significantly departs from their previous work, then the uncovering of the painting would be highly revelatory. These are two extreme scenarios, but it is easy to imagine ones that occupy intermediate points along the spectrum. Also, like duration, novelty depends on the person to whom the thing is being revealed. Suppose again that it is the same painting being revealed. If a critic's memory spans only a few minutes, then it might as well be an entirely new painting for them. With that in mind, we can say that the more novel the thing being revealed is, the more revelatory the experience is—again, all else being equal.

There may still be other factors that affect the degree to which an experience is revelatory, but the four we have considered so far—scope, clarity, duration, and novelty—are sufficient for our purposes here. Since these four factors appear to be mostly separable, we can think of them as *dimensions*. As dimensions, the four factors define a *space* of possible revelatory experiences that a person may have. An experience can be more revelatory by increasing how it scores on any of these dimensions, and in any combination. For example, you could uncover the left half of the painting for weeks and the right half for 5 seconds, while having a complex lighting scheme that makes the highly novel bottom half of the painting barely visible. That would be a strange thing to do, but it is nevertheless possible, and it would affect the overall degree to which the painting is revealed. The most revelatory experience would be one that involves viewing the full scope of a new painting with perfect clarity and with sufficient duration that would allow for its complete apprehension.

We now have a clearer idea of how revelatory experiences can come in degrees. However, so far we've only been considering revelatory experiences of things in the external world (specifically, a painting, but it is easy to see how this generalizes to the revelation of other worldly objects). We now need to turn inwards and see how we can apply this conceptual toolkit to the internal world—the human mind. We can think of this as an analytic analogue of *ekō henshō*. The goal is to see if we can make sense of psychedelic experiences as coming in degrees using the dimensions of scope, clarity, novelty, and duration.

One immediate challenge we face is that our understanding of the mind is still very much in its infancy. We have some idea about the composition of the mind—perceptions, memories, beliefs, emotions, etc.—and some frameworks for thinking about it—computationalism (Fodor 1975, Pylyshyn 1980), representationalism

---

[41] See, for example, the entry for 'Reveal' (2020) in the *Cambridge English Dictionary*.

(Dretske 1997, Lycan 1987), modularity of mind (Fodor 1983), predictive processing (Friston 2002, Hohwy 2013, Clark 2015), connectionism (Rumelhart et al. 1986, Buckner and Garson 2018), 4E cognition (Newen et al. 2018), etc. However, none of these come close to our understanding of the external world. So, we should expect progress to be slow, and we should get comfortable with uncertainty and ambiguity. Although we are not able to develop a fully general account of what it means to reveal the mind, we can develop an adequate account for specific cases. Then, based on our consideration of these cases, we may be able to see clearly enough as to how we may eventually generalize from them.

This is the method I will pursue. I'll explore how we can apply the ideas of scope, clarity, novelty, and duration to psychedelic experiences that reveal *episodic memories*. I will then suggest some plausible ways in which we may generalize from what we have learned about this specific kind of case. In the coming chapters, we will also see how these ideas can be applied to other kinds of examples. The goal, therefore, is a modest one: to demonstrate the *plausibility* that we can sensibly speak of the mind being revealed in these terms.

To get started, let's suppose that you have a memory of a time from your early childhood in which you were playing at a friend's house. Let's also suppose that although you have this memory, there is a sense in which you have lost it as well—it would be difficult for you to access it under normal circumstances. Now imagine that a part of this memory suddenly appears in your awareness in vivid detail: you can see one of the rooms that you regularly played in, with all its furniture, artwork, appliances, etc. This is a psychedelic experience since the mind is being revealed to you to some degree—that is, a hidden memory is being partly uncovered.[42] Let's now increase that degree by increasing the *scope* of the experience: imagine that instead of your memory of the room, your memory of the entire house appears in your awareness. Perhaps you can even move around in this experience, passing from room to room. If nothing else about the experience changes, we can say that this second experience is more mind-revealing because it has a larger *scope*: *more memory* is revealed in the experience.

Now consider a third experience, which is exactly like the second one, except that it is vague or fuzzy (the recollection, not the memory itself): you can remember the entire house but not at the same level of detail. This third experience has the same scope as the second, but it has less *clarity* to it, and so it is less psychedelic. In other words, it is less revealing of your memory. How does it compare to the first experience? On the one hand, the third experience has a greater scope.

---

[42] Note that this doesn't rest on the assumption that memories are stored in the brain like files in the computer. Memory recollection appears to be a fundamentally reconstructive process and can be influenced by factors that are irrelevant to the memory being recalled (such as one's present emotional state). Even though recollection is reconstructive, the information corresponding to the memory is still stored in the brain (just in a complex, distributed, and dynamic fashion). See Andonovski 2020 for a good discussion of how memory representations are stored and retrieved.

On the other hand, it has less clarity. We may not be in a position to tell which experience is more psychedelic, but there may still be a fact of the matter. For example, if we could measure the overall *informational content* of the experiences, then perhaps we could say that the more psychedelic experience is the one that contains more information.[43] This thought fits rather well with recent research that suggests that psychedelic drugs increase the "richness of conscious content" (Carhart-Harris and Friston 2019), so it has some plausibility to it. Nonetheless, even if there isn't a fact of the matter, we can still compare the third experience with the second and the second with the first. Such a partial ordering will be sufficient for our present purpose.

Let's now consider novelty. To do so, let's introduce a fourth memory-revealing experience: your memory of the room in which you ate breakfast this morning. For the sake of exposition, let's suppose that this memory appears in your awareness with the same scope and clarity as the first experience. Despite having the same scope and clarity, this fourth experience is less psychedelic because it has less novelty to it. All else being equal, our memories of recent events tend to be more accessible than our memories of more distant events.[44] This fourth experience is less novel because it is an experience that involves a part of the mind that is less novel to you. One helpful way to think about this is in terms of surprise: a sudden flashback to the room from childhood would be more surprising than a sudden flashback to breakfast this morning. Although surprise can be helpful for understanding novelty, they are not the same thing. For example, suppose that every Monday morning you relive your childhood experience of playing in the room. Since these relived experiences happen routinely, you are no longer surprised by them. Nevertheless, the experiences are still psychedelic because they aren't available at any other time: they contain information that isn't easily accessible. Your relationship to this information is like that of the art critics' to the painting that they have seen but can't recall because of their short memory span.

There is another way of understanding novelty. In the previous section, I stipulated that we are concerned with the revelation of the *unconscious* mind to the *conscious* mind. If we assume that the distinction between the unconscious and conscious mind is not binary but graded, then we can understand the novelty of a psychedelic experience in terms of how more conscious its content becomes. An experience that reveals something in the border region between the conscious

---

[43] One way of making this idea mathematically precise would be to draw upon the resources of integrated information theories of consciousness (Tononi 2004, Oizumi et al. 2014, Gallimore 2015).

[44] In memory research, it is common to distinguish the *accessibility* of a memory from its *availability*. When you are temporarily unable to recall a memory, it is temporarily inaccessible, but it is nevertheless available since the requisite information still exists. In the case of memories, we can think of the novelty of a memory-revealing experience as the inverse of the memory's accessibility: the more inaccessible the memory, the more novel its sudden appearance in awareness.

and unconscious would then be less psychedelic than an experience that reveals something that is deeply unconscious. This fits well with the idea that psychedelic drugs provide access to deep unconscious psychological material. However, we can extend that idea: an experience can be more psychedelic if what it reveals is moved more into consciousness, even if that part or aspect of the mind starts off in the border region between the conscious and unconscious. The general idea, then, is that the novelty of an experience could be understood in terms of the mental "distance" it travels.[45]

Finally, let's turn to duration. Consider two versions of the first experience: one that happens as a brief glimpse of the memory (a momentary flashback) and another that happens as a prolonged experience, allowing you to "look around" in the memory. The glimpse experience is less psychedelic than the prolonged one because it has a shorter duration (while being the same otherwise). The glimpse experience is therefore less revealing of the memory than the prolonged experience. (It's important to keep in mind that our focus is on the memory being revealed rather than on the actual details of the house, even though they may be revealed as a consequence of the memory being revealed.) Again, it is helpful to think about this in terms of information: because of the short duration, you have less ability to process the memory information being revealed. For this reason, the experience is less revelatory.

For the case of revealing an episodic memory, we see how the ideas of scope, clarity, novelty, and duration can allow us to compare experiences in terms of how psychedelic they are. In this case, an experience is more psychedelic than another if it is more revealing of the episodic memory. It can be more revealing by revealing the memory with greater scope, by revealing a memory with greater clarity, by revealing a more novel memory, or by revealing a memory with greater duration. This, in turn, gives us some useful conceptual tools for formulating hypotheses about psychedelic experiences. For example, we may hypothesize that the consumption of psychedelics tends to induce experiences involving the revelation of rich episodic memories (scope) in vivid detail (clarity) of childhood events (novelty) for periods of time that are conducive to psychotherapy (duration). If this hypothesis turns out to be true, then this would be a good sign that psychedelics are deserving of their name—that they are genuinely mind-revealing.

So far, we've been focusing on episodic memory, but there is clearly much more to the mind. The mind also contains (or consists of) beliefs, emotions, desires, perceptions, perspectives, abilities, other forms of memory (semantic, procedural, etc.), and so on. One of the assumptions underlying our explication of psychedelic experience is that the concepts of scope, clarity, novelty, and duration can be sensibly applied to these other parts or aspects of the mind. One of the promising

---

[45] In the case of a memory being revealed, we can cash this out in terms of the memory's accessibility.

signs that they do is that many, if not all, of these mental items involve *content*, and so we may be able to use the contents of these mental items to compare the different ways in which they are revealed. For example, just as we might be able to compare memory experiences in terms of their informational contents, perhaps we can do the same for revelations of beliefs, since we are familiar with the idea that beliefs have contents. As I mentioned earlier, this approach would fit well with the thought that psychedelics increase the "richness of conscious content" (Carhart-Harris and Friston 2019).[46] However, we should be open to the possibility that more than content is required to make these comparisons. For example, beliefs also have *strengths* (I believe more strongly that I have hands than I do that there will be an economic recession within the next decade). So, the strength of a belief may need to be factored into our analysis of what makes a particular belief-revelation more psychedelic than another. One way to account for this may be to understand the revelation of stronger beliefs as having more scope. However, we needn't take a stand on such issues just yet. For now, we can make do with the assumption that these details can be worked out later on if that level of precision is needed (and if the general approach proves fruitful).

We now have a better sense of how the factors of scope, clarity, novelty, and duration can be applied to the mind so that we can make sense of experiences being more or less mind-revealing—that is, more or less psychedelic. However, the idea of clarity deserves a bit more elaboration since it will be extremely important for the rest of the book. The additional detail we need is that there are two ways in which the clarity of a psychedelic experience can vary: (i) by varying in its level of *detail* and (ii) by varying in its level of *veracity*. We can think of these as two subdimensions of clarity, and they coincide with two kinds of errors that can take place within an experience: (i) errors of omission and (ii) errors of commission. An error of omission occurs when a detail is missing: for example, if some of the details of your memory of your friend's house are missing or vague. An error of commission occurs when a detail is distorted or added to the experience: for example, when you mix your memory of your friend's house with that of another house. Psychedelic experiences can involve both kinds of error and thus be lacking in clarity. All else being equal, the fewer such errors an experience has, the more accurately it reflects the mind, and the more psychedelic it is.

This point is important because psychedelic substances are known to produce bizarre, fantasy-like experiences. And for some people, this suggests that psychedelic drugs do not reveal the mind but rather *scramble* it, steering it towards delusional (and potentially harmful) beliefs. The fact that psychedelic experiences can vary in their clarity by varying in their veracity puts a halt to that argument. It doesn't follow that if someone has a fantasy-like experience, then

---

[46] Another possibility would be to use the idea of *quantity of consciousness* from integrated information theory (Tononi 2004, Oizumi et al. 2014, Gallimore 2015).

they didn't have a mind-revealing experience: it could be that they had a mind-revealing experience that was simply lacking clarity in some respects. Although a psychedelic experience that is low in clarity is not as mind-revealing as it could be, it may nevertheless be mind-revealing to some degree. The situation is a bit like looking at one's image in a "skinny" mirror. The mirror may reveal something about you—say, that you spilled coffee on your shirt—even though it creates a distorted image of your body. Psychedelic experiences may be revelatory in a similar way: you may discover something novel and true about your mind, but at the same time your mind (or your image of it) may be distorted.

The following example of a dream experience shows us how the mind can be revealed and distorted at the same time:

> Reil 1803 [. . .] quotes among others a dream reported by Lichtenberg, a German writer, who dreamed that he was relating a sad but true story to someone when a third person interrupted him to remind him of an important point, which he, Lichtenberg, had forgotten. 'Why did his fantasy', asked Reil, 'create a third person who surprised him and made him feel ashamed, how can the ego divide itself into persons, who, out of himself, produce things of which he is not aware that they were in him, and surprise him as outside wisdom?'
>
> Ellenberger 1970, pp. 127–8

In the dream, something is apparently revealed—the important point that Lichtenberg had forgotten—but through a fantasy and in a distorted form. As I mentioned earlier, dreams may not count as psychedelic experiences (in general), but it is easy to envision something like the above scenario happening during a psychedelic trip. Indeed, consider the example below of an experience induced by mescaline:

> A very curious relationship was observed between central after-images and mescaline hallucinations. One of the investigated persons, before his intoxication became manifest, carefully studied a map of a region known to him. Among his first hallucinations was a reproduction of this map, in its most minute details; but in addition to all the details of the map, a town which was actually omitted in the map appeared in its proper position in his hallucinatory representation of the map. Here was an example of a central after-image being converted into an hallucination, but into an hallucination which corrected and amplified the original object which had given rise to the central after-image.
>
> Knauer and Maloney 1913, p. 433

In this case, another memory is being revealed, but in a distorted way: the individual's memory of the town and its location was revealed by the mescaline but in the vehicle of the map's afterimage, which itself was being promoted into awareness by the drug. This is an important point: psychedelics may distort and reveal the mind simultaneously, and the distortions may be part of the revelations or even play a crucial role in facilitating them. Moreover, we also see how the question of what counts as a revelation may be nuanced. The hallucinatory representation of the map is, in a sense, more accurate than the pure afterimage. To be clear, the hallucination is more accurate in that it is a more accurate map of the world, which is an interesting point in itself. However, one may argue that the hallucination was also more accurate of *the mind* since it contained more of the individual's geographical knowledge, in comparison to the pure afterimage. The issue depends on what we decide is being revealed: the memory of the map or the individual's geographical knowledge. Perhaps the appropriate position to take is that both were being revealed, but with different levels of clarity (and scope). At any rate, we see how the clarity of a mind-revealing experience plays an important role in determining how we should think about the experience and to what degree, and in what respects, we should classify it as being psychedelic.

This point about clarity also highlights the earlier distinction between experience and inference, as well as the need to integrate psychedelic experiences with one's larger epistemic system. A psychedelic experience can be an important source of new information about one's mind, similar to how an x-ray image can be an important source of new information about one's body. However, like the x-ray image, a psychedelic experience isn't going to be 100% reliable. Indeed, no source of new knowledge is indubitable—our senses easily deceive us, witnesses and experts make mistakes, and so on. Therefore, it is important that we are mindful of this point about clarity and remember that whatever new information an experience provides, it should be integrated with, and kept in check by, the rest of one's epistemic system.[47]

With this understanding in place, we can now put everything together. Experiences can be more or less revelatory of the mind by varying with respect to four key dimensions: scope, clarity, novelty, and duration. I will call this space of revelatory experiences *psychedelic space*. An experience is more psychedelic than another if it is located deeper in psychedelic space.

This conceptual framework of psychedelic space is useful for thinking about psychedelic experiences, but it should be thought of as an incomplete model. For example, as we have just seen, the dimension of clarity can be broken down into two subdimensions, and I expect that it may eventually be useful to similarly refine the other dimensions.[48] Also, the mapping between points in psychedelic space

---

[47] It is also worth noting that while one may be especially concerned about the clarity of experiences induced by psychedelics, the concern also applies to psychedelic experiences induced by other means, including meditation. Indeed, it has recently been demonstrated that false insights—apparent revelations that are false but feel true—can be reliably induced in experimental settings (Laukkonen et al. 2020).

[48] A common question I receive is why *significance* is not a dimension of psychedelic space. The answer is that while significance may be a valuable quality of a psychedelic experience (such as when

and experiences is not one-to-one: one point in psychedelic space will represent *many* revelatory experiences. As such, we can think of a point in psychedelic space as representing an equivalence class of experiences—a set of experiences that will differ wildly in terms of their content but nevertheless be equal in terms of how psychedelic they are. There is also a question of whether the space can be used to determine how psychedelic an experience is in absolute terms. So far, we've built up the space in comparative terms: one experience being more psychedelic than another. However, if we define "normal" experiences, or one's "default" state of consciousness, as not being psychedelic at all, then we can apply a coordinate system to psychedelic space, with the origin point representing experiences that are not psychedelic in any respect. We can then understand how psychedelic an experience is with respect to the origin point of that coordinate system. To be sure, this should also be treated as a rough model (e.g. we lack units of measurement), but as we will see in the coming chapters, it can be useful to think of how such a coordinate system may transform over time, and what effects this may have on one's experiences.

There is one final question we should consider before moving on: is psychedelic space unbounded or bounded? If it is unbounded, then there would be no limit to how psychedelic one's experiences may be. If it is bounded, then there is some upper limit. This issue depends, in part, on the nature of the mind. If the mind is finite, like a painting, then an experience can only be so revealing of it—that is, there is only so much of the mind that can be revealed. Alternatively, if the mind is infinite in some way, perhaps like a fractal, then there may be no limit to mind-revelation. This matters because, for example, mystical experiences induced by psychedelics are often considered to be peak, or maximally psychedelic, states. So we will need to consider how mystical experiences relate to psychedelic space. Perhaps, for example, a mystical experience is a psychedelic experience that is maximal in scope, clarity, novelty, and duration. To answer this question, we need to develop a better understanding of mystical experiences, which will be a central task of Chapter 10.

3.5 Conclusion

We now have a clearer idea of what a mind-revealing experience is, along with two explications of the concept. The first defines whether an experience is psychedelic in binary terms, and the second, more sophisticated explication defines the *degree* to which an experience is psychedelic. Both explications have their merits, but the binary one is only superior in terms of its simplicity and convenience. It's often

---

one has a psychological insight or a creative breakthrough), it isn't a factor in how *revelatory* the experience is that isn't already captured by the other dimensions.

convenient to speak *as though* experiences are psychedelic or not, and for this purpose, the binary explication can serve us quite well. However, it lacks much of the fruitfulness of the sophisticated explication.

The second, more sophisticated explication defines the degree to which an experience is psychedelic in terms of its position in psychedelic space. An experience can be more revealing of the mind, and therefore *more psychedelic*, if it: (i) reveals more of the mind (scope), (ii) reveals the mind more clearly (clarity), (iii) reveals parts of the mind that are more deeply buried in the unconscious (novelty), or (iv) reveals the mind for a greater amount of time, so that what is being revealed can be more extensively processed by the conscious mind (duration). We've also considered the possibility that there may be such a thing as a maximally psychedelic experience. Such an experience would be one that (i) reveals the entire mind, (ii) reveals it with perfect clarity, (iii) reveals the most deeply buried elements of the unconscious, and (iv) reveals it long enough for the conscious mind to process what is being revealed.

One important point to observe is that I have left the definition of psychedelic space somewhat incomplete. For example, we don't yet know how to compare an experience that reveals a hidden desire with one that reveals a hidden memory. Such a complete account, if needed, would have to be developed at a later point. However, I think we have enough detail to see whether it is useful as the basis for a theory of those experiences attributed to psychedelics and meditation. If the theory looks promising, we can come back to the matter and fill in more of the details of psychedelic space as needed.

With the conceptual framework of psychedelic space in hand, we now have an explication of the concept of psychedelic experience, and we can now begin considering hypotheses that involve its application. That will be the task of the next chapter.

4

Hypotheses

4.1 Introduction

Now that we have a clearer understanding of the concept of psychedelic experience, we can begin exploring how we may formulate hypotheses that involve its application. That is the main task of this chapter. We will begin to turn away from the purely conceptual issues of the previous chapters and move towards developing an understanding of the phenomenon of psychedelic experience itself.

Perhaps the most salient hypothesis to consider is that so-called psychedelic drugs reliably produce psychedelic experiences. However, now that we have seen that experiences can be more or less psychedelic and that they can be psychedelic in different ways, we will need to consider how this general hypothesis can be made more specific. For example, perhaps psychedelic drugs produce experiences that are *very* psychedelic. Perhaps they also tend to produce experiences that are very psychedelic in a particular kind of way—for example, by producing experiences that are very high in scope and novelty, but not so much in duration and clarity. In addition to hypotheses that are more sophisticated in these ways, we will need to consider other complicating factors. For example, we will need to be mindful of the possibility that the experiences produced by a psychedelic may evolve over time and depend on a person's psyche, their environment, their previous history with psychedelic experiences, and so on. As we will see, we need to be quite careful whenever we try to make specific predictions about the effects of psychedelics.

Another salient hypothesis involves the claim that meditation produces psychedelic experiences. Just as with the hypothesis about psychedelic drugs, there are many complicating factors we'll need to consider here as well. Perhaps the most important such factor is that meditation, when practised systematically, has certain effects that accumulate over time. In particular, there is a common belief that whereas some of the effects of psychedelics can last for extended periods of time, the effects of meditation may be even more enduring and substantial, especially when practised regularly. Stated in terms of the conceptual framework of psychedelic space, psychedelics may temporarily take you to points that are deep in psychedelic space, whereas meditation may take you to points that are a bit closer to your default state (your origin point), but in a more enduring fashion. Said another way, meditation may tend to permanently move one's entire coordinate system deeper into psychedelic space, and psychedelics may tend to temporarily move one's experience in psychedelic space, while keeping one's coordinate system relatively fixed.[1] We will need to explore this idea more carefully so that we can formulate adequate hypotheses about the psychedelic experiences that meditation may produce.

Finally, a third hypothesis that we will need to consider concerns the possibility of *spontaneous* psychedelic experiences. These kinds of psychedelic experiences occur without any substantial intervention on the body or mind (such as consuming psychedelics or practising meditation)—they can just happen out of the blue. Again, as with the hypotheses involving meditation and psychedelics, there are complicating factors that we'll need to be mindful of. Two hypotheses we'll need to consider are that (i) spontaneous psychedelic experiences are *rare*, and (ii) they tend to be only *mildly* psychedelic. These hypotheses are important because they will help address a natural objection that some readers may have. The objection is that our explication trivializes psychedelic experiences, since it seems to imply that they happen all the time (spontaneously). However, the question of whether spontaneous psychedelic experiences are frequent or rare is an empirical matter. If they are rare, then the objection is based on a false assumption and can therefore be dismissed. Alternatively, if they turn out to be common but only mildly psychedelic, then this would reduce the objection's force. In this case, we can say that while we do have spontaneous psychedelic experiences regularly, they are only mildly psychedelic and hardly noteworthy—especially in comparison to the experiences typically produced by psychedelics and meditation. So, we'll need to explore these details in order to know where we stand with respect to this objection.

The plan for this chapter is as follows. In Section 4.2, we'll begin with the hypothesis that there are spontaneous psychedelic experiences and that they are rare and/or mild. In Section 4.3, we'll consider the various hypotheses involving psychedelic drugs. In Section 4.4, we'll examine the relevant hypotheses about the psychedelic experiences that meditation may produce. In Section 4.5, I will summarize the previous sections and discuss how the various hypotheses relate to each other. This latter task is important because it will show that there are many plausible comparative hypotheses. The most obvious such hypothesis is that psychedelic drugs tend to produce experiences that are much more psychedelic than our spontaneous psychedelic experiences. However, there are other comparisons worth considering as well. For example, perhaps psychedelic drugs tend to produce psychedelic experiences with less clarity than those produced by meditation. As another example, perhaps psychedelics make our spontaneous psychedelic experiences much more psychedelic, as opposed to simply producing new psychedelic experiences that wouldn't have occurred otherwise. By the end of

---

[1] In Chapter 6, we will see how shifts in the coordinate system correspond to increases in *mindfulness*.

the chapter, we'll have developed a sufficiently nuanced outlook that will allow us to begin thinking about the evidence more carefully.

4.2 Spontaneous Psychedelic Experiences

A psychedelic experience is spontaneous if it occurs without any substantial intervention on the body or mind. In this book, we will focus primarily on two such interventions: the consumption of psychedelic substances and the practice of meditation. However, these are not the only substantial interventions that may bring about psychedelic experiences. Other possibilities include fasting, yoga, breathwork, sensory deprivation, extreme sports, martial arts, etc. So, the basic idea here is that a psychedelic experience is spontaneous if it happens to a regular person doing regular, everyday activities. Obviously, what counts as "regular" is vague and relative to cultural norms. In some cultures, practices such as prayer, fasting, and meditation are regular activities and essential elements of a healthy life. Moreover, what counts as a regular activity can change quite rapidly—for example, the practice of meditation is becoming increasingly common in the West (and psychedelics are quickly becoming mainstream). Nonetheless, despite these complexities, this definition will suffice for our purposes here.

We have already seen some examples of spontaneous psychedelic experiences in the previous chapters: the recollection of lost childhood memories, the moment when a word comes to mind after it was stuck on the tip of your tongue, when you suddenly realize you have been attracted to someone for quite some time, and certain creative insights. There are also some potential borderline cases, such as the example of illusory motion (discussed in the previous chapter). The act of looking at a strange image that causes the illusion of motion is not the sort of thing people do during normal life. For this reason, we might not want to say that the example involves a spontaneous psychedelic experience. How we classify this sort of example is not so important, but I'd be inclined to say that it is unusual enough to not count as a spontaneous psychedelic experience.

Another potentially difficult example is that of spontaneous mystical experience. As I mentioned earlier, I will argue in Chapter 10 that we can't definitively say that mystical experiences are psychedelic. So, for now, let's stay neutral with respect to the issue of whether they are psychedelic and simply note that some mystical experiences appear to happen spontaneously. Take, for example, the following description of a mystical experience given by Douglas Shrader:

It was the summer of '71. I graduated from high school and worked through the summer as a lifeguard at a country club. It was an excellent summer—the stuff of adolescent dreams and cheap B movies—but now it was drawing to a close. I found myself walking slowly down a narrow dirt path in the densely wooded mountains of Eastern Kentucky, playing my well-worn 12-string guitar, and writing a song whose words and chords I have long since forgotten.

Suddenly, without warning, my life changed—the *world* changed—forever. In an unsolicited blinding flash—in a timeless, eternal moment that encompassed creation, annihilation, and everything that falls between the two—I was stripped bare of all my preconceptions: preconceptions about myself, about the world, and about God.

Shrader 2008, pp. 1–2

One can find many similar descriptions of mystical-type experiences throughout the literature, and it seems quite clear that they can occur spontaneously. Moreover, although they may be rare, they are likely not as rare as the frequency of their reports suggests. Since descriptions of mystical experiences often sound bizarre or incoherent, those who have had them may be wary of sharing their experiences with others.

Given the possibility of spontaneous psychedelic experiences, there are two questions that we must consider: (i) how common are they? and (ii) how psychedelic do they tend to be? These questions are important because if spontaneous psychedelic experiences are common, and just as psychedelic as the experiences produced by psychedelics, then there is a risk that our explication *trivializes* the experiences induced by psychedelics. Now, that's not necessarily a problem since Osmond may have been wrong in his hypothesis about the effects of psychedelics. That is, it is possible that the drugs in question produce experiences that are not mind-revealing but nonetheless profound and important in other ways.[2] However, based on the assumption that psychedelics do produce psychedelic experiences, it seems that there should be a way of distinguishing the experiences they cause from those that occur spontaneously. For example, if the two classes of psychedelic experience differ in terms of their frequency and/or intensity, then that would be a way to distinguish them and avoid the problem of trivialization.

On the face of it, spontaneous psychedelic experiences seem to be quite rare. For instance, flashbacks to lost childhood memories are fairly uncommon for most people. Likewise, creative insights are nowhere near as frequent as most of us would like them to be. Similarly, our emotional insights are not exactly a dime a dozen—which is one reason people spend fortunes on psychotherapy. Furthermore, spontaneous mystical experiences, although they are probably underreported, appear to be even rarer. So, although spontaneous psychedelic experiences may very well occur, it seems that they tend to be rare.

---

[2] For example, psychedelics are sometimes said to "reset" the mind, which may result in a profound experience, but this resetting may not be mind-revealing.

On the other hand, it's possible that spontaneous psychedelic experiences are far more frequent than we realize. After all, having a revelatory experience doesn't guarantee that one will recognize it as such. For example, consider someone who suddenly feels sad for no apparent reason. The sudden appearance of this inexplicable emotion could be a psychedelic experience—for instance, if the emotion has been around for a while, but the person has been too distracted to notice it. It is common for such experiences to arise during psychedelic trips, but they also happen fairly regularly during everyday life. As another example, it is not unusual for people to have seemingly random and useless ideas occur to them. It could be that these ideas normally remain hidden from awareness—say, because they are irrelevant to the task at hand—but in some circumstances, these ideas manage to break through into conscious experience. Such experiences would therefore count as spontaneous psychedelic experiences. And so, perhaps spontaneous psychedelic experiences are quite common, and we simply fail to recognize them.

Given that they may be common, we should then consider the possibility that they tend to be only mildly psychedelic. At first glance, this seems plausible. For example, memory flashbacks tend to be brief, fairly narrow in scope, and low in clarity, especially in contrast to the kind of opium-induced experience that Thomas De Quincey described. Similarly, most of us get our creative and emotional insights in small, fuzzy fragments—we only get glimpses of the solutions to our problems and of our underlying emotional states. Therefore, perhaps spontaneous psychedelic experiences are common but only mildly psychedelic.

However, if experiences like Shrader's (above) are psychedelic, then it seems that they are *very* psychedelic. Similarly, some spontaneous memory flashbacks may be very psychedelic—one famous example, which we will consider in Chapter 6, is Marcel Proust's recollection of eating tea-soaked madeleines. Furthermore, many artists, musicians, and writers speak of dry spells being broken by sudden bursts of intense creativity—when 'the muses descend', or what have you. The same goes for many a mathematician, scientist, and engineer. These exceptional periods of heightened creative output may involve the unconscious mind becoming unusually exposed to conscious awareness. It is entirely possible, then, for spontaneous psychedelic experiences to be very psychedelic.

Therefore, a combination of our two hypotheses may be true: spontaneous psychedelic experiences that are very psychedelic may be rare, while those that are mildly psychedelic may be quite common. In other words, spontaneous psychedelic experiences may be like earthquakes in that they follow a power-law distribution: the mild ones are common and hardly worth noting, and the strong ones are rare but highly noteworthy.

If this is correct, then we can see that although the explication of psychedelic experience entails that such experiences can happen spontaneously and quite regularly, there is still something distinctive about the experiences caused by psychedelics. For example, the effect of psychedelics might be that they temporarily change the shape of the distribution of spontaneous psychedelic experiences, flattening it out so that the mildly psychedelic experiences become much more psychedelic and the experiences that are very psychedelic become much more common.

4.3 Psychedelic-Induced Experiences

Let's now consider the hypothesis that the consumption of psychedelic substances tends to bring about psychedelic experiences. As stated, this is a rough heuristic that we can use to guide our thinking, but in many ways it is overly simplistic. So let's look at how it can be improved.

As we've seen, experiences vary in the degree to which they are psychedelic. So, at the very least, we need to include something about how psychedelic the experiences produced by psychedelics tend to be. A natural hypothesis is that psychedelic substances tend to produce experiences that are *very* psychedelic. Since we don't have an absolute measure for how psychedelic an experience is, we may understand this as the hypothesis that psychedelics tend to produce experiences that are *much more* psychedelic than their spontaneous counterparts. (We saw a version of this hypothesis in the previous section.)

A related hypothesis that is salient in this context is that there is a dependency on dose level: higher doses of psychedelics tend to produce experiences that are more psychedelic than those of lower doses. At first glance, this hypothesis may appear quite plausible. However, upon closer inspection, it is not so obviously true. Consider an analogy with amplifying the music that is quietly playing on a sound system. At first, as you increase the volume, you can hear the music more clearly. However, at some point, when you have increased the volume beyond the speakers' capacity, you begin to get distortion effects, and so the music becomes less clear. It is entirely possible that something similar occurs with psychedelics: beyond a certain threshold, the experiences may become *less* psychedelic as the dose level increases.[3]

Indeed, we can use the conceptual framework of psychedelic space to map out a plausible way in which this may occur. Recall that psychedelic experiences vary with respect to their scope, novelty, clarity, and duration. Increasing the dose level may make the resulting experience more psychedelic in some of these respects, but not in others. In particular, it may be that increasing the dose level tends to increase the scope and novelty of the experience but with some cost to its clarity or duration. For example, you may get a massive insight that is of fundamental importance to

---

[3] Carhart-Harris 2018 puts forward a variant of this idea in proposing that psychedelics may have their enriching (or expanding) effects on consciousness by increasing brain entropy up to a certain limit, after which consciousness may be lost.

your life, but you can't fully decipher its meaning. This loss in clarity or duration can make the overall experience less psychedelic than it would otherwise be.

A psychedelic experience can lack clarity in two ways: by lacking detail or by lacking veracity. One way in which it can lack veracity is if the mind adds new elements to the experience or distorts it in other ways. For example, in the previous chapter, we saw the story of Lichtenberg's dream in which someone reminded Lichtenberg of a point he had forgotten. The experience of remembering the point may be mind-revealing, but the experience of being reminded of it by another person may not be. Indeed, the latter appears to be a fictional artefact that was inserted into the experience by the mind. It's possible that the mind is doing this sort of thing all the time, and this tendency may be exacerbated by psychedelics.

In general, the mind appears to be highly skilled at deceiving itself. For example, consider the well-known cases of *hypnotic confabulation*, in which people construct patently false narratives to explain confusing situations they were lured into during hypnosis. Here's one such example recounted by psychiatrist Albert Moll:

> I tell a hypnotized subject that when he wakes he is to take a flower-pot from the window, wrap it in a cloth, put in on the sofa, and bow to it three times. All which he does. When he is asked for his reasons, he answers, 'You know, when I woke and saw the flower-pot there I thought that as it was rather cold the flower-pot had better be warmed a little, or else the plant would die. So I wrapped it in the cloth, and then I thought that as the sofa was near the fire I would put the flower-pot on it; and I bowed because I was pleased with myself for having such a bright idea'. He added that he did not consider the proceeding foolish, as he had told me his reasons for so acting. In this case the subject carried out an absurd post-hypnotic suggestion; he was unconscious of the constraint put upon him and tried to find good reasons for his act. Most experimenters have observed that their subjects try to find reasons for the most foolish suggested acts.
>
> Moll 1890, pp. 153–4

Hypnotic confabulations can be reliably generated in experimental settings (Cox and Barnier 2015), and there are many other scenarios in which confabulation occurs, including everyday decision-making (Nisbett and Wilson 1977). We're really good at fooling ourselves even in the best of circumstances; as Feynman 1974 famously said, 'The first principle is that you must not fool yourself—and you are the easiest person to fool'. The mind, therefore, appears to be a powerful confabulator. It constructs these narratives effortlessly and often appears to be completely convinced of them. Moreover, it seems that as we give the mind more challenging or confusing material to work with, it generates ever more creative self-deceptions.

So, while a stronger dose of a psychedelic may increase the scope and novelty of the resulting experience, it may dramatically decrease the clarity (and duration) of the experience as well. Moreover, the clarity could be reduced to such an extent that the experience becomes more mind-scrambling than mind-revealing—and, thus, more psychecryptic than psychedelic. So, we can see that it may be overly simplistic to hypothesize that stronger doses of psychedelics tend to produce experiences that are more psychedelic.[4]

A closely related complicating factor we need to consider involves the *dynamical* effects during a psychedelic trip. Indeed, we already have good evidence that there is some kind of predictable dynamical evolution of a psychedelic trip. For example, a moderate dose of psilocybin normally takes about half an hour to an hour to produce noticeable effects, and then over the next hour or so, the intensity of the experiences increases, then peaks for about half an hour to an hour, and then gradually declines again, slowly returning to a normal state over the next two to three hours. It's natural to think that this describes an evolution of the degree to which the experiences are psychedelic, but it may actually be an evolution in the *ways* that the experiences are psychedelic. For example, a trip may begin with experiences that are low in novelty and high in clarity, build up to experiences that are highly novel but unclear at its peak, and then evolve back to experiences with low novelty and high clarity. If something like this is correct, then the peak may not be the most psychedelic part of a trip. Indeed, the most psychedelic experiences of a trip may come before or after its peak.

These dynamic and dose-dependent effects may also depend on the mind of the person undertaking the psychedelic trip. Some people are more prone to fantasy and confabulation than others. Similarly, some people are more reactive and easily caught up in their thoughts. For such people, their psychedelic experiences may rapidly lose clarity as dose levels increase. And it may be that for other kinds of people—those who are less prone to fantasy, less reactive, etc.—their experiences tend to increase in scope, novelty, and duration without much of a loss in clarity. It is also possible that for some people, the effect of a psychedelic is to increase all four factors without incurring substantial trade-offs.[5] To be clear, I'm not claiming that these hypotheses are true. Rather, I am highlighting them as the sorts of possibilities that we need to keep in mind.

When the effects of psychedelics were first studied, researchers quickly recognized that the context in which the trip occurs has a dramatic impact on its qualities. This is known as the *set* and *setting* of a trip, and it covers everything from the nature of the physical environment, to the cultural environment, to the person's state of mind, to their intentions for the trip, to their physical health, etc. For example, the trip of a college student on LSD at a music festival is likely

---

[4] This possibility is closely related to the concern that psychedelic-assisted psychotherapy involves the generation of comforting delusions rather than genuine psychological insights. See Letheby 2021 for an extensive discussion of this particular concern. Here, our focus is more general and involves the effects of psychedelics that go beyond their potential therapeutic benefits.

[5] To jump ahead to later chapters (especially Chapters 6 and 9), the degree to which one is *mindful* could have a substantial impact on the nature of one's psychedelic trips.

to be very different from the experiences of a member of the Native American Church during a peyote ceremony. The cultural context of the latter may provide a conceptual framework that makes it easier to go through a psychedelic trip without a loss in clarity (or perhaps the opposite is true, for all we know). Indeed, just as we think it would be insane to open someone's body for surgery outside of a hospital setting (barring extenuating circumstances), it may be just as insane to open the unconscious mind outside of an appropriate psychological setting (see Lifshitz et al. 2018 for a discussion along similar lines).

Yet another factor to keep in mind when thinking about these hypotheses is that the class of psychedelic substances is highly variegated, and different substances can have markedly different psychological effects. For example, whereas consuming a moderate dose of psilocybin results in effects that last a few hours, inhaling a moderate dose of DMT will last for up to 20 minutes and involve experiences with a different phenomenological profile, tending towards landscapes of complex geometric patterns apparently populated with intelligent beings of some form or other. Also, although time slows down in typical DMT experiences, people still often report the experience to be too fast to "bring anything back"—especially in contrast to the experiences produced by psilocybin, ayahuasca, LSD, and mescaline. Still different yet again are the effects of inhaling 5-MeO-DMT, which is often reported to produce immediate and short-lived states of "pure consciousness".

There are also substances that can be considered borderline psychedelics or that have psychedelic effects that are dependent on how they are consumed. For example, although smoking marijuana is not often considered to produce psychedelic effects, it is commonly reported that *ingesting* it does.

MDMA is another substance that may be considered a borderline psychedelic. Indeed, there are debates about whether it is genuinely a psychedelic substance. Part of the argument against it being classified as a psychedelic is that its molecular structure and psychopharmacological effects are quite different from those of the so-called "classic" psychedelics (psilocybin, LSD, DMT, etc.). Nevertheless, there is a case to be made that although the experiences of MDMA are somewhat different from those of other psychedelics, they are still similar in that they may often be *mind-revealing* and, therefore, should be understood as psychedelic. One way of describing these similarities and differences is that a classic psychedelic *forces* elements of your unconscious into awareness, while MDMA makes it easier for you to *allow* them into your awareness. (This may be one reason why MDMA is particularly effective at treating post-traumatic stress disorder.)

The experiences produced by all of these substances may vary systematically in their scope, novelty, clarity, and duration. For example, DMT experiences may tend to have a high degree of novelty and scope, but a very low degree of clarity and duration. Reports of encounters with intelligent beings may be a sign that something highly novel is being revealed but in a scrambled way—similar to Lichtenberg's dream. Similarly, the fact that the experiences are too fast to "bring anything back" suggests that the duration of the revelatory experience is relatively low. That is, people often don't get enough time to process whatever is being revealed to them.[6] In contrast, since the gentler experiences of MDMA make it easier for people to process traumatic memories, MDMA may tend to produce experiences that are low in scope and novelty, moderate in clarity, and high in duration. As before, I'm not arguing here that these hypotheses are true (although I don't think they are implausible). The point is simply that differences of these sorts likely exist between the psychedelic experiences produced by these different substances.

So far, I have focused on hypotheses about the psychedelic experiences that psychedelic substances may tend to produce. However, we should be mindful of the possibility that these substances may have other effects in addition to their psychedelic ones, and it may be difficult for us to distinguish the effects of each type. For example, it has been suggested that psychedelics "reset" the mind (Nichols et al. 2017, Carhart-Harris 2019). Roughly speaking, the "reset" idea is that a psychedelic trip can temporarily break up the habituated mental dynamics that keep the mind trapped in suboptimal states. By temporarily breaking up the dynamics, a psychedelic can "reset" the mind and give it a chance to transition into a more optimal pattern of states (from now on I will drop the scare quotes). On the one hand, such resets may not have any mind-revealing aspects to them. On the other hand, if the mind is trapped in suboptimal states by its initial dynamics, then perhaps it is correct to say that the more optimal states are hidden from consciousness, and so by breaking up the initial dynamics, they are revealed by the psychedelic. How we answer this question will depend on our background theory of the mind. For example, if we say that the mind is nothing more than its current state and dynamics, then other states are not part of the mind, and the reset effect of the psychedelic is to *change* the mind (by changing its state and dynamics). Alternatively, if we have a broader, more *modal* understanding of the mind, then we can say that the mind is more than just its current state and dynamics and includes various alternative states and dynamics. If so, then the reset could be said to reveal these proximate mental states and dynamics, which would entail that its overall effect is psychedelic.

Alternatively, the reset effect may involve a revelation of the mind in a way that is intrinsic to the reset. For example, imagine someone who is struggling to reduce the amount of alcohol they drink every day. Let's suppose that this person drinks too much wine at night because they drink too much coffee during the day, and the reason they drink too much coffee is that they drank too much wine the night before, and so on. Clearly, this person is trapped in a suboptimal pattern of behaviour. Moreover, they can become trapped in this cycle without realizing it.

---

[6] For this reason, some researchers have worked on developing methods for slowly and continuously consuming DMT via an intravenous drip—so as to extend the duration of the experience (Gallimore and Strassman 2016).

From this person's perspective, they might consider themselves to be a "night owl" and the kind of person who needs a few drinks to fall asleep and a bucket of coffee to wake up in the morning.

A psychedelic trip may break them out of this suboptimal pattern in the form of a reset. There are two ways in which this may happen. The first is that, as a result of the trip, the person finds that they simply do not want to drink coffee and wine anymore. From their perspective, this change in their desires is inexplicable but welcomed nonetheless. The second way is that the person has an *insight* during the trip: they see that they use wine to counteract their over-caffeinated state, which leads to a hangover the next morning and the need for coffee. This insight enables the person to change their behaviour, and their newfound awareness allows them to make new decisions that help ensure their behaviour improves in an enduring fashion.

In both scenarios, there is a kind of mental reset happening. However, in the first scenario, the person doesn't have an experience that involves the revelation of the mind. In contrast, they do have such an experience (the insight) in the second scenario. We don't need to take a stand right now on which kind of scenario is more likely to result from psychedelic substances. The point is just to illustrate a kind of reset effect that does not involve mind-revelation. In this case, it would be a therapeutic, but non-psychedelic effect of a psychedelic substance.[7]

A related effect that has been proposed of psychedelics is that they temporarily increase the brain's *entropy* (Carhart-Harris et al. 2014). Roughly speaking, the idea is that the brain's functional activity becomes more chaotic and less structured, and as part of this change, different regions of the brain become more connected with each other. As with the proposed reset effect, there are various possible relationships between increases in brain entropy and mind-revealing experiences. One such relationship is that by increasing the brain's entropy, psychedelics make mental processes more random and less rigid, which, in turn, facilitates the advent of a mind-revealing experience. This causal relationship would be somewhat similar to that of psychoanalysts using free-association techniques to trigger psychological insights (Carhart-Harris 2018).

The Freudian analogy of the mind being like an archaeological dig site is helpful in this context. According to this analogy, psychoanalytic therapy is like slowly but surely excavating artefacts up from the ground. It's painstaking work, and you're not entirely sure what you're digging up. We can extend this analogy to psychedelics: the main psychological effect of these substances may be analogous to blowing up the dig site with dynamite: you get to see lots of deeply buried material (high scope and novelty), but you also create a mess in the process (low clarity), and the revelation can happen so quickly that you're not entirely sure

---

[7] For a more detailed discussion of the relationship between the mind-revelation and mind-reset hypotheses, see Swanson 2018.

what you even saw (low duration). An actual dynamite explosion is a substantial and rapid increase in entropy and thus analogous to the effect that psychedelics have on the mind.[8] Therefore, psychedelic-induced increases in brain entropy may cause mind-revealing experiences that are high in novelty and scope but relatively low in clarity and duration. Nevertheless, the significant increase in novelty and scope may be sufficiently beneficial from a therapeutic standpoint.

This analogy between psychedelics revealing the mind and dynamite being used on an archaeological dig is helpful, but we need to be careful with it as well. The explosive properties of dynamite depend on how it is used. For example, there is a big difference between controlled and uncontrolled building demolitions. Similarly, the entropy-increasing properties of a psychedelic may depend heavily on the properties of the brain it is influencing. For example, psychedelics may not increase the brain's entropy for people who are expert meditators. Such people may have so much control over their mental processes that there is no "explosive" effect from psychedelics. For them, the primary effect of psychedelics might be something else entirely.

An alternative possibility is that the order of explanation between brain entropy increasing and the mind being revealed is reversed. Perhaps a psychedelic initially causes a mind-revealing experience, which then causes a psychological reaction that corresponds to an increase in brain entropy. For example, received wisdom has it that during the very early stages of a psychedelic trip, the mind goes into "fight or flight" mode, since it can tell that something extraordinary is happening. During this stage of the trip, people often feel anxious, panicked, and even nauseous. These feelings may arise because a psychedelic experience has occurred that is high in scope and novelty but low in clarity (in that the details of what is being revealed are not yet clear). Metaphorically, a mental tectonic shift has occurred, and this can be felt consciously even though nothing in particular has yet appeared in awareness. This shift may be enough to spark psychological reactions that correspond to increased brain entropy. Alternatively, it may be that when the details appear in awareness, they spark these reactions. To put it another way, psychedelics may cause an initial experience that is the equivalent of lighting a fuse, which then causes an explosive chain reaction of psychedelic experiences.[9]

One final non-psychedelic possibility that we should consider follows from Grof's proposal about the effects of psychedelics (and which we also see in Osmond's search for an appropriate name for these substances): that psychedelics reveal the unconscious mind by *energizing* it or *amplifying* it in some way. Recall Grof's proposal:

---

[8] There is, however, an important difference: once a psychedelic trip is over, the entropy of the brain returns to its original level (or close to it).

[9] Of course, for this to make sense, we would need some neuropharmacological account of how psychedelics cause the initial disruption. One possibility may involve a disruption to thalamic gating (Vollenweider and Geyer 2001, Preller et al. 2019).

These substances function as unspecific amplifiers that increase the cathexis (energetic charge) associated with the deep unconscious contents of the psyche and make them available for conscious processing.

Grof 2009, p. xxv

The idea here is that psychedelics reveal the mind by amplifying its unconscious contents. Let's suppose for the moment that this proposal is correct (we will come back to it in more detail in the next chapter). Then, while the amplification of unconscious contents can result in some of these contents being revealed, it may also have other, *non-revelatory* effects. There are at least two ways in which this can happen.

First, perhaps some unconscious contents are amplified, but not so much that they are made available for conscious processing. Nevertheless, they may still be amplified enough to impact behaviour and thought. For instance, a traumatic memory may be amplified enough to create feelings of anxiety, but not enough for the memory to enter awareness. Similarly, unconscious associations between ideas and concepts may be sufficiently amplified to enhance the unconscious associative processing that occurs during the incubation periods of creative problem-solving (Kounios and Beeman 2015). This may happen without any of those associations ever appearing in awareness.

Second, perhaps some unconscious contents are amplified so much that they become distorted in the amplification process. This was a point we came across earlier in considering whether increasingly stronger doses lead to experiences that are increasingly psychedelic. In our analogy with the sound system, as you turn the volume up, you begin to better hear the music being played (thus revealing it). However, at some point, if you turn the volume up too much, all you get is a distorted version of the music. Some unconscious contents may be too novel or too emotionally charged to be consciously processed with any clarity, and so their amplification may result in an experience becoming more psychecryptic rather than more psychedelic.

Another factor arises when we look at psychedelics and psychedelic experiences from a different angle. Recall from the previous section that there can be *spontaneous* psychedelic experiences. The effect of psychedelics might be to make spontaneously occurring psychedelic experiences much more psychedelic than they would be otherwise. So, rather than saying that the consumption of psychedelic substances generates psychedelic experiences, it may be that this consumption causes an amplification of psychedelic experiences that are already occurring. Continuing with our analogy with the sound system, the standard view is that consuming psychedelics is like pressing the play button: music that wasn't playing begins to play. According to the alternative view, the consumption of psychedelics is like turning up the volume of the music that is already playing. Of course, it is also possible that a mixture of the two views may be true. As mentioned towards the end of the previous section, spontaneous psychedelic experiences may be like earthquakes: small ones are common, big ones are rare, and psychedelics may amplify them all.

One final factor that is relevant for our hypothesis concerns the question of *when* psychedelic-induced psychedelic experiences occur. This may seem obvious: psychedelic experiences happen during psychedelic trips. However, it could be the case that some of the experiences occur *after* the trip—like the aftershocks of a large earthquake. A slightly different version of this idea is that the spontaneous psychedelic experiences after a psychedelic trip become a little more psychedelic— as a result of the trip. For example, as we'll see in Chapter 6, people suffering from depression tend to have autobiographical memory recollections that are low in clarity (or *specificity*, in the terminology of the literature). It may be that when psychedelics successfully treat depression, these memory recollections increase in clarity (specificity) and therefore become more psychedelic.[10]

To summarize, I've argued for two crucial points in this section. The first is that simple hypotheses about the effects of psychedelics on the mind are almost certainly false—or, rather, too coarse-grained for any precise analysis of the effects. This point was recognized early on in psychedelics research, for example:

> In spite of all that may be written about drugs and their effects, there is no doubt that for these particular drugs no hard and fast predictions about their subjective effects can be made. These depend primarily on what the person is expecting or wanting to experience, upon his personal motivations, and the upon the setting in which the drug is taken. I am almost convinced that these factors are more important determinants of drug action than the true biochemical effects of the substance itself.
>
> Wilson 1974, p. 309

This point should be kept in mind as we consider the effects of psychedelics in the following chapters. It's clear that we need hypotheses that are much more careful and precise than simple hypotheses such as 'psychedelics reveal the mind'. The second crucial point is that the two hypotheses about spontaneous and psychedelic-induced psychedelic experiences may be linked in an important way. Some of the psychedelic experiences that psychedelics appear to induce may actually be spontaneous psychedelic experiences that are already occurring and which have been made *more* psychedelic by the drugs. More research needs to be done before we can assess this possibility, but it is worth bearing in mind.

---

[10] There is a nuance here that I am glossing over: it may be that the increased clarity (specificity) is a result of increased *mindfulness*. This point requires a more detailed discussion of the concept of mindfulness and how it relates to psychedelic experiences, which we will come back to in Chapter 6.

4.4 Meditation-Induced Experiences

Let's now turn to the hypothesis that meditation induces psychedelic experiences. Just as with the previous sections, this hypothesis is overly simplistic, as there are several complicating factors of which we need to be mindful.

The first is that there are many different kinds of meditation, and they have different effects on the mind. Simply speaking of 'meditation' is like speaking of 'exercise'. You can say that exercise is good for health, but if you want to say anything more substantial than that, you need to be more specific. For most of this book, we will be concerned with two specific meditative practices, which have come to be known as *focused-attention* meditation and *open-monitoring* meditation. I'll explain the details of these two practices in the next chapter. For now, though, we can make do with a rough characterization of meditation: it is the practice of sitting still, allowing the mind to settle down, and maintaining a stable state of clarity and non-reactivity. From the outside, it can look like nothing is happening when someone is meditating, but on the inside, it can be the mental equivalent of balancing on one foot for hours on end—it can be quite challenging.

Based on this understanding of meditation, we can see why it might be the sort of thing that tends to produce psychedelic experiences. Let's develop the analogy with music playing on the sound system a little further. Suppose you are at a crowded party with some music playing quietly in the background. You can hear the music over all of the noisy conversations, but just barely so. To hear the music properly, you could go to the sound system and turn up the volume. Alternatively, you could figure out a way to quiet everyone down and then listen carefully for the music. If turning the volume up is like taking a psychedelic, then getting everyone to quiet down is like meditating. Both interventions are different ways of bringing about the same outcome: you get to hear the music. This also fits well with the archaeological dig analogy. Whereas consuming a psychedelic may be like temporarily blowing up the site with dynamite, meditation is more like how Freud understood psychotherapy: it is the careful, slow, and deliberate uncovering of hidden artefacts.

These metaphors suggest a more refined hypothesis that may be plausible: meditation tends to produce experiences that are more psychedelic than spontaneous psychedelic experiences and, in comparison to the experiences produced by psychedelics, they may tend to be lower in scope and novelty and higher in clarity and duration. Roughly speaking, the thought would be that a typical session of meditation may not reveal as much of the mind as psychedelics do, and not as quickly, but what it does reveal, it reveals with greater clarity and duration. However, even this hypothesis is overly simplistic—and for several reasons.

Perhaps the most important factor to consider is *when* the meditation-induced psychedelic experiences occur. The natural thought would be that they happen *during* the act of meditation, but as we will see in the coming chapters, there's good reason to think they also happen afterward. So, just as we saw with psychedelics, the psychedelic experiences may continue after the "main event"—whether it is a psychedelic trip or a meditation session.

However, meditation is even more complicated in this regard, because there is a difference between doing a single session of meditation and implementing a sustained daily practice of meditation over extended periods of time. Again, meditation is like physical exercise in this respect. A single session of physical exercise will have measurable effects during and after the session, but a sustained practice of regular physical exercise will have rather different long-term effects. Moreover, the long-term effects will change the effects that occur during and after an exercise session—as you eventually become fitter and stronger. Analogously, meditation may have immediate, short-term, and long-term effects, and the long-term effects can eventually influence the qualities of the immediate and short-term effects.

This opens up the hypothesis space to the following sort of possibility. A person who has just begun practising meditation may have psychedelic experiences that are low in scope and novelty and high in clarity and duration, both during and immediately after the meditation sessions. Then, after continuing this practice for a while, they may start having these experiences even when they are not meditating. Eventually, they may even find that the psychedelic experiences during meditation begin to increase in scope and novelty. This can happen to such an extent that their experiences during meditation become radically different from those of their initial meditative sessions and more like the experiences one can have with psychedelics.

Of course, there is also reason to think that an extended meditation practice can have a profound impact on one's regular experience, outside of meditation. According to Buddhists, for example, if practised correctly, meditation will tend to increase one's mindfulness. The concept of mindfulness is difficult to define—despite the abundance of simple definitions found in the literature—and this is a topic we will come back to in detail in Chapter 6. For now, we can roughly think of mindfulness as a kind of clarity and freedom of mind. To the extent one is mindful, one is more aware of one's present thoughts and sensations, ruminates less about the past, frets less about the future, and experiences less involuntary mind-wandering. Although meditation may induce psychedelic experiences—for example, in the form of insights—it is also thought to increase one's mindfulness over time.

The salient possibility of meditation causing more enduring changes to a person's mental life introduces another complexity. Whereas psychedelics may temporarily move one's experience to a new point in psychedelic space, meditation may have the more enduring effect of moving the *origin* of one's entire psychedelic

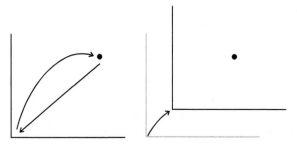

Figure 4.1 Left: A characteristic effect of a psychedelic: a large, temporary shift to a point in psychedelic space away from the origin. Right: A characteristic effect of a meditation session: a small but enduring shift in the origin of psychedelic space.

space (see Figure 4.1 for a depiction). If this is true, then we need to be mindful of a somewhat subtle point. Experiences located at the origin of psychedelic space are, by definition, not psychedelic experiences. So, if meditation moves the origin of one's psychedelic space, then this entails that some experiences that were once psychedelic are no longer psychedelic. Since it is common to distinguish between *states* and *traits* when comparing the effects of psychedelics and meditation, I will use this same terminology to describe the potential differences between these two dynamical effects. Psychedelics may tend to temporarily move your *state* (your current experience) along the dimensions of psychedelic space. And meditation may tend to move your *trait* (your disposition to have certain experiences) along the dimensions of psychedelic space.

We can imagine this difference in dynamical terms. Suppose that there is something in your mind that is slightly hidden from your awareness. Let's call it X. A psychedelic trip may temporarily reveal X to you, but once the trip is over, you may not be able to see X anymore. In contrast, a few weeks of consistent meditation may start to give you glimpses of X. And, after a year of meditation, your mind may change such that you can become aware of X whenever you choose. We will see an example of this in the next chapter—experienced meditators see more 'X's (the symbols) during attentional blink tasks than non-meditators.

If psychedelic space is bounded, then there is a limit to how psychedelic an experience can be. Therefore, if meditation moves the origin towards the upper bounds of psychedelic space, then at some point meditation will no longer induce psychedelic experiences, both in the short term and in the long term. In such a situation, the mind would be made fully accessible.[11] In this end-state, meditation may no longer be psychedelic, even though it originally was. Instead, its primary

---

[11] To be clear, this is a conceptual possibility, and there may be various constraints that prevent any human mind from achieving it. There are also some important conceptual nuances here that we will come back to in Chapter 10.

effect may be to *prevent psychecryptic experiences*—that is, to prevent the mind from concealing itself again.

It's important to note again that we are simply discussing *hypotheses*. It's entirely possible that these hypotheses are false and the situation is even more complex. For example, as we will discuss in the coming chapters (particularly in Chapter 9), there is growing evidence that psychedelics have a tendency to make people more mindful. If correct, this would mean that while psychedelics may cause one's state to shift deeper into psychedelic space temporarily, they may also cause one's trait to shift deeper into the space. Perhaps the shift in state tends to be much larger than the shift in trait. Nevertheless, there could be a non-negligible and enduring shift in one's trait (especially for a psychedelic session with a carefully designed set and setting). Similarly, as already discussed, meditation probably does more than shift one's trait deeper into psychedelic space: it may also cause temporary shifts in one's state (during and immediately after a meditation session, for example). Also, we should be aware of the possibility that the shifts, while enduring, are probably not *permanent*. The process of moving the origin deeper into psychedelic space may be a "two steps forward, one step backward" process. Indeed, given that psychedelic space consists of four dimensions, there is plenty of room to step sideways as well. However, broadly speaking, it seems reasonable to hypothesize that, over time, meditation tends to move the origin deeper into psychedelic space (and potentially towards its upper bounds, if they exist).

Finally, we should be mindful that meditative practices do not occur in an ideological vacuum, and so experiences induced by meditation can be shaped, and thus distorted, by one's school of meditative training (Sharf 1995). Although some authors argue that meditative practices expose universal structures or states of the mind (Stace 1960), others argue otherwise and point out that such practices are strongly influenced by cultural and religious expectations (Katz 1978, Nozick 1989, Sharf 2000, Thompson 2020). This is a particularly important point if there is a trade-off between novelty and clarity, such that as experiences become increasingly novel, they become increasingly distorted by one's theoretical, ethical, cultural, and religious commitments.

To summarize this section, we've seen that the relationship between meditation and psychedelic experience is quite complex and nuanced—much like the relationship between psychedelic substances and psychedelic experiences. This is to be expected, since meditation is a complex phenomenon and can affect the mind in very different ways. Perhaps the most important factor we considered is that the effects of meditation can accumulate over time and change the nature of one's psychedelic experiences. It is also worth noting that there are many other factors that I haven't discussed in this section for reasons of space. For instance, many of the factors discussed in the previous section can also apply to meditation (e.g. set and setting). Similarly, some of the factors discussed in this section will also apply to psychedelics.

Overall, the core point is that, in both cases, we are dealing with a highly complex system (the mind and its environment), a rich set of interventions (different meditative practices, and different psychedelic substances with different methods of consumption), and a rich set of outcomes (those that happen immediately, later, or over the long term, and those that vary in scope, novelty, clarity, and duration). Therefore, it is important to keep this complexity in mind as we evaluate the empirical evidence in the coming chapters.

4.5 Summary of the Hypotheses

Let's now take a step back and consider what hypotheses might be plausible given the previous considerations.

At the most basic level, we have three core hypotheses:

- H1: Psychedelic experiences happen spontaneously, during everyday life. These experiences are usually low on the psychedelic spectrum and thus not typically recognized as being "psychedelic" (but there are exceptions).

- H2: The consumption of psychedelics tends to induce psychedelic experiences and those experiences tend to be more psychedelic than the spontaneous kind, and/or it tends to make spontaneously occurring psychedelic experiences more psychedelic.

- H3: The practice of meditation tends to induce psychedelic experiences and those experiences tend to be more psychedelic than the spontaneous kind, and/or it tends to make spontaneously occurring psychedelic experiences more psychedelic.

For convenience, I'll refer to these hypotheses using various shorthands—for example, psychedelics are psychedelic (H2), and meditation induces psychedelic experiences (H3). However, it should be understood that these are mere shorthands for hypotheses that themselves are only shorthands for even more nuanced hypotheses.

We've also seen that there are reasons for thinking that psychedelics and meditation may tend to induce psychedelic experiences of different kinds. In particular:

- H4: Psychedelics tend to generate psychedelic experiences that are higher in novelty and scope but lower in clarity and duration than those induced by meditation.

Again, we should keep in mind that this hypothesis is another broad brushstroke, and there are many complicating factors. For example, six weeks of consistent daily meditation guided by a Zen master could trigger psychedelic experiences that are far more novel than those induced by a psychedelic. We also need to remember that meditation may tend to move the goal posts, and thus an experience that is quite psychedelic for you today may not be psychedelic at all after a year of intense meditation.

The potential difference between psychedelics and meditation captured by H4 will be relevant in the coming chapters. It highlights an important possibility concerning psychedelics that we need to keep an eye on: they may reveal the mind, but not all that accurately. Indeed, for some people, the real significance of psychedelics may be the revelation that the mind can be revealed rather than the revelation of particular mental contents. Thus, it may be better to think of a psychedelic-induced psychedelic experience as sometimes more of a "proof of concept" psychedelic experience. It may sound odd, but it is entirely possible that a sustained practice of meditation may ultimately be more psychedelic than the use of psychedelics (all else being equal).

So far, I have said very little about the *combination* of meditation and psychedelics. As we will see in the coming chapters, there is growing evidence that the minds of experienced meditators work somewhat differently from the rest of the population. Roughly speaking, experienced meditators appear to have more control over their minds—for example, they have better control over their attention (Jha et al. 2007, Leeuwen et al. 2009, Short et al. 2010) and better awareness and regulation of their emotions (Nielsen and Kaszniak 2006, Hill and Updegraff 2012, Teper et al. 2013, Farb et al. 2014, Lee et al. 2015). It's therefore plausible that the effects of psychedelics on the minds of experienced meditators are quite different from those they have on the minds of non-meditators. As we've seen, one of the leading hypotheses about the primary effect of psychedelics on the brain is that they increase its entropy, which is presumed to correspond to a more disordered and dynamic mode of cognition. At least phenomenologically, meditation appears to have the opposite effect by bringing clarity and stability to the mind.[12] So, it could be that brain entropy increases only occur for people who don't already have a high degree of control over their minds. If this is true (and to be clear, we don't yet know), then H4 would have to be qualified: it may only tend to be true for non-meditators. For experienced meditators, psychedelics may increase scope and novelty without significant trade-offs, such as a decrease in accuracy or clarity.

Finally, we should remember that there are many factors that have a substantial impact on the outcomes of both psychedelics and meditation, all of which we're only beginning to be able to quantify. Despite these complicating factors, there

---

[12] There is, however, some evidence indicating that meditation also increases brain entropy (Vivot et al. 2020), suggesting that more work needs to be done in translating statements about brain entropy into statements about conscious experience.

is still value in the simple hypotheses. At the very least, they provide helpful heuristics for thinking about the empirical observations we are likely to make concerning psychedelics and meditation. Moreover, many of the factors can be controlled for in experimental conditions. For example, we can provide safe and supportive environments, correlate observed effects with levels of prior experience with meditation and psychedelics, take measurements at different stages of trips and meditative practices, quantify personality types, and so on. There's a lot that we can do and a lot that we can learn. The point is just that we should be careful when making simple claims about psychedelics and meditation.

4.6 Conclusion

We've now got a good handle on the main hypotheses worth considering and how we need to be careful when drawing predictions from them. We may have mind-revealing experiences during everyday life without the consumption of drugs or the practice of meditation. However, these interventions may make our regular mind-revealing experiences *more* mind-revealing, and thus more psychedelic. Moreover, they may tend to do so in different ways. For example, the effects of psychedelics may be more explosive and temporary, with high scope and novelty and low clarity and duration, whereas meditation's effects may be more incremental and enduring, with low scope and novelty and high clarity and duration.

So far, these hypotheses have been developed based on the explication of the concept of psychedelic experience and some preliminary knowledge that we have about psychedelics and meditation. In the next chapter, we will start to look at the scientific evidence concerning psychedelics and meditation and develop a unified theory of their psychedelic effects.

5

Attention

5.1 Introduction

We have now seen the kinds of hypotheses that we can articulate using the conceptual framework of psychedelic space, with its component dimensions of scope, clarity, novelty, and duration. We have also seen how we need to be mindful of a range of complicating factors as we consider the empirical evidence for these hypotheses. In this chapter, we will look at the empirical evidence concerning the effects of psychedelics and meditation on attention.

The reason for this choice of focus is that attention plays a crucial role in determining what appears in awareness. Roughly speaking, attention functions as a kind of gatekeeper for consciousness. Depending on the circumstances, it helps promote some mental contents into awareness and keep others out. Since psychedelics and meditation both clearly have a profound impact on awareness— and are often said to "expand consciousness"—it stands to reason that they may do this by having some important effect on attention. Indeed, in the case of meditation, this couldn't be clearer. As we will see, meditation involves the training of attention, and there is growing scientific evidence that this training works. In the case of psychedelics, however, the situation is less clear. Because of the effects that psychedelics have on awareness, it seems reasonable to expect that these effects occur via some effect on attention. However, the theory and evidence are less definitive than they are with respect to meditation. So, one of the central goals of this chapter is to develop this theory in more detail and highlight the empirical evidence that currently exists in support of it.

The key idea will be that whereas meditation gives us more control over our attention, psychedelics free up our attention so that more of it is available for allocation to our various mental contents and processes. The two interventions— practising meditation and consuming psychedelics—are clearly different, but they nonetheless result in various mental contents and processes receiving more attention than they otherwise would. This extra attention helps lift these contents and processes out of unconsciousness and bring them into the light of conscious awareness. My proposal, then, is that meditation and psychedelics induce mind-revealing experiences via these effects on attention.

If correct, this theory will provide us with a unified account of how psychedelics and meditation reveal the mind. It will also point the way to how we may further develop our understanding of these interventions and their interactions.

For example, the act of meditating during a psychedelic trip may have important and novel effects on consciousness and well-being as a result of it enabling a skilful control of the attentional surplus afforded by the psychedelic. As such, the experiences that one has while meditating during a psychedelic trip may be more psychedelic than the experiences one has as a result of meditation or psychedelics alone. We already have a sense of why this might be the case: the improved control over attention due to meditation may bring more clarity and duration to the experiences, and the extra attention made available by the psychedelic may make the experiences more novel and greater in scope. If this is correct, then such hybrid experiences are more psychedelic because they get the best of both interventions: more clarity and duration in conjunction with more novelty and greater scope.

To get started in developing this theory, it will help if we first examine what we know about attention in general. After that, in Section 5.3, I'll explain how meditation can be understood as a practice for training attention and discuss the evidence for thinking that this training can give rise to psychedelic experiences. In Section 5.4, I will focus on psychedelics and the effects they may have on attention. As I mentioned, the situation with psychedelics is less definitive than it is with meditation. This is in part because there is simply less research on psychedelics and attention. Nevertheless, I'll argue that the evidence we do have is supportive of the hypothesis that they free up one's attentional resources.

Let's begin by getting some basic facts about attention on the table.

5.2 Attention

Although William James famously said that everyone knows what attention is (James 1890, ch. 11), some have argued that no one knows what it is (Hommel et al. 2019), that it doesn't exist (Anderson 2011), and that it is a sterile concept (Lollo 2018). Moreover, there are also several competing accounts of attention and its role in human cognition. In what follows, I'm going to remain as neutral as possible on such issues, with the minimal commitment that for our level of analysis, the term 'attention', when used with appropriate care, can be a convenient way of referring to a cluster of related phenomena and processes. As such, much of what I say can be translated into one's own view of attention.

Early attention research was dominated by the *spotlight* metaphor for visual attention, which was first proposed by Posner et al. 1980. According to this idea, attention functions a lot like a spotlight: it selects features in a particular region that is limited in scope, but can nevertheless move around somewhat freely. When the spotlight of attention selects some features, they appear to us in a more vivid or enhanced way—we see more of their details, for example. While this metaphor enjoyed some popularity, it was quickly replaced by more sophisticated accounts. For example, Eriksen and Yeh 1985 proposed that attention is more like a *camera zoom lens* in that it has a focal region that can change in location and size, and as the focal region increases in size, the resolution of detail decreases. So-called *gradient* models introduce a further complexity by allowing for a more continuous change between the focal region and the rest of the visual field, where the gradient of change depends on task type and other contextual factors (Downing 1988, LaBerge and Brown 1989). Although there are differences between these models, what they have in common is that attention takes the form, or involves the application, of a *limited cognitive resource*. If that resource becomes more concentrated in one region, then it must become less concentrated elsewhere. The idea that attention is a limited resource that can enhance cognitive processing will be important in the following sections.[1]

It's natural to think of attention in terms of our sensations—for example, you are attending to these words as you read them. However, as William James observed, in addition to perceptual attention, we also have what he called *intellectual* attention: attending to different states or processes in your *mind* (James 1890, p. 416). This distinction between perceptual and intellectual attention has also come to be known as *external* and *internal* attention (Chun et al. 2011, Fortney 2019). For example, internal attention is at work when you shift your focus to your present emotions or when you focus on your memory of dinner last night. Although we normally think of attending to things in the external world (people, menus, smells, music, etc.), we can also attend to things in the internal world (emotions, memories, desires, ideas, etc.).

There is also a subtlety regarding external attention that will be important to keep in mind as we work through the coming sections. Although we usually think of ourselves as attending to things in the external world, there is a sense in which this isn't actually what happens. Instead, attention selects (or enhances) our *representations* of things in the world. This point is made particularly vivid by the fact that our attention can appear to act upon stimuli *retroactively*. Sergent et al. 2013 and Thibault et al. 2016 demonstrated this by cueing attention to the location of a fleeting stimulus shortly *after* the stimulus was presented to subjects. When their attention wasn't cued in this way, subjects were not aware of the stimulus, but they were aware of it (after it was gone) when the stimulus was cued. The explanation for this result is that the mind's representation of the stimulus is still active even after the stimulus has disappeared and that by focusing attention on the stimulus' location, some attentional resources are indirectly allocated to the

---

[1] There is some debate about the underlying nature of this resource and the mechanisms by which it is allocated. For example, attentional resources might involve metabolic energy (Kahneman 1978), a capacity for reentrant processing (Lollo 2018), the readying of limited metabolic resources in the form of adaptive gain modulation (Bruya and Tang 2018), or the optimization of precision expectations that selectively weight some prediction errors over others (Hohwy 2013). In what follows, we won't need to take a stand on such issues, so we can remain neutral with respect to them.

mind's representation of the stimulus. This indirect allocation can then activate the representation enough for it to appear in conscious experience.

To be sure, when we attend to an object in the world, it doesn't *seem* like this is what is happening. Instead, it appears as though we are attending to the object itself and not our representation of it. Although it seems like this is what we are doing—and although it is reasonable for us to *speak* in this way—attention is nevertheless operating on our mental *representations*.[2] This will be important later on for two closely related reasons. First, just as attention can enhance our awareness of things in the world by enhancing our representations of them, psychedelic experiences can be world-revealing as a result of being mind-revealing—that is, by having a mind-revealing experience, one can become more aware of the world. Second, experiences that may seem like they are only world-revealing may, in fact, also be mind-revealing. For example, if you become aware for the first time of some details of a familiar building, this may be because those details were previously perceived unconsciously and have now become consciously perceived. In other words, there is an intimate connection between mind-revelation and our experience of the world, and this point about attention operating on our representations of things in the world will help us make sense of this.

Attention is also often likened to a filter that helps us manage our limited cognitive resources. At any given moment, the world in our immediate vicinity contains a vast array of objects and properties that are potentially crucial to our interests and survival. However, we have limited cognitive resources and therefore lack the ability to process this overabundance of information. The brain's solution to this problem is to devote some of its cognitive resources to the task of prioritizing. As part of this prioritizing system, attention up-selects some of the available information for enhanced processing and down-selects some of it for reduced processing.[3] So, the selecting or enhancing effect of attention has two sides to it: an amplifying one and an inhibiting one. Both require limited attentional resources to be spent, and both help the brain optimize its limited cognitive resources.

There are many different processes that help determine which subsets of information are chosen for amplification or inhibition, but one such process involves the use of *salience maps*. The key idea here is that the brain has some prior expectations about what kinds of signals are likely to require extra processing—a sudden blast of sound, a subtle glance from a potential love interest, a new pain sensation, a gut instinct, etc. Salience maps can change over time and respond to context (particularly those involving meditation and psychedelics), but they

---

[2] I've expressed this point in terms of representationalism simply out of convenience. The general point about attention is compatible with other views, and we could instead, for instance, make reference to *presentations* or *mental states*.

[3] For an account of attention that makes the prioritizing function central, see Watzl 2017.

are typically rigid enough to function as an initial "best guess" as to which representations or sensations should be prioritized.

The relationship between attention and awareness is closely related to this idea of attention functioning as a prioritizing filter. It's an open question as to why we have awareness, but it seems to have something to do with the need for a kind of ultra processing of some information—perhaps especially information that relates to planning, behaviour, and decision-making (Baars 1993). As many scholars have observed, this kind of ultra processing is costly (Gilbert 1999, Kahneman and Frederick 2002), and so it makes sense that the brain would have a system in place that ensures it is used wisely. Attention appears to play an integral role in this system. Indeed, some have argued that attention is both necessary and sufficient for awareness (Brigard and Prinz 2010). This view may seem plausible at first glance. After all, how can you attend to something you are not aware of? And how can you be aware of something to which you are not attending? However, there is evidence that attention and awareness are, in fact, distinct but interrelated phenomena (see Lopez 2022 for a recent review and discussion). We needn't get into these details here. All we need for our purposes is that there is some kind of a strong, positive connection between attention and awareness. Specifically, in what follows, I will assume that in general, if some attention is allocated to a mental representation then, all else being equal, that representation is more likely to appear in awareness or feature in awareness more vividly.

It is worth noting that the term 'attention' can waver somewhat ambiguously between attentional resources and the *control* over how those resources are allocated. For example, when we say that someone has good attention, we normally don't mean that they have good (or a lot of) attentional resources. Rather, we mean that they have good *control* over their attention. Similarly, an attention deficit disorder doesn't necessarily involve a deficit in a person's attentional resources but rather a deficit in their *control* of those resources (Hallowell and Ratey 2021). However, we also talk about someone *paying* attention, or *focusing* their attention, or having divided or diffused attention. In such cases, 'attention' is more naturally interpreted as referring in some way to the person's attentional resources.

A distinction is also made between *endogenous* and *exogenous* attention.[4] Endogenous attention is a form of attention that is goal-driven and moved around or maintained voluntarily, while exogenous attention is stimulus-driven and moved around involuntarily, such as when you hear an unexpected loud noise. It is not altogether clear whether these are two different kinds of attention or if they are merely two different ways of *orienting* one's attention. Relatedly, while there appears to be some degree of generality to our attentional resources, there is also some complexity in how they are allocated across different kinds of tasks

---

[4] The endogenous/exogenous attention distinction often goes by other names, such as top-down/bottom-up, voluntary/involuntary, or executive/stimulus-driven; however, there may be subtle differences in how these terms are used.

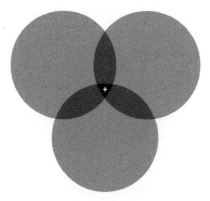

Figure 5.1 An example of how attention can affect appearance (due to Tse 2005). Keep your eyes fixed on the white cross and shift your attention to one of the discs. You'll notice that the disc becomes darker. After a few moments, you may notice your attention involuntarily wander around to the other discs, also making them darker.

and modalities, and it may be that we have multiple pools of semi-segregated attentional resources.[5]

One final fact about attention that will be relevant for the coming sections is that our attention affects how things appear to us. In a seminal paper, Carrasco et al. 2004 demonstrated that attention affects appearance—specifically, that attention can increase the apparent contrast of our perceptions. Indeed, using an example developed by Tse 2005, we can see this at work for ourselves. Look at the cross in the image in Figure 5.1 and, while keeping your eyes still and fixed on the cross, direct your attention to any one of the grey discs. If you're like most people (this example doesn't work for everyone), you'll notice that your selected disc becomes darker in appearance. This example illustrates how focusing your attention on an object can increase the apparent contrast of your perception of that object. In a subsequent paper, Fuller and Carrasco 2006 showed that focusing attention can increase the apparent *saturation* of our perceptual experience, and they also found that focusing attention did not affect apparent *hue*. Thus, it appears that attention alters some features of the visual field but not others. Carrasco and Barbot 2019 suggest that this difference may be explained in terms of the structure of these properties: hue is a metathetic dimension, and contrast and saturation are prothetic dimensions. Combined with the assumption that attention amplifies or enhances elements of the mind, this then explains the difference in effects: contrast and saturation are properties that can be enhanced, whereas hue is not such a property.[6]

---

[5] See Young and Stanton 2002, Peelen et al. 2004, Wahn and König 2017, and Keefe and Störmer 2021.

[6] Fuller and Carrasco 2006 also observed that while attention didn't change the apparent hue, it did increase subjects' abilities at hue *discrimination*. This again fits well with the hypothesis that attention is an enhancer of cognitive processing.

Of course, much more could be said about what we know (and don't yet know) about attention. However, we now have enough to consider what effects meditation and psychedelics may have on a person's attention.

5.3 Meditation

Let's start with meditation and how it can reveal the mind by improving our control over our attentional resources. There are two forms of meditation that will be especially important here. They are known by different names, but I'll follow the standard terminology that has emerged in the scientific literature on meditation: *focused-attention meditation* and *open-monitoring meditation*. Very briefly, focused-attention meditation consists of gently focusing your attention on something for a sustained period of time, while open-monitoring meditation consists of simply observing your thoughts and sensations.

Typically, when you first learn how to meditate, it makes sense to begin with focused-attention meditation. You can use anything as the focal point of your attention, but a convenient choice is to focus your attention on your breath. If you've never done it before, try it out. I guarantee that you'll notice at least one thing very quickly: although it may seem like a simple thing to do, this exercise is actually quite difficult. As William James noted, 'there is no such thing as voluntary attention sustained for more than a few seconds at a time' (James 1890, p. 397). Our attention loves to wander, despite our best efforts to prevent it from doing so.

In fact, you may have experienced this effect when you tried to focus your attention on one of the grey discs in Figure 5.1. When you first focus your attention on one of the discs, that disc becomes darker in its appearance. However, something else soon happens: one of the *other* discs becomes darker. Although you are trying to focus your attention on your chosen disc, your attention soon wanders away to one of the other discs, and that other disc then appears darker. The nice thing about this example is that we can, in a sense, *see* our attention wander around. However, our attention also wanders in other, less obvious ways—especially when it comes to our thoughts, feelings, and emotions—and meditation can help us become aware of this.

Indeed, when you first become aware of your attention escaping your control, there's a sense in which you get your first *success* at meditation.[7] In noticing your loss of focus, you get a glimpse of how your mind moves on its own. Your *second* success can come immediately after the first, when you refocus your attention. In doing that, you have done the equivalent of exercising a mental muscle. As you

---

[7] Indeed, this first success is a mini psychedelic experience that reverses a mini psychecryptic one that snuck up on you as you forgot to pay attention to your breath.

keep doing this, you get better at noticing when you lose focus, and better at refocusing. It's just like physical training. Over time, you increase in skill and strength: the skill of catching your attention starting to wander and the strength necessary to pull it back and hold it in place.[8]

Once you have developed your ability to stabilize your attention via focused-attention meditation, it can then make sense to introduce yourself to open-monitoring meditation. With this second form of meditation, you don't have to worry about keeping your attention focused on some point. Instead, you simply observe your thoughts and sensations as they naturally come and go. As before, this is much harder than it sounds. When you practise open-monitoring meditation, you quickly notice that it is quite difficult to *only* observe your thoughts and sensations: they have a tendency to suck you into them—very similar to how you can become engrossed in a good book or movie. The goal of open-monitoring meditation is to notice your thoughts come and go and to not react to them. It gets interesting pretty quickly, and sometimes it can feel like your mind is deliberately working against you. It is not uncommon to be suddenly flooded with memories of urgent tasks or be bombarded with creative ideas with the feeling that you absolutely must write them down before they're forgotten. And so on. It is almost as though your mind doesn't want to be seen—like a threatened squid squirting its ink into the water. All of this is okay. The practice of open-monitoring meditation involves observing this mental activity and letting it pass, or evolve, on its own accord without getting caught up in it.

What do these meditative practices have to do with psychedelic experiences? Very briefly, these practices bring a kind of stability and clarity to the mind that allows you to better observe it. Steve Jobs described this process quite nicely:

> If you just sit and observe, you will see how restless your mind is. If you try to calm it, it only makes it worse, but over time it does calm, and when it does, there's room to hear more subtle things—that's when your intuition starts to blossom and you start to see things more clearly and be in the present more. Your mind just slows down, and you see a tremendous expanse in the moment. You see so much more than you could see before.
>
> Steve Jobs, quoted in Isaacson 2011, p. 134

One neat feature of this description is that it also allows us to see how meditation might relate to the four dimensions of psychedelic space described in Chapter 3. When 'your intuition starts to blossom' and you 'hear more subtle things', the

---

[8] The "strength" metaphor is not entirely appropriate here since it implies that the focusing of attention must involve some sort of strenuous effort, whereas the practice of focused-attention meditation concerns *gently* focusing your attention.

novelty of your experience increases. When you 'start to see things more clearly', the *clarity* of your experience increases. When 'your mind just slows down', *duration* increases. When 'you see a tremendous expanse', the *scope* increases. Finally, and in totality, when 'you see so much more than you could see before', you have had an experience that is more mind-revealing than before. In other words, you have had an experience that is *more psychedelic.*[9]

It is not uncommon to find similar descriptions of meditation given by Buddhists. For example, Tsongkhapa, a Tibetan Buddhist monk living in the late fourteenth and early fifteenth century, used an analogy that is very similar to the one I gave of a painting being revealed (in Chapter 3). Tsongkhapa was concerned with the fact that meditation practice needs both the ability to observe the mind (*sati*, which we will discuss in the next chapter) and the development of *stability* in that observation (*samādhi*):

> To draw an analogy, in order to examine a hanging tapestry at night, if you light an oil-lamp that is both radiant and unflickering, you can vividly observe the depicted images. But if the lamp is either dim, or—even if it is bright—flickers due to wind, you would not clearly see the forms.
> Tsongkhapa, *Small Exposition of the Stages of the Path to Enlightenment*[10]

In this analogy, the brightness of the light corresponds to the dimensions of clarity and scope, and the flickering of the light corresponds to the dimension of duration (inversely). Thus, the best way to see the tapestry is to have a bright light shine consistently from the lamp. The point of the analogy, of course, is that the same is true for observing the hidden mind. You need to have both the ability to see things in the mind clearly and the ability to maintain sustained awareness of them.

We don't need to appeal to the authority of Steve Jobs and Tsongkhapa to see how meditation may reveal the mind via its effects on attention. We can also see how this follows from first principles by using the definitions of focused-attention and open-monitoring meditation and what we know about attention.

We can begin with a fact that we can all observe for ourselves: in general, it is very hard to stay focused. Indeed, as I mentioned earlier, William James observed that it is impossible to maintain sustained attention on anything for more than a few seconds—and we also saw this effect in action with the changing luminosity of the grey discs. A few pages later, James continues:

> [...] the faculty of voluntarily bringing back a wandering attention, over and over again, is the very root of judgment, character, and will. No one is *compos sui*

---

[9] As we will see in the next chapter, when this change in experience settles down and becomes more enduring, your *mindfulness* increases.

[10] Wallace 1998.

if he have it not. An education which should improve this faculty would be *the* education *par excellence*. But it is easier to define this ideal than to give practical directions for bringing it about. The only general pedagogic maxim bearing on attention is that the more interest the child has in advance in the subject, the better he will attend.

James 1890, p. 401

Although James is correct that having control over one's attention is an incredibly valuable skill, he was mistaken about the difficulty of giving practical instructions for developing it. The instructions for focused-attention and open-monitoring meditation are fairly easy to give, and these practices do, in fact, develop the ability to control one's attention (we'll see evidence of this in a moment). So, let's see why we should think that these two forms of meditation may have beneficial consequences for attention.

First, let's consider focused-attention meditation. The most basic thing we know about this form of meditation is that it focuses and stabilizes attention. And from the previous section, we know that there is an important connection between attention and awareness. Simply put, by focusing attention on mental representations, those representations are more likely to appear in awareness, or, if they are already in awareness, then they will appear more vividly. It makes sense, then, that the ability to focus and hold one's attention could be used to reveal parts or aspects of the mind, or to see them more clearly. In terms of the camera-lens model of attention, focused-attention meditation helps you do two things: (i) hold the camera in one place for a sustained period of time, and (ii) focus the lens with high precision.[11]

Second, let's consider open-monitoring meditation. The basic instruction of open-monitoring meditation is to sit still and just observe whatever appears in your awareness. As with pretty much anything else in life, when you take the time to look, you start to see things you didn't see before. It's not surprising, then, that open-monitoring meditation reveals parts or aspects of the mind. However, there is more to open-monitoring meditation than this. Open-monitoring doesn't just consist of *observing*: it consists of *just* observing. That is, the point is to observe and *not react* to whatever appears in your mind. A reaction directs attentional resources to whatever it is you are reacting to. Since attention is a limited resource, this moves attention away from the task of observing and into the reaction. This means that when you are reacting, you are not looking as well as you could be. This entails that by *just* looking, you are able to see even more than if you were looking and reacting. In other words, by directing attentional resources to the task

---

[11] The camera-lens model is just a useful metaphor, and we could equally use one of the other models mentioned in Section 5.2. We can also state the point directly in terms of properties of the distribution and dynamics of attentional resources.

of observation and diffusing that attention throughout the mind, you can bring more of the mind into awareness than you would otherwise.

The attentional skills developed through focused-attention and open-monitoring meditation can also be combined in various ways and used to support other meditative and contemplative practices. For example, suppose you become quite skilled at both forms of meditation. In doing so, you unlock a kind of superpower: instead of *just* looking, or looking *and reacting*, you can now look *proactively*. For example, you might start by just looking, and then feel something pop up that interests you—say, a vague idea for a solution to a problem at work. If you wish, you can use your focused-attention skills to concentrate your attention on that idea. In doing so, you can uncover the details of that idea, or see the idea more clearly, or give yourself more time to comprehend the idea, or become aware of something else that may lie behind the idea. Of course, you can do this without becoming skilled in these forms of meditation. However, the point is that it is much easier to do this, and it can be done more efficiently, if you are so skilled.

In short, by practising these two forms of meditation, you are repeatedly practising how to focus, diffuse, stabilize, and shift your attention at will. And the underlying thought is that the more you practise controlling your attention with meditation, the better you get at controlling your attention in general. Of course, there is more to the practice of meditation than this, but the basic idea of developing one's faculty of attention captures a core aspect of these meditative practices (particularly during the early stages of one's practice).

We should now turn from thinking about attention and meditation in terms of first principles and start examining the scientific evidence to see if any of this is actually true. If these ideas about attention and meditation are correct, then we should be able to observe improvements in attention as a result of meditation. This appears to be the case: we now have a substantial number of studies that show that meditation results in a variety of improvements to attentional control. Cásedas et al. 2020 and Sumantry and Stewart 2021 provide helpful systematic reviews and meta-analyses of these studies, and Jha 2021 provides a nice overview of this area of research. Since this literature is now quite large, I will focus primarily on studies that bear on our main interest: how meditation expands *awareness* via its effects on attention.

To begin, it is worth observing that there is growing evidence that meditation improves executive control over attention. For example, Leeuwen et al. 2012 examined the effects of focused-attention and open-monitoring meditation on the allocation and dynamics of spatial attention. They did this by examining how both kinds of meditation interact with the *global precedence effect*. This is the effect by which global properties of an object in the visual scene tend to dominate our attention over local properties. For example, consider the object displayed in Figure 5.2. When presented with that object and asked to quickly identify the small/local numbers (the '3's), people struggle more than when they are asked to identify the big/global number (the '2'). In other words, it is

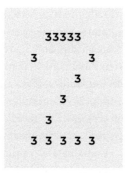

Figure 5.2 An example of the global precedence effect: it is easier to see the big '2' than it is to see the smaller '3's.

easier to see the big '2' than the small '3's. However, Leeuwen et al. found that meditators proficient in focused-attention meditation showed faster responses when identifying local numbers than when identifying global numbers. Moreover, after completing a 4-day open-monitoring meditation retreat, the same meditators showed no difference in response times. This is evidence that focused-attention meditation concentrates attention and that open-monitoring meditation diffuses or distributes it more evenly across the scene. Meditators proficient in both kinds of meditation also had a reduced global precedence effect and were faster at identifying both local and global numbers. This indicates that such meditators have more control over the allocation of their attentional resources.

The empirical result that meditation improves our control over attention shouldn't be surprising—it's analogous to finding out that weight training increases physical strength. However, the downstream effects of this improvement are more interesting. For example, meditation has been observed to reduce the *attentional blink effect*. One example that demonstrates this effect involves subjects being presented with a series of mostly black letters on a grey background in quick succession and having to perform two identification tasks. The first task is to report when a white letter appears. The second task is to report whether an 'X' appears after the white letter. People are good at identifying the white letter, but if an 'X' appears soon after the white letter, people tend to miss it. It's as though their attention 'blinks', resulting in a mini psychecryptic experience.

Several studies have shown that meditation reduces attentional blink, causing people to see the 'X' more frequently. For example, Slagter et al. 2007 found that 3 months of intensive vipassanā meditation training—a combination of focused-attention and open-monitoring meditation, but giving more weight to the latter[12]—reduced attentional blink (both within and between subjects). Leeuwen et al. 2009 also found that long-term practitioners of focused-attention and

---

[12] Strictly speaking, there is no one practice that is "vipassanā meditation", and instructions vary across traditions and instructors. What they have in common, though, is that they tend to place more

open-monitoring meditation exhibited reduced attentional blink when compared to both age-matched non-meditators and younger non-meditators (attentional blink is known to increase with age). Fabio and Towey 2018 also found that long-term meditators had reduced attentional blink in comparison to a matched control group. Coming back to intervention studies, Roca and Vazquez 2020 found that after 8 weeks of meditative training (30–45 minutes of daily practice), *emotional attentional blink* (two faces are presented in rapid succession and the emotion of the second face is not recognized) was significantly reduced. Similarly, Wang et al. 2022 found that 8 weeks of meditative training reduced attentional blink (and reductions correlated with increased mindfulness and reduced reactivity).[13] In general, the explanation for the attentional blink effect is that too much of one's attentional resource gets devoted to the first task and one can't shift it fast enough to the second task (Slagter et al. 2007, Leeuwen et al. 2009). Correspondingly, the explanation for why meditation reduces attentional blink is that it improves the efficiency of allocating and reallocating attentional resources.

What's particularly interesting about these results, at least for the present context, is not so much the effect on *attention*, but rather the effect on *awareness* (that comes as a result of the effect on attention). These results suggest that meditation makes it easier to see something that is hidden in the unconscious— namely, the mental representations of the 'X's that don't normally make their way into awareness. This may seem like a strange description of the results, but note that attentional blink doesn't occur because you blink your eyes: the 'X' still hits your retina and sends a signal to your visual cortex, etc. Indeed, it has been observed that the second stimulus can have a priming effect on the identification of a third stimulus (Visser et al. 2005, Zivony et al. 2018). Put another way, there is a representation of the 'X' in your mind, but it remains unconscious— it doesn't appear in your awareness. Because meditation improves the efficiency in the allocation of your attentional resources, more attention is able to be allocated to the unconscious representation and thus increase the chance of it appearing in your awareness. When this happens, you have a mini psychedelic experience: the representation that would normally be hidden in the unconscious is revealed.

A closely related effect that meditation has on awareness via attention involves the phenomenon of *inattentional blindness*. As mentioned in Chapter 3, inattentional blindness occurs when a cognitive task is demanding of attentional resources (such as counting the number of passes of a basketball between players). In such a condition, there is a tendency for people to fail to notice unexpected stimuli (such as a person dressed in a gorilla suit dancing in the background).

emphasis on cultivating mindfulness (*sati*) and less on cultivating concentration (*samādhi*), while recognizing that these two faculties go hand-in-hand (see next chapter).

[13] See also Vugt and Slagter 2014 and Colzato et al. 2015 who report potential differences in attentional blink between short sessions of focused-attention and open-monitoring meditation.

Given that this lack of awareness is due to attentional resources being consumed and prioritized by the cognitive task, we should expect meditation to reduce the inattentional blindness effect.[14] Indeed, Hodgins and Adair 2010 found that regular meditators (approximately 10 hours per week, on average) had reduced inattentional blindness, when compared with infrequent meditators (approximately 0.4 hours per week, on average), but the difference did not reach statistical significance. Hodgins and Adair suggest that this may have been due to the fact that the cognitive task they used was unusually demanding.[15] In a later study, Schofield et al. 2015 found that 7 minutes of a variant of open-monitoring meditation (openly attending to one's sensory experience while eating raisins) reduced inattentional blindness compared to a control group (who listened to 7 minutes of interesting facts about raisins). Pandit et al. 2022 also found that an 8-week mindfulness-based intervention (MBI) programme reduced inattentional blindness in 13 neurosurgeons (compared to controls). Altogether, this evidence indicates that by changing how attentional resources are allocated, meditation reduces inattentional blindness (thus expanding awareness). However, these are the only such studies so far (to my knowledge), and the effect observed by Hodgins and Adair 2010 was not statistically significant. Therefore, more work needs to be done before we can know with confidence that the effect is real.

Another example of meditation affecting awareness comes from Carter et al. 2005, who investigated the *binocular rivalry* effect for Tibetan Buddhist monks. As we saw in Chapter 3, binocular rivalry occurs when one image is presented to one eye and a substantially different image is presented to the other eye (Wheatstone 1838). Instead of seeing a mixture of the two images, as might be expected, one sees a regular oscillation between the two images, with one image being dominant for about 2–4 seconds and then the other image coming to dominate for a similar period of time. However, some people occasionally experience a *mixed percept* of the two images. Mixed percepts are often not precisely defined, but two common forms of them are (i) an overlay of the two images and (ii) a patchwork-like integration of the two images. Carter et al. found that during and after sessions of focused-attention meditation, the monks experienced extended durations of percept dominance (during which one image remains dominant in visual experience). Interestingly, Carter et al. also found that some of the monks experienced longer durations of the mixed percepts than normal. In a more recent study, Katyal and Goldin 2021 found that long-term meditators were able to

---

[14] As also mentioned in Chapter 3, it has been found for some experimental setups that although subjects are not aware of the unexpected stimulus, it nevertheless undergoes substantial unconscious processing (Moore and Egeth 1997, Mack and Rock 1998, Wood and Simons 2019, Kreitz et al. 2020, Nobre et al. 2020).

[15] It is worth noting that the performance on the task was higher for meditators and that Hodgins and Adair also found that the frequent meditators experienced less *change blindness*, indicating another respect in which meditation can expand awareness.

extend the durations of mixed percepts following 20 minutes of a form of focused-attention meditation. Katyal and Goldin also reported that some of the meditators experienced prolonged periods during which the two images separated (so that they were no longer mixed, and also neither image was dominant).

How is this relevant to psychedelic experience? Although it is never described this way in the literature, it follows from our explication of psychedelic experience that binocular rivalry is, in fact, a repeating sequence of simultaneous psychedelic and psychecryptic experiences. When one image dominates the visual field, the other image is *hidden* from awareness and then, after a few seconds, it is *revealed* in experience, while the first image is *concealed*. In the case of mixed percepts, things are a bit more complicated. When the mixed percept is a patchwork, then *parts* of each percept are revealed, with neither percept being fully revealed. When the mixed percept is an overlay, then both percepts are revealed, although they partly obscure each other. In the rare case of separation of the two images, both percepts are fully revealed (assuming this isn't due to a failure in setting up a stimuli rivalry).

When we frame binocular rivalry in this way, we see that the effects reported by Carter et al. 2005 and Katyal and Goldin 2021 are cases of meditation modulating spontaneous psychedelic experiences. When the duration of a dominant or mixed percept is extended, this counts as the duration of a psychedelic experience being extended. In this respect, the psychedelic experience becomes slightly more psychedelic since *duration* is one of the dimensions of psychedelic space. In the case of the overlay mixed percepts, the increased duration may also count as an increase in *scope*, assuming that the alternative experience would typically be one of a dominant percept (with a cost to clarity). The increase in scope corresponds to both percepts being revealed instead of only one being revealed. Finally, the prolonged experiences of image separation may count as the most psychedelic since they involve increases in duration, scope, and clarity (since neither percept is partly obscured by the other as is the case in overlay mixed percepts). In all cases, the novelty of the experience is, arguably, constant, since the two primary percepts are equally concealed—on average, for typical subjects, and given the experimental designs.[16] As before, more work needs to be done to confirm these results, but so far it appears that meditation can induce experiences that are more revealing of the two percepts.

Srinivasan and Singh 2017 found a somewhat similar effect when they studied the colour afterimage experiences of meditators with extensive practice in *sahaj samadhi* meditation, a form of focused-attention meditation. Srinivasan and Sing observed that meditators experienced the afterimages for longer periods of time and with greater visual clarity when compared to a control group

---

[16] Priming one of the percepts would be a way of making the other more concealed.

of non-meditators. This fits well with the thought that meditation induces psychedelic experiences that are higher in clarity and duration in comparison to spontaneous psychedelic experiences. They also found that decreasing the scope of attention had a positive effect on the duration and clarity of the afterimage experiences. This also fits well with the hypothesis that attention is a limited resource and that meditation improves control over its allocation. In a later paper, Srinivasan et al. 2020 found that meditators had more control over their perceptual experience when viewing a bistable image (a Necker cube) when compared to controls, demonstrating another way that control over attentional resources can impact visual awareness.

In another visual imagery study, Kozhevnikov et al. 2009 sought to examine the effects that different meditative techniques have on the ability to generate and sustain mental imagery. They found that 20 minutes of *deity meditation*—which is a form of focused-attention meditation that directs attention to an internally generated image of a deity—increased performance in image-maintenance and spatial tasks for experienced meditators. Kozhevnikov et al. interpret this result in terms of deity meditation developing one's capacity to access visuospatial memory resources. They propose that this happens because the brain has latent resources that can be consciously activated by focusing attention on them, and this appears to be what is happening during deity meditation. If correct, this would involve a different form of mind-revelation, whereby latent cognitive resources and visual processes are revealed (instead of particular visual representations being revealed).

Together, these studies indicate that meditation can reveal hidden visual representations and processes of the mind by increasing the efficiency with which attentional resources are allocated and reallocated. However, the effects that meditation has on awareness via its effects on attention are not limited to visual experience. Several other studies have shown that meditation also increases awareness of other elements of the unconscious mind. Below are three examples.

First, Fox et al. 2012 found that subjects experienced in *vipassanā* meditation had greater introspective accuracy than novice meditators. Fox et al. measured a form of introspection in terms of the subjective assessments of the clarity and intensity of tactile experiences that could be objectively validated. They also found that introspective accuracy correlated with the total number of hours of meditation experience. As Fox et al. pointed out, their result is important because introspection is generally regarded as unreliable (Nisbett and Wilson 1977). In line with this, they found that general introspective accuracy was indeed low. In other words, we generally have poor introspective accuracy, but this can be improved over time with sustained meditative practice. Fox et al. understand this improvement in terms of meditation's effects on attention, since *vipassanā* meditation involves paying close attention to one's inner experience, including one's bodily sensations. In a randomized controlled trial study, Mirams et al. 2013 found a similar effect:

6 days of body-scanning meditation (a form of focused-attention meditation with an element of open-monitoring) significantly reduced tactile misperceptions and increased sensitivity during a somatic signal detection task.[17]

Second, Strick et al. 2012 sought to test the hypothesis that a form of focused-attention meditation, which they call "Zen meditation" (*susokukan*; focusing attention on the breath and counting each exhale), provides greater access to the unconscious mind. They did this in two experiments. First, they examined participants' performance on a remote associates test (a standard method for measuring creativity). In such a test, a participant is presented with three words and must come up with a fourth related word. Strick et al. found that subjects who meditated for 20 minutes before the test performed better than those who did not. This was a sign that meditation facilitated access to the unconscious mind, where ideas for the fourth word are presumed to be generated. However, it was possible that meditation was having an effect on the unconscious mind itself—for example, by making it more associative rather than by making it more accessible. To control for this, Strick et al. conducted a second experiment in which they subliminally primed participants with a word, such as 'spring', and then measured how likely they were to use the primed word in response to a subsequent task, such as 'Name one of the four seasons'. They found that subjects who had meditated for 20 minutes were more likely to use the subliminal prime as their response. Strick et al. also understand this observed effect in terms of attention: participants' focusing their attention increased the degree to which they processed the subliminal percept, making it more available to their awareness (ibid. pp. 1479–80).

Third, and finally, several studies have shown that 10–20 minutes of focused-attention meditation causes increases in estimations of time periods *after* the meditation session (Kramer et al. 2013, Droit-Volet et al. 2015, Singh and Srinivasan 2019). And Droit-Volet et al. 2018 found *decreases* in estimations of time periods *during* sessions of two kinds of focused-attention meditation (replicating an earlier result by Droit-Volet and Heros 2016). The authors of these studies all explain their results in terms of meditation's effect on attention and the attentional-gate model of time perception (Zakay and Block 1995). This model consists of a pacemaker, an accumulator, and an attentional gate linking the two. The pacemaker produces a series of pulses, which can be captured by the accumulator when the attentional gate is open. When more attention is directed to time, the gate is opened wider, and so more pulses are captured by the accumulator, resulting in increased estimations of duration. The explanation, then, is that after a session of meditation, it is easier to allocate more attentional resources to time perception and thus reveal

---

[17] There are other studies using different methods of measuring bodily awareness with mixed results. Treves et al. 2019 performed a meta-analysis of such studies and found an overall positive effect that was small but still significant.

more of the pacemaker pulses to the accumulator. In contrast, *during* a session of meditation, there are fewer attentional resources available for time perception, and so the attentional gate closes, thus concealing more of the pacemaker pulses from the accumulator. These two effects are hypothesized to result in the meditation-induced overestimations and underestimations of time periods.

One important question concerning the effects of expanded time perception is whether they amount to psychedelic experiences. On the one hand, it seems that they do not since the accumulator of the attentional gate model presumably operates outside of awareness, and so the "revelation" of additional pulses after meditation is an unconscious one. If we assume, as we did in Chapter 3, that psychedelic experiences involve revelations of unconscious material to conscious-ness, then the opening up of the attentional gate won't amount to an experience that is psychedelic. On the other hand, it could be argued that the additional pulses do make their way into conscious processing, and it is just that they are not experienced as discrete pulses—the concomitant change in one's experience would be one of there being "more time" in a continuous sense. It could also be argued that an experience of time expansion may also count as psychedelic because the expansion involves the revelation of other mental contents—for example, one may become aware of more of one's sensations. Overall, it is difficult to answer the question definitively, but there does seem to be a case for treating experiences of expanded time perception as psychedelic.

We've now seen several studies that indicate that meditation reveals hidden parts or aspects of the mind via its effects on attention. In addition to these studies, there is a more general theory that is based on neuroimaging results and known as *the brain theory of meditation* (Raffone et al. 2019). Very briefly, this theory has two core premises. The first is that the human brain has a strong energetic limitation: approximately only 1% of neurons in the cortex can be firing at an elevated level at any given time (Lennie 2003, Tomasi et al. 2013). The second premise is that meditation develops the ability to use that 1% more efficiently. In short, the brain theory of meditation says that we have a limited amount of cognitive processing power, and meditation helps us to use it more efficiently. This fits well with the hypothesis that meditation improves our ability to control the allocation and dynamics of our attentional resources. Our attentional resources draw from the limited pool of energy and help with the efficient allocation of that energy to other cognitive tasks.

The scientific research on meditation is still quite nascent, so we should be cau-tious about what conclusions we draw from it (Dam et al. 2018a, 2018b, Davidson and Dahl 2018). However, the evidence that we have so far seems to align well with the theory: focused-attention and open-monitoring meditation (and related meditation practices lying between the two) improve our ability to efficiently allocate our attentional resources and this, in turn, facilitates the revelation of parts or aspects of the mind that would otherwise remain concealed from awareness.

Overall, the evidence indicates that meditation expands the sphere of awareness via its effects on attentional resources.[18]

5.4 Psychedelics

As we saw in the previous two chapters, one prominent idea about the psychological effects of psychedelics is that they are *unspecific amplifiers of the mind*. According to Stanislav Grof, this accounts for why psychedelics are effective in assisting psychotherapy: they help amplify undercurrents of the unconscious psyche and bring them into conscious awareness.

In Chapter 2, we also saw that Osmond expressed a similar idea when he introduced the hypothesis that psychedelics reveal the mind. Recall that some of the other terms he considered were: *psychehormic*, mind-rousing; *psychezymic*, mind-fermenting; and *psycherhexic*, mind bursting forth. Therefore, although Osmond settled on 'psychedelic', to capture the idea that these substances have the *effect* of revealing the mind, it seems that he was also considering the *psychological processes* by which they might do this. Although not stated explicitly, his idea appeared to be that psychedelics reveal the mind by rousing, or energizing, it in some way.

Let us call this the *Osmond-Grof hypothesis*: psychedelics cause psychedelic experiences by amplifying the mind or energizing it, so that elements of the unconscious appear in conscious experience. This hypothesis is conceptually distinct from, but compatible with, Huxley's 1954 idea of a "reducing valve", which we find instantiated in contemporary neuroscientific models, such as the cortical-striatal-thalamic-cortical (CSTC) model (Vollenweider and Geyer 2001) and the REBUS model (Carhart-Harris and Friston 2019). The initial motivation for this hypothesis comes from anecdotal psychedelic trip reports and decades of observations of psychedelic-assisted psychotherapy sessions (Grof 2009). The hypothesis definitely has some intuitive appeal—and perhaps some readers will even think that it is obviously true. Nevertheless, it is another hypothesis that could easily be false, and so we need to evaluate it as such.

However, in order to do that, we first need to make the hypothesis more conceptually precise. As currently stated, the hypothesis relies too heavily on metaphors and vague terms: amplification, rousing, fermenting, energizing, etc. So, it would be useful if we could express the hypothesis in terms that are more recognizable to cognitive science. There are different ways to do this. For example, we could think about making sense of these terms within computational or predictive processing frameworks. Or we could try to reduce them to something observable at the neural level. These are reasonable strategies that we could pursue—and they are already

---

[18] See also Jha 2021 for an excellent discussion of meditation's effects on attention.

being pursued in the scientific literature. However, I think a more natural starting point, given our purposes, is to understand the hypothesis using concepts that are abstract enough to cut across most models and frameworks while at the same time precise enough so that we can begin evaluating the hypothesis with respect to the evidence we already have.

The concept of *attention* appears to be an ideal candidate in this regard. As we saw in Section 5.2, attention is often said to have an "amplifying" or "enhancing" effect on mental representations.[19] We also know that attention plays a fundamental role in determining what appears in our conscious experience and in shaping its character. Moreover, attention has a general domain of applicability. We can attend externally, to sights, sounds, tastes, etc. And we can attend internally, to thoughts, desires, emotions, memories, etc. This generality of attention may help explain the high phenomenological variability of psychedelic experiences. So, it seems plausible that psychedelics may produce their distinctive effects on awareness by having some impact on attention.[20] Moreover, since it is clear that meditation has its effects on awareness via its effects on attention, this idea gives us an appealing theoretical symmetry (see Figure 5.3). It also paves the way for

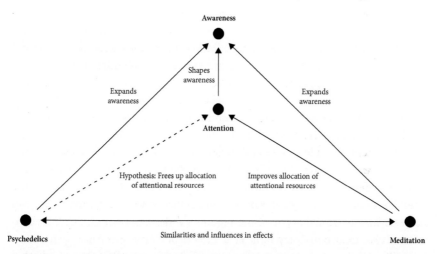

Figure 5.3 A unified theory of the psychedelic effects of psychedelics and meditation in terms of their impact on attentional resource allocation.

[19] Some philosophers even argue that attention is a particular kind of amplification (Fazekas and Nanay 2021).

[20] It is also worth noting that attention plays a central role in current neuroscientific accounts of the effects of psychedelics, such as the CSTC and REBUS models (Vollenweider and Geyer 2001, Carhart-Harris and Friston 2019). Attention figures as prediction error weighting in the predictive processing framework of the REBUS model (although, see Ransom and Fazelpour 2020 for criticism of this point), and the arousal and allocation of attentional resources has been associated with the thalamus (e.g. Schiff et al. 2013), which has been dubbed as the 'gateway to the mind' (Ward 2013) and is a key element of the CSTC model.

a unified understanding of the effects of meditation and psychedelics and how these interventions interact with one another (Heuschkel and Kuypers 2020, Payne et al. 2021). Indeed, since attention is a cognitive process over which we have some voluntary control, choosing it as a central concept of our precisification of the Osmond-Grof hypothesis may also result in some *practical* value—in that we might learn how to better navigate the experiences that psychedelics tend to induce. Nevertheless, since psychedelics and meditation clearly can have different effects on consciousness, their precise effects on attention are also likely different in some way. So, if we are to understand the Osmond-Grof hypothesis in terms of attention, we need to determine the effect that psychedelics have on attention such that this effect explains their effects on awareness, as well as the similarities and differences between those effects and those of meditation. The question, then, is: what effect do psychedelics have on attention?

One salient possibility is that psychedelics cause temporary increases in the attentional resources that are available for allocation. This idea would fit well with the intuition behind the Osmond-Grof hypothesis, since more available attentional resources would mean that more representations and processes in the mind can be amplified. It also fits well with the thought that psychedelics expand consciousness, given the close connection between attention and awareness. Having more available attentional resources would mean that more unconscious representations and processes can be brought into awareness. Moreover, for those representations and processes that are already conscious, an increase in available attentional resources would allow them to appear in an enhanced way to us—more vividly, intensely, etc. In short, this idea that psychedelics somehow increase one's available attentional resources seems to fit well with the common phenomenological descriptions that people give of their psychedelic trips.

If we accept this idea, then the next question we need to answer is *how* psychedelics might have this effect. One possibility is that psychedelics somehow *create* new attentional resources by lifting the metabolic constraints on the brain. For example, some studies have found evidence suggesting that psilocybin increases metabolic activity in some regions (Vollenweider et al. 2017, Vollenweider 1998, Gouzoulis-Mayfrank et al. 1999) but may also cause reductions, depending on the measurement technique (PET, ASL, and BOLD) and whether global signal regression is used (Carhart-Harris et al. 2012, Lewis et al. 2017). Another possibility is that psychedelics free up existing attentional resources by disrupting the patterns of their allocation. This would be a natural implication of the entropic brain hypothesis and of the REBUS model (Carhart-Harris et al. 2014, Carhart-Harris and Friston 2019). More specifically, several studies have indicated that psychedelics change the brain's functional connectivity—particularly in relation to the *salience network* (SN), the *default mode network* (DMN), and the *dorsal attention network* (DAN)—in a way that would suggest that the attentional resource allocation system is disrupted.[21] In particular, the DMN is associated with mind-wandering and task-free mental processes (Mason et al. 2007, Christoff et al. 2009, Scheibner et al. 2017), and spontaneous activity within the DMN is known to be anti-correlated with spontaneous activity in task-positive networks (TPNs), including the DAN, which are engaged when attention is focused on a task (Fox et al. 2005). This would suggest that one way by which psychedelics may free attentional resources involves a disruption of the usual functioning of the DMN and its functional connectivity with these other networks. So, the attentional resources consumed by DMN-related cognition, such as worrying and rumination, are released and allowed to flow more freely.

Interestingly, focused-attention meditation and open-monitoring meditation have been associated with reductions/disintegrations in DMN activity (Tomasino et al. 2013, Brewer et al. 2011, Garrison et al. 2015, and Scheibner et al. 2017). Also, focused-attention meditation has been observed to strengthen the usual DMN-TPN anti-correlation, while another kind of meditation—known as *non-dual awareness meditation*, which involves a collapsing of the subject/object distinction—has been found to weaken the anti-correlation (Josipovic et al. 2012). Moreover, the strength of the DMN-TPN anti-correlation has been found to increase during engagement with an attention-demanding task and to be associated with increased intraindividual variability (Kelly et al. 2008), which is an index of the efficiency by which attention is regulated (Stuss et al. 2003, Bellgrove et al. 2004). Altogether, these results suggest that different meditative practices have specific effects on the DMN and its functional connectivity with other regions of the brain, and that these effects are involved in the improvements in attention regulation that are due to meditation.

The fact that meditation has these closely related effects on the DMN points to the possibility of unifying the effects of psychedelics and meditation at three different levels of analysis: (i) both induce psychedelic experiences, (ii) both do so by changing the allocation of one's attentional resources, and (iii) both do this, at least in part, by changing the usual functioning of the DMN and its functional connectivity with other brain networks.[22] Furthermore, there is growing evidence that psychedelics can bring about long-lasting increases in *mindfulness*.[23] The concept

---

[21] For example, see Carhart-Harris et al. 2012, Lebedev et al. 2015, Palhano-Fontes et al. 2015, Carhart-Harris et al. 2016, Sampedro et al. 2017, Müller et al. 2018, Pasquini et al. 2020, Madsen et al. 2021, Doss et al. 2021, Daws et al. 2022, and especially Stoliker et al. 2023. Also, psychedelic-induced disruptions to cortico-striato-thalamo-cortical (CSTC) feedback loops (Vollenweider and Geyer 2001, Preller et al. 2019) may also be indicative of a release of attentional resources from their usual patterns of allocation.

[22] However, we needn't be committed to the view that this is the *only* way that these interventions release attentional resources. It could be that disrupting these networks is just one, perhaps particularly effective, way of freeing up attentional resources.

[23] For example, see Thomas et al. 2013, Soler et al. 2016, Sampedro et al. 2017, Soler et al. 2018, Domínguez-Clavé et al. 2019, Smigielski et al. 2019, Uthaug et al. 2019, Mian et al. 2020, Uthaug et al.

of mindfulness is an important one and requires its own detailed analysis (which we will address in the next chapter). For now, we can make do with the observation that meditation is thought to promote mindfulness via its effects on attention. This points to a fourth commonality between psychedelics and meditation—that is, that they can give rise to long-lasting increases in mindfulness.

This unification of psychedelics and meditation should not be taken to entail that they amount to the same intervention on the brain/mind. Psychedelics and meditation clearly have differences between them, with perhaps the most obvious being that the effects of meditation tend to be more gradual, enduring, and controllable, while the effects of psychedelics tend to be more dramatic, temporary, and uncontrollable. (However, for such statements, it is crucial to keep in mind the qualifications discussed in Chapter 4.) It should also be noted that the above unification does not entail these are the *only* effects of psychedelics and meditation, nor does it entail that these are the only ways by which they may reveal the mind. And we should remember that there are different practices of meditation and different kinds of psychedelics. For example, it is sometimes thought that MDMA facilitates mind-revealing experiences by functioning as a kind of "mental anaesthetic", making it easier for people to engage with psychological content that would otherwise be too painful for them to approach. This way of revealing the mind appears to be quite different from the typical process of, say, a psilocybin trip, but it also appears to be similar in some respects to the non-reactivity developed via open-monitoring meditation. (There are also some notable similarities between MDMA and loving-kindness and compassion meditative practices.) Therefore, while there may be an important unification between psychedelics and meditation—particularly with respect to their effects on attention—it is important to recognize that there are differences, and the full relationship is likely to be quite complex.

To summarize, we now have a plausible interpretation of the Osmond-Grof hypothesis: psychedelics cause psychedelic experiences by temporarily freeing up attentional resources so that they are available for novel allocations throughout the mind. Exactly how the released attentional resources are allocated will depend on many factors specific to the particular context and, in some ways, be highly unpredictable. However, it also seems reasonable to tentatively assume that, without some external intervention, the reallocation will tend to be somewhat random.[24] This is the 'unspecific' component of Grof's idea that psychedelics are unspecific amplifiers of the unconscious. We also see this idea in Osmond's

2020, Davis et al. 2020, Madsen et al. 2020, Murphy-Beiner and Soar 2020, Oorsouw et al. 2022, and Søndergaard et al. 2022; and see Radakovic et al. 2022 for a meta-analysis.

[24] Randomness and unpredictability are not necessarily identical. For example, for a given individual undergoing a psychedelic trip, their attentional resources may be non-randomly attracted towards a traumatic memory from their childhood, even though it may be virtually impossible for us to forecast this outcome before the trip with any reasonable accuracy. And attentional resources becoming more random in their allocation may have predictable consequences, such as them flowing into the visual field and causing all sorts of visual effects (which we will discuss in a moment).

consideration of the terms *psychelytic* (mind-releasing) and *psycherhexic* (mind bursting forth) as appropriate names for psychedelics. The hypothesis, then, is that psychedelics create a surplus of attentional resources that tend to flow somewhat freely and unpredictably onto various mental representations and processes. By having this effect on attentional resources, psychedelics amplify parts of the mind into awareness that would otherwise remain hidden in the unconscious. The typical randomness and unpredictability of this released flow of attentional resources, along with the domain generality of the attention system, would also go some way in accounting for the phenomenological variability of psychedelic experiences.

We now have a plausible and more precise interpretation of the Osmond-Grof hypothesis. Let's call it *the attentional-resource hypothesis*. Is there any evidence for (or against) it?

At first glance, it might seem that the available evidence speaks against the hypothesis. Although there are not yet many studies that directly investigate the attentional effects of psychedelics, the few that do exist all point in the same direction: psychedelics appear to *impair* attention.[25] This result may seem like bad news for the attentional-resource hypothesis.

However, this line of reasoning is mistaken. The effect of freeing up attentional resources differs from that of improving attention. The latter necessarily involves having better *control* over attentional resources, whereas the former does not.[26] The freeing up of attentional resources *can* lead to an improvement in attention, but it can also easily lead to a deterioration. It depends, in part, on: which constraints are removed (or diminished), which ones remain, which new ones are imposed (if any), and one's prior ability to control one's attention.[27] For example, for an individual who already lacks good control over their attention, a sudden freeing up of a large amount of attentional resource (from a high dose, say) would likely lead to a chaotic stream of experiences. In contrast, an individual who already has good control over their attention and only has a small amount of attentional resource freed up (from a small dose, say) would likely have a rather different stream of experiences—perhaps even one in which attentional performance is *enhanced*.[28] In addition to this point about control, there will also be differences in effects due to differences in how attention tends to be allocated before it is disrupted by psychedelics. In general, what happens to attentional performance

[25] For example, see Gouzoulis-Mayfrank et al. 2002, Hasler et al. 2004, Carter et al. 2005, Vollenweider et al. 2007, and Quednow et al. 2012.

[26] It is worth noting that ADHD has recently been characterized not in terms of not having enough attention, but rather as having too much attention and not enough control over it (Hallowell and Ratey 2021).

[27] Other aspects of the set and setting will also be relevant, but for the present discussion, we can make the simplifying assumption that they have been controlled for.

[28] The anecdotal evidence regarding the use of psychedelics to enhance performance in extreme sports and martial arts aligns with this hypothesis (Oroc 2011).

when attentional resources are freed from their usual constraints will depend heavily on the details of the situation, and so no easy prediction can be made.

Nevertheless, we may be able to tentatively make the general, coarse-grained prediction that if psychedelics do, in fact, free up attentional resources, then unless the allocation of those resources is somehow controlled, attentional performance will likely be diminished. Without some form of guidance, the newly unleashed attentional resources could end up anywhere in the mind—one's emotions, memories, financial concerns, plans for the future, etc., or one's representations of the external environment, with its sights, sounds, smells, etc. And as the salience of these things fluctuates, the attentional resources would flow throughout the mind accordingly. As Carter et al. 2005 note in a study on the effect of psilocybin on attention: 'impaired attentional performance may reflect a reduced ability to suppress or ignore distracting stimuli rather than reduced attentional capacity'. Therefore, studies investigating attentional performance will not necessarily speak for or against the hypothesis. To evaluate the hypothesis, we need a way of separating these two factors (the control of attention and the amount of available attentional resource). To my knowledge, we currently lack any solid evidence along these lines, but there are some considerations that appear to be favourable to the hypothesis.

One such consideration concerns the effects of low doses of psychedelics on visual experience and those that tend to occur during the early and later stages of psychedelic trips. In such situations, we might reasonably expect that attentional resources are freed up, but not so much as to cause (or correspond to) deteriorating effects. Moreover, since we know that the focusing of attention has particular local effects on visual appearance (Section 5.2), it would make sense to predict that psychedelics, in these contexts, might have similar effects on visual experience, but in a global fashion. For example, since we know that focusing attention on an object enhances its apparent saturation and contrast and leaves its hue unaffected (Carrasco et al. 2004, Tse 2005, and Fuller and Carrasco 2006), it seems reasonable to expect that psychedelics may tend to have this effect on the entire visual field (for low doses and early/late stages of trips). While psychedelics may not lead to a focusing of attention on anything in particular, they may allow for more attentional resources to flow through the entire visual field, thus making *everything* appear more saturated and higher in contrast.

There is some evidence that psychedelics have these effects on visual experience. From early on, researchers studying the effects of psychedelics noted the drugs' effects on vision. Although the hallucinations caused by psychedelics often received the most discussion, these researchers were careful to comment on other types of visual effects. For example, Knauer and Maloney 1913 reported that visual sensibility was substantially increased by mescaline, that visual acuity was incontrovertibly enhanced by the drug, and that visual hyperesthesia was objectively demonstrated for colour. They also reported that subjective sharpness of object contours—that is, contrast—was enhanced, but they could not demonstrate this objectively (they didn't explain why). After describing how mescaline made his visual perceptions more vivid and caused a tremendous increase in the clarity of his kinaesthetic sensations, Samuel Fernberger accounted for these changes in terms of attention and the revelation of normally unnoticed stimuli:

> My state, at this period, can best be described as a supernormally clear focus of attention (which, however, was very rapidly changing) with practically no background of consciousness. The increase in clearness was quite evident in sensory modalities other than the kinaesthetic. I was aware of throat-noises when a person a number of feet away from me swallowed; of color shadows in a magazine cover, and the like; in a word, of stimuli which are normally well above the sensory threshold but which usually pass unnoticed.
>
> Fernberger 1923, p. 269

Klüver 1928 systematized a large number of anecdotal reports from early investigations into the effects of mescaline (including those of Knauer and Maloney 1913) and concluded that while hue is not systematically altered by mescaline, other visual properties—such as saturation, brightness, and illumination—are all systematically and substantially increased (pp. 24–6). He noted that while there is some variation in these effects (pp. 33–4), the enhancement of contrast is a particularly robust effect (p. 35). These observations fit well with the result that focusing attention enhances saturation and contrast but leaves hue unaffected.

Aldous Huxley also famously commented on these visual effects of mescaline:

> First and most important is the experience of light. Everything seen by those who visit the mind's antipodes is brilliantly illuminated and seems to shine from within. All colors are intensified to a pitch far beyond anything seen in the normal state, and at the same time the mind's capacity for recognizing fine distinctions of tone and hue is notably heightened.
>
> Huxley 1956, p. 89[29]

To be sure, these effects are not limited to mescaline. From his extensive practice in LSD-supported psychotherapy during the 1960s, Stanislav Grof reports that 'LSD makes colors very bright, penetrating, and explosive, as well as enhancing and deepening light and color contrasts' (Grof 2009, p. 98). Hartman and Hollister 1963 also reported that both psilocybin and LSD enhance the subjective experience of colour: afterimages were described as containing more colours, and the drugs enhanced the experience of flicker-generated colours. Oster 1966

---

[29] Recall that while Fuller and Carrasco 2006 found that focusing attention did not change apparent hue, it did increase hue sensitivity, fitting well with Huxley's observation.

similarly reported LSD to enhance colour saturation and other aspects of visual perception. In general, people frequently report that psychedelics intensify their sensory experience and make them aware of qualities of sensory experience that they weren't aware of before (Silverman 1971).

This evidence from early investigations into the effects of psychedelics aligns with the hypothesis that psychedelics disrupt the usual allocation of attentional resources and result in additional resources flowing into the visual field, thus increasing the vividness of one's visual experience of the world. It is important to note, however, that there is little evidence in support of the claim that perceptual *accuracy* is increased. A number of studies indicate that low-level perception is either left unchanged or impaired by psychedelics (Carlson 1958, Edwards and Cohen 1961, Hartman and Hollister 1963). More recent studies are relatively more difficult to come by, but some work has been done. Carter et al. 2004 found that psilocybin impaired high-level but not low-level motion perception. Kometer et al. 2011 note that psychedelics are commonly reported to increase brightness, and found via high-density EEG that they enhance P1 amplitude, which is associated with stimulus brightness (Proverbio and Zani 2002). Clearly, more research needs to be done before we can draw any strong conclusions about the effects of psychedelics on (veridical) perception (for helpful reviews of the literature, see Kometer and Vollenweider 2018 and Aday et al. 2021).

One observation that doesn't line up so neatly with the hypothesis is that it is not uncommon for psychedelics to change the apparent hue of objects. However, such changes in hue appear to be local in nature, occurring for individual objects and not for the entire visual scene. As a result, these local changes in hue might be due to higher-level effects on visual perception and thus involve interpretive elements to them.[30] Once attentional resources make their way up to higher levels of perception and cognition, it is difficult to predict the particular effects on vision. Indeed, we know that increases in apparent brightness from local increases in attentional resources are dependent on scene interpretation (Tse 2005). So, we should expect that similar effects will occur under psychedelics and that they will become more substantial and involve higher-level interpretive effects, as dose levels become higher or as the setting engenders unusual interpretations of the sensory input.[31]

Another line of evidence we ought to consider in this context concerns the modulation of binocular rivalry by psychedelics. As we've seen already, binocular rivalry involves changes in awareness of visual stimuli that can be modulated by

---

[30] From the perspective of predictive processing, increasing attention to a signal (e.g. because it has high expected precision) can cause the errors to propagate higher in the hierarchy and result in substantial changes to one's visual perceptions.

[31] In this regard, it is worth noting the role attention plays in creating synaesthetic experiences (Rich and Mattingley 2013).

attention. So, this is a natural place to look for evidence that could confirm or disconfirm the attentional-resource hypothesis.

To date, there have been three studies exploring the effects of psychedelics on binocular rivalry. Frecska et al. 2003 found that ayahuasca slowed down rivalry rates and that subjects who had doses higher than the median dose experienced longer durations of mixed percepts. Carter et al. 2005 found that psilocybin also extended durations of both dominant and mixed percepts (but the latter effect was not statistically significant). In a follow-up study, Carter et al. 2007 found that psilocybin caused a significant increase in durations for both dominant and mixed percepts.[32]

What are we to make of these results? On the one hand, they appear to line up with the results concerning meditation and binocular rivalry. They also fit what we'd expect to see if psychedelics made experiences more psychedelic by pushing them deeper into psychedelic space. For example, as before, longer experiences of mixed percepts can be understood as increases in scope and duration.

On the other hand, it's not immediately clear how these results speak to the attentional-resource hypothesis. For example, if the hypothesis is understood as entailing that the two percepts receive more attention than they otherwise would, then it seems we should have expected the switching rates to increase and the durations of percepts to decrease. This is because other studies have shown that drawing attention away from the binocular rivalry task causes switching rates to slow down and durations of percepts to increase (Paffen et al. 2006, Alais et al. 2010). Moreover, Zhang et al. 2010 have observed, using EEG signals as proxies for the percepts, that when attention is strongly drawn away from the percepts, the anti-correlation that usually exists between the signals for the individual percepts disappears, suggesting a convergence on mixed percepts that lie outside, or only faintly within, the subject's awareness. Reviewing these studies and the rest of binocular rivalry and bistable perception literature, Dieter et al. 2016 propose that drawing attention away from the binocular rivalry task reduces the apparent contrast of the percepts, which reduces the urgency for the visual system to reconcile the conflicting inputs, which, in turn, slows down the rivalry rate (and extends the percept durations). In the extreme case, when attention is fully drawn away from the task, there is no need to resolve the conflict, and the system allows for the mixed percept to be dominant while also leaving it outside of awareness (in line with the observations of Zhang et al. 2010).

If correct, this looks like it spells trouble for the attentional-resource hypothesis. The body of evidence suggests that psychedelics draw attentional resources *away* from the percepts rather than to them. This is especially plausible given that

---

[32] The difference between these two results is likely due to a slight difference in method: in the first study, subjects were asked to report mixed percepts only if they considered them non-transitional, and in the second study, subjects were asked to report the mixed percepts no matter what.

psychedelics are known to cause all sorts of other disturbances to conscious experience, such as activating old memories, triggering emotional insights, etc. These disturbances can be quite distracting, and it would be natural to expect that they draw attention away from the rival percepts. To this point, Carter et al. 2007 found a significant positive correlation between the slowing down of binocular rivalry and a reduction in subjectively reported *vigilance*, a measure of sustained attention.

Although this alternative hypothesis is appealing in some respects, it also can't be the full story. This is because, on this view, as attention is drawn away from the percepts, they reduce in contrast and eventually fade from awareness. Although the Frecska et al. and Carter et al. studies do not report how vividly the percepts appeared to the subjects, it is implausible that they were fading from awareness. So, something more must be going on.

One explanation might be that the freeing up of attentional resources is global or holistic in nature. That is, it is not just that some attention is allowed to move away from cognition normally associated with the DMN and SN and then flow into the visual field. Rather, it may be that attention is allowed to flow more freely *in general*. If correct, this would mean that local constraints on attention are also relaxed, including those associated with the binocular rivalry task. In particular, if there is a constraint that limits how much attention can be given to each percept simultaneously, then, when that constraint is relaxed, each percept would be able to receive more attention and thus be amplified into awareness with the observed patterns. Such an explanation would fit neatly with the entropic brain hypothesis and the REBUS model, as well as the altered beliefs under psychedelics (ALBUS) model, which permits the strengthening of beliefs in addition to their weakening (Safron 2020).

There is also some indirect evidence worth considering. Some people appear to be more disposed than others to see mixed percepts. In particular, Antinori et al. 2017 found that people who score higher on the core personality trait of *openness* tend to see mixed percepts more frequently than other people. Psychedelics have been observed to cause long-lasting increases in openness.[33] Openness has also been associated with the ability to flexibly allocate attentional resources (Swift et al. 2020).[34] Together, these three results fit well with the hypothesis that psychedelics allow for a more flexible allocation of attentional resources, which involves a relaxation of the usual constraints on those resources during binocular rivalry, thus allowing for mixed percepts to appear in awareness.

---

[33] For example, see MacLean et al. 2011, Lebedev et al. 2016, Nour et al. 2017, Bouso et al. 2018, Erritzoe et al. 2018, Erritzoe et al. 2019, and Madsen et al. 2020.

[34] Openness has also been associated with reduced inattentional blindness (Kreitz et al. 2015) and reduced attentional blink (MacLean and Arnell 2010, but also see Kranczioch and Thorne 2013).

Let's now come back to the more general point that psychedelics increase the amount of attentional resource that is available for allocation. So far, we have been focused on how this effect will manifest in low-level visual experience. What other kinds of effects should we expect from the hypothesized effect on attentional resource?

If psychedelics do increase available attentional resources, then the observed effects will likely not be limited to the lower levels of perception. As doses become stronger, we should expect to see higher-level effects of attention on perception. Because of the complex interpretative effects mentioned earlier, it is difficult to predict what these will be, but some broad brushstroke predictions may be possible. For example, while some ability to control attentional resources is still retained, it should be possible to focus those resources on bringing desired images into one's visual experience—much like what is done during deity meditation, as we saw in the previous section. Knauer and Maloney 1913 reported that such effects occur. In fact, they note that these effects seem to only occur after period of sustained concentration on the intended image and are not perfect. For example:

> In addition to its delay this self-suggested representation was not a precise reproduction, but merely a distorted effigy of the vision which was desired. Thus, while watching a panorama of a danseuse on a stage, one of us attempted to picture a shoe. He repeated to himself all of the separate parts of a shoe, and endeavored by concentration to bring up an hallucinatory image of a shoe. The danseuse continued to dance undisturbed for some time, and then suddenly and unexpectedly there appeared a gigantic misshapen shoe, seemingly molded in plaster, and colored green.
>
> Knauer and Maloney 1913, pp. 431–2

The effect of the psychedelic here appears to be an enhancement of voluntary mental imagery. Some effort of focusing attention is required, but it appears that mental imagery is produced that would not have otherwise been possible. This would suggest that the psychedelic is allowing more attentional resource to be devoted to production of the intended image.[35] In this regard, it is worth noting that ayahuasca has been observed to treat non-congenital aphantasia (Santos et al. 2018) and that psychedelics in general are commonly reported to enhance mental imagery (Studerus et al. 2012).

More generally, the onset of complex hallucinations (non-veridical, complex mental imagery; see ch. 7) also makes sense if we embed the attentional-resource hypothesis within the predictive processing framework. One way such hallucinations can arise is if an unusual amount of attention is directed (voluntarily or

---

[35] Thus providing a clear case of cognition penetrating perception (cf. Firestone and Scholl 2015), albeit under unusual conditions.

involuntarily) to an object of perception. On the predictive processing framework, this increase in attention would result in predictive errors being propagated further up the hierarchy than would normally be appropriate (provided that the priors are accepting of them). This, in turn, would cause the revision of higher-level priors that would otherwise have remained unchanged (as before, this picture could fit naturally within the REBUS model).

So far, we have been considering sources of possible evidence for—or against— the attentional-resource hypothesis with respect to the known effects that psychedelics have on the visual field. Although these visual effects can be striking, and although the research on attention in general has long been dominated by a focus on visual attention, we should also consider other kinds of effects that may arise from a disruption of attentional resources. In the coming chapters, we will consider other notable examples, including memory recollections (Chapter 6), creative insights (Chapter 8), psychological insights and increases in mindfulness (Chapter 9), and mystical experiences (Chapter 10). For now, we will consider two final arguments.

The first argument stems from how psychedelics affect the perception of time. Psychedelics are well known to cause experiences of time slowing down.[36] If attentional resources are made more freely available and some of them make their way to the attentional gate between the pacemaker and accumulator (as described before), then we should expect to see a slowing down of perceived time. At that abstract level of analysis, the evidence fits well with what we would expect to see. Based on a differential effect that psilocybin had on the reproduction accuracy of short and long duration intervals, Wittmann et al. 2007 argue that the observed alterations to time perception are due to disruptions to cognitive and working memory rather than a disruption to the pacemaker-accumulator clock. However, it should be acknowledged that the opposite effect may also occur—although they appear to be less common, there are documented cases of psychedelics causing subjective time to flow more rapidly (Kenna and Sedman 1964). This may be due to individual differences in how attention is normally allocated. So, for some individuals, the effect of disrupting attention may result in the attentional gate receiving less attentional resource.

The second (and final) argument concerns how psychedelics disrupt the complex phenomenological structure of attention. In particular, psychedelics appear to regularly disrupt the phenomenal *transparency* and *opacity* of one's experience (Lyon and Farennikova 2022). To see this, let's first consider an easy example of how these notions apply to regular experience. Imagine you are enjoying a comedy sitcom, laughing along with the jokes and relating to some of the characters in the show. Now suppose that your attention is suddenly drawn to the show's laugh

[36] For example, see Kenna and Sedman 1964, Fischer and Mead 1966, Wittmann et al. 2007, Wackermann et al. 2008, and Yanakieva et al. 2018.

track. This shift in your attention has a remarkable effect on your experience of the show: suddenly, the jokes don't seem as funny, and the whole show has a feeling of artifice to it—you may even have the experience of the characters being replaced by the actors that play them. This change in your experience is due to an increase in phenomenal opacity (Metzinger 2003, Vervaeke and Ferraro 2016).[37] Before the change, there was a sense in which you were seeing through the actors to the characters, or hearing through the laugh track to the intended humour of the jokes. Once you notice the laugh track, it can be difficult to shake off this phenomenological change; however, most people eventually forget about the laugh track and return to the world of the show, again laughing at the jokes and empathizing with the characters. This eventual change is an increase in phenomenal transparency.

Such changes in transparency and opacity are intimately bound with our attentional system and have a substantial impact on how we experience the world. To take another example: when you learn how to ride a bike, you begin interacting with the bike in a predominantly opaque mode: you are thinking about the pedals, the handle bars, the seat, the breaks, etc. At some point, when you become familiar with these parts of the bike, they "disappear" and you enter a kind of *union* with the bike. Around this time, you start to ride the bike with ease, and you begin to be aware of other features of the world *through* the bike—for example, bumps in the road, or the traction of the surface. These notions of phenomenal transparency and opacity can apply to almost any part or aspect of the mind. In general, increases in opacity can be characterized as a kind of "stepping back" from experience and taking on a more analytical or "distant observer" relation to it. Various meditative practices have been understood as facilitating the ability to make this kind of shift (Vervaeke and Ferraro 2016). In contrast, increases in transparency involve a "plunging" into experience, taking on a more involved, engaged relation to it. Increases in transparency tend to involve increases in meaningfulness and connection, and a kind of union with the objects of experience—the sort of unity with experience that arises in flow states. In extreme cases, this culminates in a mystical experience (see Chapters 9 and 10) whereby one is no longer in a relational stance with respect to anything and is instead simply *being*—in a state of knowing-by-identity (Forman 1999). Increases in opacity tend to involve the opposite kind of change—meaning tends to be stripped out of experience, and one becomes more disconnected from its elements.[38]

[37] See also Polanyi 1966 who describes the same types of changes in attention and awareness, though using different terminology.

[38] This book can be seen as an exercise in increasing phenomenal opacity with respect to the experiences induced by psychedelics and meditation. The explication given in Chapter 3 in terms of psychedelic space takes a representational step back from the experiences in question, abstracting away from their contents, so that they can be viewed from a broader and more flexible perspective. (Thanks to Martijn Schirp for pointing this out to me.)

Letheby 2021 has argued that the primary mechanism by which psychedelics have their therapeutic effects is that they cause increases in phenomenal opacity. For example, someone who is stuck in depressive rumination can be jolted out of the stream of such thoughts and experience them as *mere* thoughts. This person then has the mental space to examine those thoughts and change them, potentially leading to an improvement in their well-being. However, while psychedelics do cause such increases in opacity, it is clear that they *also* cause substantial—and often radical—increases in transparency. This can be seen in the qualitative descriptions of psychedelic sessions. For example, people often report feeling more connected and more "at one" with all sorts of things, including one's self, one's body, other people, music, nature, the universe, and God—or getting lost in visual hallucinations, sounds and music, physical sensations, and so on. To quote a few examples from the qualitative descriptions recorded in the literature:

> It was like being inside of nature, and I could've just stayed there forever—it was wonderful. All kinds of other things were coming, too, like feelings of being connected to everything, I mean, everything in nature. Everything—even like pebbles, drops of water in the sea . . . it was like magic. It was wonderful, and it wasn't like talking about it, which makes it an idea, it was, like, experiential. It was like being inside a drop of water, being inside of . . . a butterfly's wing. And being inside of a cheetah's eyes.
>
> Belser et al. 2017, p. 371

> I felt that I was part of the music and I was in the music, it was me. It was it just me listening to music. I was the music. I was the drum, or the flute, or the violin, and I was really part of that.
>
> Belser et al. 2017, p. 374

> Before I enjoyed nature, now I feel part of it. Before I was looking at it as a thing, like TV or a painting. You're part of it, there's no separation or distinction, you are it.
>
> Watts et al. 2017, p. 534

> [It] just opens you up and it connects you . . . it's not just people, it's animals, it's trees—everything is interwoven, and that's a big relief . . . I think it does help you accept death because you don't feel alone [. . .] That's the number one thing—you're just not alone.
>
> Swift et al. 2017, p. 499

> The part that continues to stick out for me was 'knowing' and 'seeing' and 'experiencing' with every sense and fiber of my being that all things are connected.'
>
> Griffiths et al. 2008, p. 19

And, summarizing the effects on visual experience, Belser et al. 2017 write:

> These complex visualizations are not merely interesting scenes painted on the proscenium curtain of the theater of the mind. Rather, among study participants, these visions served as principle organizing motifs of subjective experience with multifold vectors (e.g. audiovisual, relational, autobiographical, spiritual, epistemological, ontological). Such visions were often deeply coded with layers of meaning by participants.
>
> Belser et al. 2017, p. 379

Similar descriptions and summaries can be found throughout the literature. Indeed, it would seem that increases in transparency might be more characteristic of the effects of psychedelics than increases in opacity are. Moreover, their tendency to increase transparency may provide a better explanation for the therapeutic efficacy of psychedelics, especially since many of the conditions they are effective in treating involve *disconnection* in various forms (Carhart-Harris et al. 2018) and since psychedelics have traditionally been combined with shamanic or tantric practices. At any rate, the important point for our present argument is that psychedelics appear to cause *both* effects, and this amounts to another way in which psychedelics disrupt our usual patterns of attentional resource allocation—either by increasing transparency and/or increasing opacity. Psychedelics appear to allow attentional resources to flow more freely "back" and "forward" through the mind's hierarchies of representations and associations. This point also lines up neatly with the observation that the practices of mindfulness-oriented traditions involve learning how to make *both* kinds of shift, and even simultaneously (Vervaeke and Ferraro 2016). Therefore, we have another point of contact with meditation (and other mindfulness practices), which focuses on the deliberate change in how attention is allocated throughout the mind.

Let's now take stock. In general, it is difficult to make specific predictions about the effects of freeing up attentional resources: the observed effects will depend on how attention ends up being allocated, and this will depend on the individual and their context. However, roughly speaking, we should expect more things to appear in awareness and also for things to appear in awareness more vividly: emotions will be intensified, sounds will be more distinctive, smells will be stronger, memory recollections will be more frequent and immersive (Chapter 6), creative and psychological insights will be more frequent and novel (Chapters 8 and 9), and so on. There are also likely to be general phenomenological changes in the structure of experience, such as the slowing down of the perception of time and increases in the opacity and transparency of mental representations. Moreover, it is likely that many of these effects will tend to happen simultaneously and thus bewilder those experiencing them (especially if one is new to such experiences). That is, if more attentional resources are flowing freely throughout the mind, then we should expect lots of things to appear vividly in conscious experience at the same time. This, of course, fits well with common reports of psychedelic trips. In general, the experience of an individual will become richer but also potentially more chaotic or unpredictable (depending on the situation), which aligns with the hypothesis that psychedelics temporarily increase the brain's entropy (Carhart-Harris et al. 2014 and Carhart-Harris 2018).[39]

Clearly, more research needs to be done—both empirical and philosophical—before we can conclude that the attentional-resource hypothesis is correct. However, given what we know about awareness, attention, the relevant brain networks (SN, DMN, and DAN), meditation, binocular rivalry, and the perception of time, it does appear to have some plausibility to it. On the other hand, if evidence comes in that renders the hypothesis unlikely, it can then be used to challenge the widespread notion that psychedelics expand awareness. In other words, if it is true that psychedelics expand awareness, then given the close connection between attention and awareness, we should expect that they correspondingly expand or increase attention in some way. If it turns out that psychedelics don't have such an effect on attention, then we'll need an alternative explanation for how they can expand awareness. If such an explanation is not forthcoming, the notion that psychedelics expand awareness would not look so plausible.

5.5 Conclusion

We do not yet know exactly how psychedelics and meditation have their effects on consciousness, and it is likely that these effects are produced by multiple psychological processes and mechanisms. However, I have argued that attention likely plays a substantial mediating role in both cases. With respect to meditation, it is safe to say that this has now become the consensus view (for example, see Jha 2021). The case involving psychedelics is less definitive, but I have argued that it is nevertheless quite plausible.

If correct, this unification of psychedelics and meditation in terms of attention explains why it is common for people to develop an interest in meditation after having had some experience with psychedelics (Simonsson and Goldberg 2022). It also explains why psychedelics and meditation tend to induce experiences that are rather different from one another but are still of the same kind: they involve different ways of enhancing hidden parts or aspects of the mind and promoting them into one's awareness (or heightening one's awareness of them). The unification in terms of attention also explains why the two methods for bringing about

---

[39] As before, it is important to keep in mind the qualifications set out in Chapter 4. It is entirely possible for the experience to involve an equanimous state of attention, especially if the person in question is meditating or has cultivated a high degree of mindfulness.

psychedelic experiences may have synergistic effects and complement each other (Heuschkel and Kuypers 2020, Payne et al. 2021). Psychedelics may provide new and valuable "raw material" to work with during meditation, and meditation may help one better manage the attentional resources freed up by psychedelics.

Finally, the unification also gives us a relatively precise interpretation of the Osmond-Grof hypothesis, which says that psychedelics are nonspecific amplifiers, or energizers, of mental representations and processes. I have argued that this hypothesis can be understood in terms of psychedelics releasing attentional resources, which then flow somewhat freely (i.e. nonspecifically) throughout the mind (unless they are directed otherwise). Thus, we can understand psychedelics as being mental amplifiers, since allocating more attentional resources to a mental representation increases the probability that it will appear in awareness or, if it is already in awareness, that it will feature in awareness more vividly. This, in turn, explains the common report that psychedelics "expand consciousness" and supports the hypothesis that they reveal the mind.

6
Memory

6.1 Introduction

In the previous chapter, we considered how attention may play an important role in the underlying processes by which meditation and psychedelics cause psychedelic experiences. Many meditative practices involve the direct training of one's attentional system, and we saw that these practices can result in empirically observable effects (often of a beneficial kind). I also argued that one of the primary effects of psychedelics is that they disrupt one's attentional system, thus causing one's attentional resources to flow more freely throughout the mind. As a result, both of these interventions cause some parts and aspects of the mind to receive more attentional resources than they otherwise would. Given the close connection between attention and awareness, we therefore have a strong case for the hypothesis that meditation and psychedelics produce psychedelic experiences— understood as mind-revealing experiences—via their effects on attention.

In this chapter, we will consider the effects that meditation and psychedelics have on *memory*. In particular, we will examine the evidence that these two interventions may produce psychedelic experiences by revealing hidden memories— that is, memories that are *available* but *inaccessible*.[1] There are three main reasons to focus on memory.

The first reason is that we are all familiar with experience of a hidden memory being revealed to us. Consider, for instance, the situation when a word was stuck on the tip of your tongue and the feeling of suddenly remembering it. Or consider what happens when you encounter a distinctive smell that triggers a memory flashback to some event in your childhood. In both cases, a memory was partly hidden from your awareness, then something changes, and the memory suddenly appears in your conscious experience. Because these experiences are so common, they provide a convenient template that we can use to extrapolate to the memory-revealing experiences induced by meditation and psychedelics.

The second reason is that the revelation of hidden memories gives us a nice way of testing the hypothesis that meditation and psychedelics reveal the mind. One general problem with testing this hypothesis is that it is often difficult to determine whether something hidden in the mind is revealed, or instead created in the moment. For example, consider the last time you had an emotional or

---

[1] For discussions of this distinction, see, for example, Tulving and Pearlstone 1966 and Habib and Nyberg 2008.

creative insight. Was the insight already lurking in your unconscious for some time before it showed up in your conscious experience? Or did your mind generate it in that very moment? It's difficult to say.[2] In contrast, it should be easier to objectively determine whether a memory is revealed since memories, by their very nature, are stored in the mind and can be reasonably expected to have some degree of correspondence with the external world. Although there are constructive aspects to the recollective process that shouldn't be ignored, we know we can test, in at least some respects, whether a memory is genuinely stored in the mind (e.g. consider all the exams we make students take at schools and universities). Memory, therefore, provides us with a convenient way of testing the hypothesis that meditation and psychedelics reveal the mind. If they do, then we should be able to find evidence that they help people access memories that they otherwise wouldn't be able to recall.[3]

The third reason is that focusing on memory provides us with a convenient way of introducing an important concept that we haven't yet properly addressed: the concept of *mindfulness*. Mindfulness is often defined in terms of attention (or awareness), but as we will see, such a definition only scratches the surface of mindfulness. It turns out there is a deep connection between mindfulness and memory that will be useful for us to explore. I will also argue that there is a subtle and important connection between mindfulness and psychedelic experience—and, in particular, that we can understand mindfulness as the inverse of a *psychecryptic state* (a concept I introduced in Chapter 3). Given how widespread attentional definitions of mindfulness have become, this connection between memory and mindfulness may be counterintuitive to some readers. To help ease those readers into the coming discussion, it is worth noting now that the literal meaning of the original Pali term for mindfulness, *sati* (*smrti*, in Sanskrit), is 'memory'. To be sure, there is more to mindfulness than memory (as many Buddhists will be quick to point out), but it is worth emphasizing this important connection because it is so often lost in discussions of mindfulness. Indeed, the connection between mindfulness and memory can help us appreciate why mindfulness is so important. As John R. Anderson noted:

Memory is involved in almost everything we do, but most of the time we think of ourselves not as remembering but rather as doing something else.

Anderson 2007, p. 122

---

[2] But not impossible (Siegler 2000).

[3] These first two reasons are philosophically safe in that they help us connect psychedelic experiences to common sense and science. A less safe, but philosophically interesting, reason for focusing on memory stems from Plato's theory of *anamnēsis* and the role that beauty plays in reminding us of what the soul has previously seen (e.g. in *Symposium* and *Phaedrus*). I won't pursue this line of thought here, but it is worth noting that it aligns with the feeling of "coming home" that people report having with psychedelics and some meditation practices.

Memory plays a fundamental role in everything from perception and emotion to the use of our skills, decision-making, planning, and our behaviour in general. This is a big part of the reason for why mindfulness is so important.

The plan for this chapter is as follows. In Section 6.2, we will sort out some basic conceptual and terminological issues and survey some of relevant scientific evidence regarding memory. In particular, we will revisit the idea that we can have *spontaneous* psychedelic experiences in the form of memory flashbacks and review the connections between attention and memory, which will help us understand why meditation and psychedelics may have an impact on memory. In Section 6.3, we will unpack the notion of mindfulness and examine the evidence that meditation can reveal hidden memories. In Section 6.4, we will then examine the evidence that psychedelics also reveal hidden memories. Finally, we will conclude in Section 6.5.

6.2 Remembering

Before we get going, there is some terminology that we need to sort out. The terms 'remembering', 'recollecting', and 'memory' are often used interchangeably, but they can also be used to indicate different things. For example, imagine you are sitting for an exam and come across a question to which you know the answer but cannot remember at that moment. Another way of describing this scenario is that you do remember the answer, and it is just that you cannot *recollect* it. The entry for 'Remember' in the *Cambridge English Dictionary* is explicit about this ambiguity: 'remember: to be able to bring back a piece of information into your mind, or to keep a piece of information in your memory'. We also sometimes use the term 'remember' to refer to the mental state of holding a memory in awareness—such as when you reminisce with an old friend about the time you first met. These ambiguities can make precise discussions of memory a little challenging because we often need to distinguish three aspects of remembering: (i) having an item in mind (as a memory), (ii) being able to bring that item into awareness, and (iii) actually having it in awareness. Unfortunately, the usual methods of fixing this sort of issue—for example, introducing new technical terms—would only replace one awkwardness with another. So in what follows, I will make do by being clear about which sense of remembering is being used.

With that terminological issue clarified, let us come back to the idea that some of our everyday memory recollections are psychedelic. This idea might be counterintuitive to some readers because it is commonly assumed that psychedelic experiences can only be caused by the consumption of psychedelic substances. However, recall from Chapter 2 that a psychedelic experience is just a mind-revealing experience, regardless of how it is brought about. Another reason why some readers may have the intuition that only psychedelics cause psychedelic experiences is because if psychedelics are deserving of their name, then they tend to cause experiences that are *very* psychedelic. This is especially so when we compare them to our spontaneous psychedelic experiences, which tend to be only *mildly* psychedelic. In other words, the experiences that psychedelics induce stand out to us more vividly in a way that our spontaneous psychedelic experiences do not.

However, there are some important exceptions. While it is true that our usual recollections tend to be only mildly psychedelic (if at all), this is by no means always the case. Some people's experiences with their memories are quite different from those of the rest of us (we will see a famous example in a moment). And we all occasionally have recollective experiences that are more psychedelic than usual. These experiences, for instance, often happen when we come across some rare olfactory cue—the aroma of a particular dish being cooked, the smell of a perfume, etc.—that is linked to an old memory. When this happens, the memory, in all its richness, floods our consciousness. This is because our olfactory receptors have unusually direct connections to the hippocampus (Mouly and Sullivan 2010), which is associated with autobiographical and episodic memories (Bird and Burgess 2008). It seems that memories can lie dormant in the mind for decades, even if they are never, or rarely, remembered. In some cases, this is because they are difficult to activate with an environmental cue—since the pathways by which they may become activated weaken over time. However, since the olfactory activation pathways are unusually direct, coming across the right smell can trigger such a memory and cause it to rush into one's awareness.

We can see this phenomenon at work in Marcel Proust's famous description of his recollection of eating tea-soaked madeleines as a child (in his novel *In Search of Lost Time*). Although quite long, it will be useful to see his description in detail:

[...] I raised to my lips a spoonful of the tea in which I had soaked a morsel of the cake [a madeleine]. No sooner had the warm liquid mixed with the crumbs touched my palate than a shiver ran through me and I stopped, intent upon the extraordinary thing that was happening to me. [...]

I drink a second mouthful, in which I find nothing more than in the first, then a third, which gives me rather less than the second. It is time to stop; the potion is losing its virtue. It is plain that the truth I am seeking lies not in the cup but in myself. [...] I put down the cup and examine my own mind. It alone can discover the truth. But how? What an abyss of uncertainty, whenever the mind feels overtaken by itself; when it, the seeker, is at the same time the dark region through which it must go seeking and where all its equipment will avail it nothing. [...] So that nothing may interrupt it in its course I shut out every obstacle, every extraneous idea, I stop my ears and screen my attention from the sounds from the next room. [...] I place in position before my mind's eye the still recent taste of that first mouthful, and I feel something start within me, something that leaves its resting-place and attempts to rise, something that has been anchored at a great depth; I do not know yet what it is, but I can feel it mounting slowly; I can measure the resistance, I can hear the echo of great spaces traversed. [...]

But its struggles are too far off, too confused and chaotic; scarcely can I perceive the neutral glow into which the elusive whirling medley of stirred-up colours is fused [...]

Will it ultimately reach the clear surface of my consciousness, this memory, this old, dead moment which the magnetism of an identical moment has travelled so far to importune, to disturb, to raise up out of the very depths of my being? I cannot tell. Now I feel nothing; it has stopped, has perhaps sunk back into its darkness, from which who can say whether it will ever rise again? Ten times over I must essay the task, must lean down over the abyss. And each time the cowardice that deters us from every difficult task, every important enterprise, has urged me to leave the thing alone, to drink my tea and to think merely of the worries of today and my hopes for tomorrow, which can be brooded over painlessly.

And suddenly the memory revealed itself. The taste was that of the little piece of madeleine which [...] my aunt Léonie used to give me, dipping it first in her own cup of tea or tisane. The sight of the little madeleine had recalled nothing to my mind before I tasted it; perhaps because I had so often seen such things in the meantime, without tasting them [...] that their image had dissociated itself from those Combray days [...]

And as soon as I had recognised the taste of the piece of madeleine soaked in her decoction of lime-blossom [...] immediately the old grey house upon the street, where her room was, rose up like a stage set to attach itself to the little pavilion opening on to the garden which had been built out behind it for my parents [...] and with the house the town, from morning to night and in all weathers, the Square where I used to be sent before lunch, the streets along which I used to run errands, the country roads we took when it was fine. And [...] in that moment all the flowers in our garden and in M. Swann's park, and the waterlilies on the Vivonne and the good folk of the village and their little dwellings and the parish church and the whole of Combray and its surroundings, taking shape and solidity sprang into being, town and gardens alike, from my cup of tea.

Proust, In Search of Lost Time

There is obviously a lot in this description, and I have trimmed many of Proust's interesting detours. However, it is clear that although the experience was not drug-induced, it is a *psychedelic* experience, in which a deeply hidden memory is revealed in particularly vivid and rich detail.

We might wonder, though, whether this really is an example of spontaneous psychedelic experience. Although there is no mention of any psychedelic substances, we can see in Proust's description several references to meditative techniques. He drew his attention away from distractions, then focused it on the initial experience of drinking the tea, and repeated this process several times (ten, according to him). Moreover, he is aware of, and is able to resist, the default tendency to give up 'the cowardice that deters us from every difficult task' and which would encourage him to 'think merely of the worries of the today and my hopes for tomorrow'. This style of thinking has been associated with the default mode network (DMN), and, as we saw in the previous chapter, focused-attention and open-monitoring meditation have been observed to reduce/disintegrate its activity. So perhaps Proust's experience wasn't so spontaneous and was induced by him intentionally maintaining a meditative or meditative-like state.

On the other hand, there does not appear to be any evidence that Proust practised meditation. It seems that he was just unusually talented at observing and describing his mind. In light of that, it is perhaps more fitting to think of his psychedelic experience as a spontaneous one. After all, the experience was initially brought about via an external trigger—namely, the taste of the tea-soaked madeleine. Alternatively, it might be best to classify the experience as a borderline case lying somewhere between being spontaneous and meditatively induced.

Regardless, Proust's experience serves to highlight how some of our memory recollections can be more psychedelic than others without the assistance of psychedelic substances. Indeed, Proust's description of the memory coming to mind reads somewhat like a psychedelic trip report. More importantly, we can see how it scores high on all of the dimensions of psychedelic space. Although the experience starts off low in *clarity* ('the memory starting as a shiver and then partly rising up from the darkness so that it can be scarcely perceived'), it eventually bursts into his awareness ('the clear surface of his consciousness') in spectacularly rich and vivid detail. Similarly, the *scope* of the memory appears to be quite high. The memory isn't just of him eating the tea-soaked madeleine, it is also of 'the old grey house upon the street', 'the good folk of the village', 'the whole of Combray and its surroundings', and so on. The *duration* of the experience also appears to be quite high, since despite it being large in scope and high in clarity, Proust was able to record the experience in his beautifully detailed prose. In other words, the experience was sufficiently long in duration for him to turn it into a famous passage of literature. Finally, the *novelty* also appears to be high, for, as Proust says, the memory was an old and dead moment that had been long residing in the very depths of his being. Jonah Lehrer describes Proust's experience in similar terms:

Proust's memory is hauntingly specific and completely unexpected. His memory of Combray, cued by some chance crumbs, interrupts his life, intruding for no logical reason, 'with no suggestion of its origin'. Proust is shocked by his past.

Lehrer 2007, p. 90

Moreover, in the full passage, it is clear that more than just a memory of Combray is being revealed: there is a cluster of emotions, desires, and an underlying sense of self that is being brought forth as well.[4] Since the experience scores high on all of the dimensions, it is located deep in psychedelic space, and therefore it counts as being very psychedelic.

Proust is likely an outlier when it comes to memory recollections.[5] Many of us typically don't have recollections that are so high in scope, clarity, novelty, and duration. Nevertheless, we can all recognize *some* degree of similarity between his experiences and our own. Most of us have had the experience of coming across a scent that triggers the sudden recollection of a memory from childhood—one that seems like it had been completely lost to us, until that very moment. In many cases, these experiences are barely psychedelic—for example, you might catch a vague glimpse of freshly baked cookies. In other cases, these experiences can be much more psychedelic—for example, you might remember in vivid detail helping make the cookies and then enjoying their deliciousness while watching cartoons.

These observations help mitigate some of the initial counterintuitiveness of the claim that some of our memory recollections are psychedelic experiences. Typically, such experiences are only mildly psychedelic (and barely noteworthy), and it is only the more intense recollections, such as Proust's, that are highly psychedelic. And even those recollections may not be as psychedelic as those that are facilitated by meditation and psychedelic substances. It is also worth emphasizing that only those recollections that involve *hidden* memories count as psychedelic experiences. Regular recollections of easily accessible memories, such as what you had for breakfast this morning, do not count as psychedelic experiences.

Let's now turn our focus to some of the scientific knowledge we have about memory, which will be crucial as we consider whether meditation and psychedelics give us greater and more reliable access to our memories.

Perhaps the most important fact for us to know in this regard is that a surprising number of our memories are *false memories*. That is, we have experiences in which we think we are remembering something that happened to us that in fact did not. There is an experimental paradigm known as the Deese-Roediger-McDermott (DRM) paradigm that clearly demonstrates how we can have false memories. In a typical DRM experiment, subjects are presented with a list of words that are closely related to a *lure* word, which is not on the list. For example, for the lure word *sleep*, the list of words would look like this:

bed, pillow, night, yawn, sheets, tired, blanket, pyjamas, rest, dreams

---

[4] Indeed, it could be argued that the full passage indicates that Proust had a *mystical-type experience* (see Chapter 9).

[5] Another kind of outlier is mnemonist Solomon Shereshevsky, who had an unusually vast memory, as reported by Luria 1968.

Subjects are presented with these words and then asked to remember as many of them as possible. People tend to "remember" the lure just as often as they remember the other words on the list. You might think that this is because they are guessing that the lure word is on the list based on their memory of the other words. However, about half of the time people report that they remember *seeing* the lure word. In other words, these people believe in an experience that never actually happened to them. It seems that a substantial number of people confabulate an experience of seeing the word and then perceive that as a real memory. In Roediger and McDermott's words: 'the results reveal a powerful illusion of memory: people remember events that never happened' (Roediger and McDermott 1995, p. 803).

This false memory effect will be important later because there is a natural concern that psychedelics do not induce the recollection of real memories and instead only produce fantasies that *seem* like recollections. So, we should keep in mind that we are susceptible to false memories even when not under the influence of psychedelics. Moreover, as we will see in the next section, there are now several studies on how meditation may impact false memories on the DRM paradigm. There is also evidence that DRM false memories increase when attention is divided (Shah and Knott 2018), thus providing another link between attention and psychedelic (and psychecryptic) experiences. The DRM paradigm therefore provides us with a useful tool of investigation as we consider the question of whether psychedelics and meditative practices reveal hidden memories.

The next basic fact about memory concerns attention and *involuntary autobiographical memories* (IAMs). These are memories about one's life that appear in awareness without any attempt to deliberately recall them, and they are quite common in everyday life (Berntsen 1996). The initial stage of Proust's recollection of eating tea-soaked madeleines is an example of an IAM. Involuntary memories are important for our purposes because they appear to be the kind of memory recollection that psychedelics and meditation often trigger. Moreover, there is a growing body of research indicating that they are affected by changes in how attentional resources are distributed. If psychedelics and meditation impact how attentional resources are allocated throughout the mind, then we should be able to observe these two interventions having effects on the involuntary recollection of autobiographical memories. This connection with attention can, therefore, help us determine more clearly how changes in attentional resource allocation may reveal the mind—in this case, by revealing hidden autobiographical memories. The literature on attention and IAMs is quite involved, so we will make do with two of the major takeaways.

First, it appears that diffusing attention increases the frequency of IAMs. It has been proposed that this happens because diffusing attention (i) enhances the unconscious processing of environmental cues, (ii) facilitates the spreading of subsequent activation through memory networks, (iii) reduces the usual relevance screening that memories must pass before they enter awareness, and (iv) draws attentional resources away from metacognitive processing, thus making it more difficult for environmental cues to be registered as memory triggers.[6] However, Barzykowski and Niedźwieńska 2018 found that while focusing attention on demanding tasks reduces the number of IAMs (in line with (ii) above), it also reduces the frequency of *other* mental contents (that are not IAMs), allowing the relative *density* of IAMs in conscious experience to increase. Barzykowski and Niedźwieńska propose that this is because autobiographical memories are more automatic, and therefore more robust, than other mental contents, and so they are less affected by increases in cognitive load.

These results suggest that the effects that psychedelics and meditation have on IAMs may be somewhat nuanced. For example, they suggest that, by diffusing attention, open-monitoring meditation will tend to increase the occurrence of IAMs. However, they also suggest that while focused-attention meditation should decrease the occurrence of IAMs, it will also increase the relative density of IAMs, thus potentially giving the *appearance* that focused-attention meditation triggers IAMs. The upshot is that both forms of meditation may have the appearance of inducing IAMs that would otherwise remain unconscious. Similarly, by diffusing attention, psychedelics may increase the occurrence of IAMs while also decreasing their density relative to other mental contents. Moreover, by also impairing metacognition and reducing meta-awareness, psychedelics may create the impression that even more IAMs occur than they otherwise would. The upshot is that psychedelics may simultaneously enhance environmental suggestibility (in line with the received wisdom concerning set and setting), while also clouding the individual's awareness of this suggestibility, making it seem as though more memories are appearing "out of thin air".

The second major takeaway concerns the accessibility of autobiographical memories. Barzykowski and Staugaard 2018 found that IAMs are often highly accessible in that they tend to be intense, unusual, recent, and rehearsed. They argue that this observation fits their *threshold hypothesis* for IAMs, which says that: (i) a memory needs to pass a threshold of activation in order to reach consciousness, (ii) the ease in which this happens is the memory's *accessibility*, and (iii) those memories that make it into awareness involuntarily tend to have higher accessibility, as evidenced by salient properties such as emotional intensity, importance, unusualness, recency, rehearsal, and vividness (Ritchie et al. 2006, Barzykowski and Staugaard 2016). The threshold hypothesis explains why we are not constantly bombarded with IAMs during normal experience. For a memory to make it into awareness,

---

[6] For example, see Berntsen 1998, Kvavilashvili and Mandler 2004, Ball and Little 2006, and Vannucci et al. 2019.

it has to be substantially activated, or perhaps have some kind of "special access pass" based on its task relevance. The thought, then, is that many of our memories are lying dormant, never active enough to reach awareness spontaneously, never deliberately retrieved, and never activated by environmental cues.

Barzykowski et al. 2019 develop the threshold hypothesis further, arguing that there is a universal pool of autobiographical memories from which memories can be retrieved voluntarily or involuntarily. An arbitrary memory selected for voluntary retrieval will tend to be low in accessibility and require a concerted effort to locate and sufficiently activate. Conversely, the typical memory that appears in awareness involuntarily will likely have been already close to the threshold. Such memories will therefore have distinctive properties that tend to draw attentional resources, as Barzykowski et al. point out:

> In order to reach one's consciousness, each memory has to pass an awareness threshold and the ease with which this happens is known as the accessibility of the memory. For example, it may be easier for an emotionally intense memory to pass the awareness threshold because such a memory property may be especially good at drawing one's memory-related attention.
>
> Barzykowski et al. 2019, p. 34

In addition to being good at drawing attention, some memories may also not require much attention to pass the threshold. To use an analogy, we can think of autobiographical memories as like mouse traps and attentional resources as like mice. Some mousetraps are rusty and therefore can only be triggered by a big, heavy mouse. Other mousetraps are more easily triggered—some so much that they will snap shut even in the absence of a mouse. Mousetraps also vary in terms of how they are baited: some are much more attractive to mice than others. And so with memories: some are "rusty", some get triggered by nothing, and some require certain kinds of "baits". This variation in the properties of memories explains, along with the threshold hypothesis, why some memories are more likely to be triggered as IAMs and why attention plays a key role in this process.

The upshot, then, is that if psychedelics and meditation change how attentional resources are allocated throughout the mind, and if the threshold hypothesis is correct, then these interventions should have observable effects on autobiographical memories, particularly in the form of IAMs. For example, since open-monitoring meditation diffuses attention, we may see that this form of meditation tends to induce involuntary autobiographical memories. Similarly, if psychedelics free up the amount of available attentional resource, then this would have a similar effect to diffusing attention: more dormant memories receive more attention than they otherwise would.

6.3 Meditation

Let's now consider the reasons we may have for thinking that meditation induces psychedelic experiences that involve the revelation of hidden memories.

We've already seen one reason for thinking that meditation may reveal hidden memories: attention and memory are closely related cognitive faculties, and we know that meditation has various positive effects on attention (Chapter 5). So, it's reasonable to expect that meditation also has positive effects on memory via its positive effects on attention. We'll see later that there is some evidence in favour of this idea.

However, it is also worth exploring the connection between meditation and memory independently of attention. This is because there is good reason to think that the connection between meditation and memory is actually quite a deep and subtle one. While it is common to think about meditation primarily in terms of attention (as we did in the previous chapter), there's a sense in which meditation is more concerned with memory than it is with attention. One way to see this is by considering the trait of *mindfulness* that many meditative practices are intended to cultivate. It turns out that there is an important relationship between mindfulness and memory. Moreover, by appreciating this relationship, we will begin to see another that will be important in the coming chapters: the relationship between psychedelic experience and mindfulness. Very briefly, a psychedelic experience involves the revelation of some hidden part or aspect of the mind, and the development of mindfulness involves removing the *hiddenness* of various parts and aspects of the mind (without necessarily bringing them into awareness). We will come back to this in more detail later. For now, let's start with the concept of mindfulness itself.

A common definition of mindfulness says that it involves maintaining a state of non-judgemental attention to the present moment (Kabat-Zinn 1994). This is sometimes known as a *bare-attention* definition of mindfulness. According to this definition, you are not being mindful if you are thinking about the past or future, or if you are thinking about anything (including the present) in judgemental terms. That is, you are being mindful when you are paying attention only to the present moment in a non-judgemental fashion. We can see how the two forms of meditation that we have been considering might promote this trait. Focused-attention meditation can help you maintain a state of paying attention to the present moment by developing your ability to focus and stabilize your distribution of attentional resources. And open-monitoring meditation can help you pay attention in a non-judgemental way, by developing your ability to notice your reactions to various thoughts and sensations, as well as by reducing the speed at which those reactions occur and the power they have on your general state of mind.[7]

---

[7] This is a rough characterization, and there is more to be said about both forms of meditation. For example, focused-attention meditation also involves non-judgemental attention, and both forms of meditation interact with each other as one's practice deepens.

While this definition gets something right about mindfulness and can be useful to help one get started with meditation, it isn't entirely adequate for our purposes. As several scholars have pointed out, the definition doesn't fit well with traditional understandings of the concept.[8] Specifically, the process of bringing attention non-judgementally to the present moment is not necessarily best thought of as mindfulness itself, but rather it can also be usefully thought of as a *method* for helping one to achieve mindfulness (Dreyfus 2011, p. 52). The point is that the method of bringing attention non-judgementally to the present moment helps one break free from compulsions to think in certain ways—to worry about the future, lament the past, avoid discomforts of the present moment, etc. Roughly speaking, developing mindfulness involves increasing one's cognitive flexibility and stability—or one's cognitive *freedom*—so that it is easier for the mind to be in a state that is appropriate for its circumstances. For example, while fretting about the future is not being mindful, deliberately and efficiently planning a course of action can be. In other words (and still roughly speaking), mindfulness is less about bare attention and more about whether you are in control of your mind. One way to reconcile the two ways of thinking about mindfulness is to identify the former with what we may call *state* mindfulness and the latter with *trait* mindfulness, and then the natural thought would be that by repeatedly cultivating the former, one gradually develops the latter (see Kiken et al. 2015 for discussion of a similar distinction drawn in the research literature).[9]

At this point, you might wonder what all this has to do with memory. Cognitive flexibility and stability seem like good things, and it is clear that they are different from bare attention, but they don't have an obvious link to memory. What, then, does mindfulness have to do with memory? Quite a lot. In fact, memory is an *essential* aspect of mindfulness. To see this, we need to examine the origins of the concept.

It makes sense to begin with the etymology of the term 'mindfulness'. The term was first introduced in Davids' 1881 translation of the Pali word *sati*, which literally means 'memory'. The reason why Davids chose 'mindfulness' instead of 'memory' as a translation for *sati* is that the Buddhist concept of *sati* is not the concept we typically have in mind when we think of memory. The term 'mindfulness', with its Christian roots of meaning 'paying attention to others' needs' and 'paying attention to one's surroundings', does a better job of conveying the concept. However, it also doesn't fully capture the concept since it misses the memory aspect of *sati*. This can be confusing, and it can be tempting to demand clarity here. Which is it? Is *sati* memory, or is it about paying attention in a certain way? In typical Buddhist

---

[8] For example, see Bodhi 2011, Dreyfus 2011, Gethin 2011, and Purser and Milillo 2015.
[9] In fairness to Kabat-Zinn, he is well aware of these subtleties, and I think his decision regarding how to define mindfulness for a Western audience was a good one—especially given his primary objective, which was to bring mindfulness into therapeutic practices in a way that is acceptable for various kinds of stakeholder. See Kabat-Zinn 2011 for his perspective on this issue.

style, the answer is 'both' and that 'they are kind of the same thing' (it can also depend on who you ask).

We can see this dual aspect of *sati* in the definition of the concept that Buddha is said to have given to his *bhikkhus* (monks, or devotees):

> And what, bhikkhus, is the faculty of mindfulness? Here, bhikkhus, the noble disciple is mindful, possessing supreme mindfulness and discretion, one who remembers and recollects what was done and said long ago. He dwells contemplating the body in the body... feelings in feelings... mind in mind... phenomena in phenomena, ardent, clearly comprehending, mindful, having removed covetousness and displeasure in regard to the world. This is called the faculty of mindfulness.
>
> Samyutta Nikāya, V:48:10[10]

As various Buddhist scholars have observed, this definition has two parts to it. The first part says that mindfulness involves remembering and recollecting what was done and said long ago. That is clearly about memory. The second part says that mindfulness is about contemplating things as they are and not evaluating them. That is clearly about paying attention in a certain way. But, again, these seem like different things. The puzzle, then, is how the two parts of the definition can be reconciled.

One potential solution comes from Davids' observation that *sati* came to take on a more specific meaning:

> Etymologically *Sati* is Memory. But as happened at the rise of Buddhism to so many other expressions in common use, a new connotation was then attached to the word, a connotation that gave a new meaning to it, and renders 'memory' a most inadequate and misleading translation. It became the memory, recollection, calling-to-mind, being-aware-of, certain specified facts. Of these the most important was the impermanence (the coming to be as the result of a cause, and the passing away again) of all phenomena, bodily and mental. And it included the repeated application of this awareness, to each experience of life, from the ethical point of view.
>
> Davids 1910, p. 322

This understanding of *sati* emphasizes the aspect of mindfulness that involves the remembering of certain facts or ideas, especially that of impermanence. Mindfulness, then, might be understood as the ability to remember and hold in mind various important ideas, including the importance of paying attention to things

---

[10] Bodhi 2000, p. 1672.

in a particular way. Analogously, according to the original Christian concept of mindfulness, we may say that mindfulness involves remembering to pay attention to the needs of others.

That helps somewhat in solving our puzzle, but it only captures one layer of the connection between mindfulness and memory. Mindfulness is not just about remembering ideas or facts. It's also about *the nature of the mind* that can recollect well:

> The word *smrti* (Pali *sati*) comes from the Sanskrit root *smr*, which means to remember and keep in mind. The word itself can refer to the act of remembering and keeping in mind, as well as to what is kept in mind. [...] Within the Buddhist context, this word has usually a related but more restrained meaning and refers to the *quality of the mind* when it is recollecting or keeping in mind an object.
>
> Dreyfus 2011, p. 45 (emphasis added)

On this understanding, mindfulness is not about the remembering of a specified fact, but about the quality of mind that is recollecting or keeping in awareness some mental object (or no mental object).

But what, exactly, is the quality? Bodhi's 2011 analysis of *sati* clarifies it thus:

> [...T]o establish mindfulness is not to set about remembering something that occurred in the past, but to adopt a particular stance towards one's present experience. I characterize this as a stance of observation or watchfulness towards one's own experience. One might even call the stance of *sati* a 'bending back' of the light of consciousness upon the experiencing subject in its physical, sensory, and psychological dimensions. **This act of 'bending back' serves to illuminate the events occurring in these domains, lifting them out from the twilight zone of unawareness into the light of clear cognition.** [...] We might characterize mindfulness in this sense, in the simplest terms, as *lucid awareness*. [...] I believe it is this aspect of *sati* that provides the connection between its two primary canonical meanings: as memory and as lucid awareness of present happenings. *Sati* makes the apprehended object stand forth vividly and distinctly before the mind. When the object being cognized pertains to the past—when it is apprehended as something that was formerly done, perceived, or spoken—its vivid presentation takes the form of memory. When the object is a bodily process like in-and-out breathing or the act of walking back and forth, or when it is a mental event like a feeling or thought, its vivid presentation takes the form of lucid awareness of the present.
>
> Bodhi 2011, pp. 25–6 (emphasis added)

On this understanding of mindfulness, we begin to see how it is closely connected with the idea of psychedelic experience, since it involves lifting elements of the mind out of the unconscious and into awareness ('the light of clear cognition'). In other words, to be mindful involves having the ability to call things into awareness. With mindfulness, one can not only remember what was done and said long ago, but also become aware of details about the present moment that are available in the unconscious mind.

However, mindfulness is not just about bringing parts or aspects of the mind into awareness, it is also about *holding them* in awareness indefinitely—whether they be memories, present sensations, thoughts, etc. Because of this, mindfulness is sometimes said to involve *retention* or *not-forgetting* and therefore also has a connection with *working memory* (Dreyfus 2011).[11] A point closely related to this is that mindfulness involves seeing the things in one's mind *as they are*—'feelings in feelings...mind in mind...phenomena in phenomena'—without them being contorted by 'covetousness and displeasure'. Mindfulness thus involves a kind of mental *clarity*—a lucid awareness—that is extremely important. Using our explication of psychedelic experience, we can see that mindfulness involves the prevention of psychecryptic states and experiences. That is, it helps protect against states and experiences in which items of present experience are, or become, concealed in some way—for example, by sliding back into the twilight of unawareness or by becoming distorted by desires, prior expectations, conceptualizations, and so on.

Thus, we arrive at a simple way of expressing this understanding of mindfulness in terms of the conceptual framework of psychedelic space. Recall, from Chapter 4, the idea of one's default state—one's trait—moving along the dimensions of psychedelic space (as opposed to one's experiential state doing so). When this happens, all psychedelic experiences become less psychedelic. This is because they are now less revelatory, in that some parts of the mind have become *less hidden*, even when they are outside of awareness. In other words, some parts of the mind become easier to bring into awareness. This gives us a way of defining mindfulness: one is mindful to the extent that one's trait (the origin of one's coordinate system) is located deep in psychedelic space.[12] This gives us the connection between psychedelic experiences and mindfulness to which I alluded earlier: both can be defined in terms of the dimensions of psychedelic space. This point will be useful in later chapters, and especially in Chapter 9, when we consider the relationship

[11] One subtlety worth noting here concerns the distinction between concentration (*samādhi*) and mindfulness (*sati*), which are mutually reinforcing of each other and are such that the cultivation of one requires sufficient support from the other. Thus, one may argue that while *sati* does involve retention, this is actually a feature of its supporting *samādhi*. This subtlety won't matter for our purposes.

[12] In terms of the distinction between trait and state mindfulness, this definition is for the former and not the latter. However, state mindfulness also has an interesting connection with psychedelic experience: cultivating state mindfulness during meditation practice will involve a psychedelic experience since it will involve the revelation of something (e.g. the present moment), including awareness itself (sometimes this is described as acquiring 'awareness of awareness').

between psychedelic experiences and well-being. For now, though, our primary focus is memory.[13]

Defining mindfulness in terms of psychedelic space helps us see how the notion of memory is deeply and intricately embedded in the notion of mindfulness and the practice of meditation. With respect to hidden memories of past events, shifting one's trait deeper into psychedelic space increases one's ability to 'remember and recollect what was done and said long ago'. This is clearly in alignment with the first part of Buddha's definition of mindfulness. However, the connection with memory is broader than this. This is because we don't just remember events; we also remember ideas, principles, lessons learned, plans of action, etc.—even ways of being. All of these things also tend to become easier to call to mind when one's origin shifts deeper into psychedelic space. Correspondingly, mindfulness increases. The Buddhist scholar, Bruce Alan Wallace, has noted this more general connection with memory:

> In addition to its connotation of 'retrospective memory', *sati* also refers to 'prospective memory', which enables us to remember to do things in the present and future [. . .].
>
> Wallace 2006, p. 61

Understood this way, increases in mindfulness can have practical benefits. However, many Buddhists believe that the full import of mindfulness only comes from its integration with the rest of Buddhist practice (particularly the Noble Eightfold Path). As Thanissaro argues:

> [. . .] the practice of mindfulness is most fruitful when informed by the Buddha's own definition of right mindfulness and his explanations of its role on the path. As he defined the term, right mindfulness (*sammá-sati*) is not bare attention. Instead, it's a faculty of active memory, adept at calling to mind and keeping in mind instructions and intentions that will be useful on the path. Its role is to draw on right view and to work proactively in supervising the other factors of the path to give rise to right concentration, and in using right concentration as a basis for total release.
>
> Thānissaro 2012, p. 7[14]

---

[13] As an aside, it is worth noting that there is a method for improving access to memories that is similar to mindfulness and has also been observed to have positive effects of mindfulness. This is the *method of loci*—or the "memory palace" method—and has been observed to be an effective method for mood regulation among depressed subjects (Dalgleish et al. 2013, Werner-Seidler and Dalgleish 2016). This method is somewhat like mindfulness in that it enhances access to memories, but one important difference is that the method of loci is used to recall content-specific items (for example, mood-lifting memories), whereas mindfulness is not. As mentioned in the main text, mindfulness is also more than just remembering past events—for example, it also involves lucid awareness of one's present sensations.

[14] *Right view* and *right concentration* are two other elements of the Noble Eightfold Path. Roughly speaking, having right view involves being aware of the consequences of one's thoughts and actions,

As mindfulness increases, alternative ways of being become more available—forgotten ones are remembered and new ones are therefore also more easily developed using remembered instructions and intentions (see also Levman 2017).

What about the strong emphasis on seeing things as they are, with lucid awareness? This is the second part of Buddha's definition of mindfulness. This aspect of mindfulness is also captured in terms of shifting one's trait deeper into psychedelic space, but this time with respect to the dimension of clarity (particularly the lack of distortion). We can also see this in Bodhi's discussion of this aspect of mindfulness:

> Nevertheless, despite my reservations about the use of 'bare attention' as an alternative expression for *sati*, if we consider how mindfulness is to be practiced in the system laid down in the *Satipatthána Sutta*, we can find considerable support for the idea that the initial task of *sati* is to 'keep to a bare registering of the facts observed' as free as possible from distorting conceptual elaborations. The problem, as I see it, is not with conceptualization itself, but with conceptualization that ascribes erroneous attributes to the objects and the experiential act itself.
>
> Bodhi 2011, p. 32

In other words, the point is not just to be able to call things to awareness and hold them there, but also to be able to see them clearly, as they truly are. It's this aspect of mindfulness that the clarity dimension of psychedelic space captures.

Overall, it looks like the concept of mindfulness can be usefully illuminated in terms of shifting one's trait deeper into psychedelic space. We also see, now, how the memory aspect of mindfulness relates to the cognitive flexibility and stability that meditation is said to develop. The flexibility is the ability to bring things to awareness as they are needed or desired, due to a shift of one's trait along the dimensions of scope, clarity, and novelty. And the stability involves the ability to hold these things in awareness, due to a shift in one's trait along the duration dimension of psychedelic space.[15]

To summarize, just as we have reason to expect meditation to have observable effects on attention, we also have reason to expect that meditation should have observable effects on memory. Obviously, the above discussion of mindfulness has landed on some grander themes, such as one's progression along the path of enlightenment, and such topics are not yet well studied by cognitive science. Nevertheless, the discussion has also involved more measurable predictions. For

---

and having right concentration involves maintaining focused attention in a way that leads to certain states of absorption known as *jhanās*.

[15] Some Buddhists may wish to separate the dimension of duration from the others in this analysis of mindfulness. For them, duration corresponds to the stability of attention that is *samadhi* and mindfulness (*sati*) corresponds to the dimensions of scope, clarity, and novelty.

example, if the practice of meditation increases one's mindfulness, then it should facilitate 'remembering and recollecting what was done and said long ago'. And it turns out that there is a growing body of scientific evidence in support of this, which we will now examine.

Before we dive into that literature, a point of clarification is needed: only part of scientific literature on meditation and memory is relevant to our purposes. This is because memory involves the encoding, consolidation, and retrieval of information, and our focus is just on the *retrieval* aspect of the memory. Many of the studies on meditation and memory focus on encoding and consolidation, or they don't allow us to easily distinguish meditation's effects on them from those it has on retrieval. Since our focus is on whether meditation induces psychedelic experiences with respect to revealing hidden memories, I will limit the discussion to those studies that allow us to clearly discern the effects that meditation has on the retrieval aspect of memory.[16]

One cluster of results, starting with Williams et al. 2000, involves autobiographical memory, depression, and mindfulness-based cognitive therapy (MBCT). Prior research had shown that people suffering from depression tend to have overly general autobiographical memories. That is, when presented with a cue and asked to recall a specific event related to it, depressed subjects tend to only be able to recall minimal summaries of the cued events from their pasts. For example, when presented with the cue 'kindness', someone with depression will tend to give a general response, such as 'my grandmother was always kind to me', rather than mention a more specific event, such as 'my grandmother complimented me on my artwork one afternoon'. In terms of psychedelic space, these memories are low in clarity because they lack specificity.[17] Williams et al. 2000 hypothesized that 8 weeks of MBCT, which involves focused-attention and open-monitoring meditation, should increase memory specificity. One reason they gave for this expectation was as follows:

> MBCT explicitly focuses on allowing mental contents to occur without judging them or trying to suppress or avoid them, thus potentially reducing the tendency to truncate the memory retrieval process as a means of regulating affect.
> Williams et al. 2000, p. 151

In line with this expectation, Williams et al. found that the MBCT programme increased memory specificity. This fits well with the hypothesis that meditation can help make autobiographical recollections more mind-revealing by increasing their clarity (with respect to detail).

---

[16] The reader who is interested in the general effects that meditation has on memory may wish to see Levi and Rosenstreich 2019 for a comprehensive review.

[17] Memory specificity is also referred to as *memory precision* (e.g. Berens et al. 2020).

In a later study, Hargus et al. 2010 investigated whether 8 weeks of MBCT would increase the specificity of memories that depressed patients had of their last *crisis day*, which was defined as the last day they felt suicidal or wanted to harm themselves. Subjects were randomly assigned to a group that received MBCT in conjunction with treatment as usual (TAU) or a TAU-only group. MBCT had a non-significant increase in memory specificity, but the TAU-only group had a significant decrease, resulting in a significant difference between the two groups. Although this study didn't show an *increase* in specificity due to MBCT, the results of the study indicate that the MBCT prevented a decrease in specificity.

In another related study, Heeren et al. 2009 found that MBCT increased memory specificity for non-depressed subjects (compared to matched controls). They modified the MBCT programme to remove depression-related content and found that the modified training resulted in a significant increase in memory specificity as well as an increase in cognitive flexibility, which partially mediated the increase in memory specificity. Their proposed explanation for the effect is that overly-general memory is more cognitively accessible than specific information because it automatically attracts and captures attentional resources and, by increasing cognitive flexibility, MBCT reduces this automatic capturing of attentional resources, freeing them up to uncover more specific memories. Heeren et al.'s observed effect and their proposed explanation for it fit well with the hypothesis that meditation helps make autobiographical recollections more psychedelic (as a result of increased mindfulness) by increasing their clarity with respect to detail, as well as the hypothesis that meditation achieves this by increasing the control and efficiency of attentional resource allocation.[18]

Another cluster of results centres around a study by Wagstaff et al. 2004a, which examined whether a short session of focused-attention meditation would improve the recollection of details involving the funeral of Princess Diana, an event that took place 5 years before the date of the study. Subjects were assigned to four groups: meditation with and without eyes closed, and no meditation with and without eyes closed. In the meditation conditions, subjects were given 1.5 minutes of focused-breathing meditation instruction and were asked to continue this breathing exercise while they answered questions about the funeral. Wagstaff et al. found that the meditators recalled more correct details and fewer incorrect ones than the non-meditators. The effect was also stronger for the eyes-closed group.

Several other studies have also found that the same focused-attention meditation intervention can enhance memory recollection. Wagstaff et al. 2004b found that the intervention improved subjects' recognition of faces they had been shown

---

[18] Rice et al. 2015 found the same effect in a group of young adolescents but it was not statistically significant. Also see Dominguez et al. 2022 for a recent review of the relationship between mindfulness and specificity of autobiographical memories.

10 minutes prior to the meditation session. Hammond et al. 2006 also found that the same focused-attention meditation intervention improved recollection of a 30-second film that the subjects had seen two days earlier. Wagstaff et al. 2011 found similar effects and, moreover, that focused-attention meditation reduced the errors caused by the deliberate introduction of misinformation by experimenters. This suggests that meditation not only increases access to one's memories, but also that it reduces the distortions of memories that would occur otherwise. Overall, these results indicate that a short session of focused-attention meditation can improve access to memories by increasing the scope and/or clarity of recollective experiences.

These two clusters of results support the hypothesis that we are considering: that meditation can reveal the mind by revealing hidden memories. A third cluster of results stems from an initial study that indicated that meditation doesn't always have a positive effect on memory. Wilson et al. 2015 found that 15 minutes of meditation increased DRM false memories while leaving correct recalls unchanged. They described the form of meditation they studied as "mindfulness meditation", which they defined as focusing attention on one's breath without judgement (p. 1568) and which can therefore be understood as a form of focused-attention meditation. However, they also describe their "mindfulness meditation" intervention as observing without judgement or reaction whatever comes to mind (p. 1571), which is a form of open-monitoring meditation. Therefore, it isn't entirely clear what kind of meditation was used, but it was likely a *vipassanā*-like mixture of focused-attention and open-monitoring meditation. At any rate, one important point about the meditation session was that it was conducted *before* the encoding of the experiment, and so it is possible that the meditation session impaired the encoding process rather than the retrieval process. Indeed, this is what Wilson et al. originally hypothesized—that the non-judgemental aspect of meditation should make subjects less discerning between mental content resulting from external stimulation and mental content that is internally generated.

Following up on this result, Calvillo et al. 2018 examined the effect that 3 minutes of mindfulness meditation had on DRM false memory rates when it was conducted before and after encoding (just prior to retrieval). They found that when the meditation was conducted before encoding, there was no effect on false memory rates, conflicting with the result of Wilson et al. 2015. One possible explanation for the conflicting results was that Calvillo et al. only used 3 minutes of meditation, whereas Wilson et al. used 15 minutes. So it could be that 3 minutes is not enough to generate an effect. However, Calvillo et al. also observed that 3 minutes of mindfulness *after* encoding resulted in a *decrease* in false memory rates. This suggests that 3 minutes is indeed enough to have an effect, which fits well with earlier studies that relied on only 1.5 minutes of focused-attention meditation.[19] Calvillo et al.'s results therefore give further support to the hypothesis that meditation enhances the ability to remember—this time by reducing distortions of the recollective experience and thus increasing its clarity.

Although our focus is on the effects that meditation has on retrieval, it is worth noting that it could be objected that while 3 minutes are enough to have an effect on retrieval, they are not enough to have an effect on encoding. However, Baranski and Was 2017 sought to directly replicate Wilson et al.'s study, using 15 minutes of the same meditation instruction prior to encoding, and found no increase in false memory rates. It is also worth noting that Shah and Knott 2018 found that *dividing* attention at recall increased false memories on the DRM paradigm. While this was not a study on meditation, it fits well with the other studies that show the focusing attention at recall reduces false memories. More recently, Sherman and Grange 2020 and Wendt et al. 2021 both failed to replicate Wilson et al.'s result after introducing several methodological improvements to the experimental design. Again, in both studies, the meditation session occurred before encoding, not after. Overall, these new results indicate that the Wilson et al. 2015 original result doesn't replicate and that meditation after encoding and just prior to retrieval may improve the ability to remember.

Altogether, we have three clusters of results that support the hypothesis that meditation can reveal the mind by revealing hidden memories. MBCT programmes appear to increase scope and/or clarity of memory recollections; a short session of focused-attention meditation appears to also increase the scope and clarity of recollections of both recent and old memories; and a few minutes of mindfulness meditation appears to enhance the clarity of recollective experiences, thus making people less susceptible to DRM false memories.[20] Therefore, things are looking good for the hypothesis; however, we should keep in mind that the research is still young and undeveloped[21] and hardly spans the range of effects that meditation may have on memory recollections. The above discussion is also not a comprehensive review of the literature on meditation and memory (for such a review, see Levi and Rosenstreich 2019). There are several other studies that have observed positive effects of meditation on memory[22] but some suggest these positive effects are not universal, especially when encoding effects are accounted for (Crawley 2015, Konjedi and Maleeh 2020). However, these studies often don't

---

[19] Lloyd et al. 2016 also found a similar effect, but they didn't use the DRM paradigm.

[20] It is not clear how much effects involving the DRM paradigm represent real-life cases of false memory (Ost et al. 2013), so we should be careful not to conclude that meditation reduces false memories in general.

[21] For example, to be more confident in the drawn conclusions, we would need to have replication studies that include active control conditions.

[22] For example, Vugt et al. 2012, Lykins et al. 2012, Xu et al. 2014, Boccia et al. 2015, Brown et al. 2016, Rosenstreich 2016, Alberts et al. 2017, Rosenstreich and Ruderman 2017, Kral et al. 2018, Basso et al. 2019, Nyhus et al. 2019, and Nyhus et al. 2020.

allow us to easily separate the effects that meditation may have on encoding and consolidation from those it may have on retrieval.

Curiously, so far there has been little research on meditation and involuntary autobiographical memories (IAMs), despite the growing literature on this kind of memory recollection and attention (Section 6.2) and meditation's known effects on focused and diffused attention (Chapter 5). Nevertheless, the concepts that researchers are using to study IAMs are very close to those used to describe focused-attention and open-monitoring meditation. For instance, Barzykowski et al. 2019 draw a distinction between *intention* and *monitoring*. Intention, in their usage, is the intention to retrieve a memory that matches a specific cue, which they argue narrows the range of memory content that can be reported. Monitoring, on the other hand, involves watching the stream of consciousness and looking for contents that match certain requirements—for example, a memory that arose involuntarily. Based on their results involving these concepts, Barzykowski et al. argue that:

> [...] intention and monitoring are two main mechanisms of autobiographical memory retrieval which, by lowering the awareness threshold, influence the frequency of retrieving highly vs poorly accessible memories. Put differently, intention and monitoring are cognitive tools that enhance access to memories with low levels of accessibility.
>
> Barzykowski et al. 2019, p. 44

While intention and monitoring are distinct from focused-attention and open-monitoring meditation, we can see how they are closely related. Open-monitoring meditation should develop one's ability to monitor for involuntary autobiographical memories (and other mental contents), and focused-attention meditation should develop one's ability to focus attentional resources on memory contents that match a given cue. To date, studies have not yet been done to confirm this— although there is some anecdotal evidence that meditation can uncover deeply buried memories of traumatic life events (Miller 1983). Interestingly, Fujino et al. 2018 found that open-monitoring meditation reduces the involvement of brain regions in memory function in such a way that suggests that it increases detachment from a spontaneously arising autobiographical memory. In line with this result, Isham et al. 2022 found that an online version of MBSR programme resulted in increases in non-reactivity to involuntary and voluntary autobiographical memories.

Overall, more research is clearly needed, but the available evidence suggests that meditation may help make memory recollections more psychedelic and/or bring about recollective psychedelic experiences that are more psychedelic than regular memory recollections. In addition to improving the efficiency and control over the allocation of attentional resources, it appears that meditation can also facilitate the retrieval of memories. It does this by bringing more memories into awareness than would otherwise be possible, or by bringing them into awareness more clearly by enhancing the detail of recollections and by reducing the mind's tendency to generate false memories and details.

6.4 Psychedelics

Let's now see if there is any reason to think that psychedelics reveal the mind by revealing hidden memories. Recall that this is an important test case for the general hypothesis that psychedelics induce mind-revealing experiences. The revelation of hidden memories is perhaps the best place to consider when searching for clear empirical evidence in favour of this hypothesis. This is because it is difficult in general to objectively determine whether something was already present in the mind prior to it appearing in conscious experience. For example, while some creative ideas may be generated and incubated outside of awareness (Chapter 8), some ideas may be generated in the very moment we become aware of them. In contrast, because memories have external checks—that is, they should line up with past events to some degree—it is easier to evaluate whether a particular memory recollection is a genuine recollection or a confabulation created in the moment. As we saw in the previous section, one can design experiments to test whether a particular intervention (in that case, meditation) can improve memory recall.

However, whereas the case for meditation revealing hidden memories is fairly strong (keeping in mind that the research is still nascent), the case for psychedelics having this effect is less clear. This is in part due to the fact that the effects of psychedelics are much more uncontrollable in nature. For example, while it is fairly straightforward to have someone complete a DRM task after having meditated, it is much more difficult to have them perform such a task when emotionally charged mental contents are flooding their conscious experience—as often happens during psychedelic sessions. As many authors have noted, the contents that psychedelics tend to reveal (if this is what they, in fact, do) tend to be highly personal in nature and tied to the individual's motivations and life history. This makes it more difficult (though not impossible) to test the hypothesis that psychedelics reveal hidden memories.

Another difference between psychedelics and meditation in this respect is that we have lacked a strong theoretical reason to expect that psychedelics reveal hidden memories. Whereas with meditation, there is good theoretical reason to think that it will facilitate access to hidden memories (via its association with mindfulness and attention), we have lacked the same kind of theoretical basis for expecting that psychedelics may reveal hidden memories. And since research is often guided by theory, this may be another reason why we lack the appropriate studies.[23] However, given what we know about involuntary autobiographical memories (IAMs) and their relationship with attention (from Section 6.2), it seems we should be able to start building such a case for psychedelics and explain why they would reveal hidden memories.

For instance, recall Barzykowski and Staugaard's threshold hypothesis for IAMs. The central idea behind this hypothesis is that there is a threshold of accessibility that memories must pass before they can enter awareness as recollective experiences. The accessibility of a memory is determined by several factors, such as its recency, the unusualness of the event that it is about, how often it is rehearsed, and whether it has been cued by a stimulus. Based on this hypothesis, IAMs should tend to be memories that are generally high in accessibility and therefore need only a small increase in activation to get them over the threshold and into awareness. Combined with the Osmond-Grof hypothesis that psychedelics amplify elements of the unconscious, this would suggest that we should see more IAMs appear in awareness during psychedelic sessions. Moreover, it would also suggest that such memories would normally be lower in accessibility if psychedelics are causing substantial amplifications. In other words, if psychedelics are substantially amplifying unconscious memories, then we should see some that are far below the threshold of accessibility suddenly appear in awareness during psychedelic trips. Such memories should fit a low-accessibility profile—for example, they are not often rehearsed, not easily cued, old, and perhaps repressed or suppressed. In addition, it seems we should also expect that psychedelics not only get some memories past the threshold and into awareness, but they also push some memories *way* past the threshold, so that they appear more vividly and fully in awareness than memories normally do.

A similar argument can be put forward if we use the attentional resource interpretation of the Osmond-Grof hypothesis (Chapter 5), which says that by disrupting the attentional system, psychedelics free up attentional resources for reallocation throughout the mind. Recall that one of the main drivers of IAMs is the distribution of attentional resources. A natural prediction, then, is that if more attentional resources are free to be allocated to memories that exist below the threshold of accessibility for awareness, then some of them may be sufficiently activated to pass the threshold for awareness. That is, if psychedelics free up attentional resources, then we should see more memories receive more attentional resources and, thus, more of them making it past the accessibility threshold and into awareness. Similarly, we should see some memories appear more vividly and completely in awareness than they otherwise would.

---

[23] Of course, the situation is changing rapidly as psychedelics research accelerates. However, while proposals about psychedelics have existed since the 1950s and 1960s (e.g. psycholytic therapy), it is only fairly recently that we've began to see accounts, such as the REBUS model (Carhart-Harris and Friston 2019), that connect the pharmacological action of psychedelics with their psychological and phenomenological effects by way of a general theory.

We saw earlier, in Chapter 3, what such an experience would look like in de Quincey's description of his experiences with opium:

> The minutest incidents of childhood, or forgotten scenes of later years, were often revived: I could not be said to recollect them; for if I had been told of them when waking, I should not have been able to acknowledge them as parts of my past experience. But placed as they were before me, in dreams like intuitions, and clothed in all their evanescent circumstances and accompanying feelings, I *recognized* them instantaneously. [...] Of this at least I feel assured, that there is no such thing as *forgetting* possible to the mind [...].
>
> Quincey 1821, p. 581

Although opium is not normally considered a psychedelic, this is the sort of memory-revealing experience that we should expect to see from psychedelics if the threshold and Osmond-Grof hypotheses are true. We see that old memories that de Quincey could not have recollected otherwise appeared in vivid detail in his experience. Moreover, this appears to have happened so regularly that he became convinced that forgetting is impossible. In the language of cognitive science, this corresponds to the idea that memories are always *available* and merely become *inaccessible*. While such an extreme statement is likely false, the essential idea is that we can, in principle, remember much more than we think we can. And certain substances, such as opium, may make it easier to recall memories that we normally would find difficult or impossible to recollect.

Reports that psychedelics, such as LSD and psilocybin, have such effects on memory are widespread in the literature on psychedelic-assisted psychotherapy. For example, it was observed early on that LSD can facilitate the recollection of childhood memories:

> One of the striking things about LSD treatment is the way in which the majority of the patients regress into childhood and appear to remember things which were apparently forgotten. In a number of cases it has been possible to ascertain from other sources that the events described by the patient did, in fact, happen, and this has been confirmed by some of my colleagues.
>
> Sandison 1959, p. 498

Not only are the memories revived by the psychedelic, but they are reanimated in particularly vivid and detailed form (Sandison et al. 1954, Frederking 1955). Moreover, as Sandison 1959 reported, in some cases, their accuracy can also be objectively verified. Consider, for example, Grof's account of a parent reacting to her daughter's childhood memory being revealed during an LSD treatment session:

Dana, a patient with rather severe and complicated neurotic symptomatology, relived in one of her LSD sessions a traumatic episode from infancy that she tentatively located at the end of her first year of life. She described in great detail the interior of the room where this event happened to the point of being able to draw the elaborate pattern of embroidery on the bedspread and tablecloth. Dana's mother was independently asked to give her description of the room in question. When confronted with the material from the patient, she was absolutely astonished by the accuracy of the account concerning the traumatic event as well as its physical setting. Like many other parents confronted with such relivings, she found the idea of her daughter's having such reliable access to the circumstances of her early childhood rather startling and embarrassing. It activated in her strong guilt feelings and a tendency to apologetic explanations. She could not understand the mechanism by which this early memory was recovered. The description of the room was photographically accurate, even in the most minute detail, and its authenticity was unquestionable because of the very unusual character of the furniture and some of the objects involved. The room had a mirror of quite extraordinary design, the crucifix on the wall was an unusual piece of work, and the embroidery and furniture had very specific features. In this case, there did not seem to exist a possibility that this information could have been transmitted by some other means. Before the patient was two years old, the family left this house; shortly afterward, it was condemned and torn down. The interior decoration of the room was not part of their new life; Dana's mother gave away many of the things that formed the setting of the relived incident. There were no photographs of the room or of any of the described pieces, and the mother did not remember ever having mentioned any of the objects in front of the patient.

Grof 1975, pp. 65–6

Indeed, this effect that psychedelics can have on memory would naturally explain some of the therapeutic benefits of psychedelics. Although their psychotherapeutic value is multifaceted, their tendency to promote the recollection of old memories appears to be a noteworthy component of their psychotherapeutic profile. For example, the uncovering of such memories may bring about a cathartic release of emotion, or it may provide valuable information about the past that would be difficult or even impossible to obtain otherwise. This natural fit with psychotherapy and the psychotherapeutic value of psychedelics suggests that psychedelics may reliably reveal hidden memories.

Reports of similar experiences can also be found outside of the psychotherapy literature. For example, in one of the earliest studies on whether psychedelics enhance creative problem-solving, Harman et al. 1966 reported that some subjects experienced unusual recollections of previously acquired knowledge:

[... It] brought about almost total recall of a course that I had had in thermody-
namics; something that I had never given any thought about in years.

Harman et al. 1966, p. 18

If such an effect can be reliably induced, then a practical consequence is that
psychedelics may enhance creative problem-solving by enhancing access to parts
of one's knowledge base that are usually hidden from conscious access.

Let's take stock. Overall, the anecdotal evidence suggests that psychedelics
induce psychedelic experiences in which hidden memories are revealed. Moreover, such experiences appear to score higher than usual with respect to the
dimensions of psychedelic space. This is perhaps most obviously so with respect
to the dimension of novelty, since psychedelics seem to be uncovering deeply
buried memories. However, it also appears that scope and clarity are high, given
the remarkable amount of information contained in the experiences. And duration
also seems to be high, given that the experiences can be reported with sufficient
precision and detail to allow for verification. However, we should be careful in
thinking that such effects are uniform. At the very least, there appears to be some
variation in clarity with respect to distortion since the memories often appear in
alternative representational forms. For example:

A patient often re-experienced repressed events with such vividness and force
that they were described as having been 'relived'; at the same time, he could
witness these incidents with some detachment. Occasionally, the patient could
recognize his problems even when they appeared in symbolic form. More frequently it was necessary to interpret the unconscious material as it arose. Such
interpretations, which in conventional psychotherapy might have had devastat-
ing effects, appeared to be accepted without difficulty.

Eisner and Cohen 1959, p. 617

In such cases—in which the memories appear in symbolic form and require
interpretation—it seems that the memories are revealed with less clarity than they
could be otherwise.

Although the anecdotal evidence that psychedelics can reveal hidden memories
is quite compelling, it should be emphasized that it *is* anecdotal and, because
of this, there are many important questions left unanswered. For instance, we
don't know *how often* psychedelic-assisted psychotherapy sessions produce these
revealed-memory experiences. Perhaps for every session like the one reported in
the earlier quote by Grof, there are hundreds of other sessions during which no
genuine memories are revealed. While Sandison and Grof informally report that
memory-revealing experiences are common, we currently lack good, objective
measures of their true frequency.

One noteworthy study in this direction involved a small trial of LSD-supported psychotherapy by Busch and Johnson 1950. They reported that 5 out of 8 patients experienced LSD-enhanced access to apparent memories. Below are their notes on the 5 patients:

- Patient 22: She was able to recall her childhood vividly.
- Patient 24: Better able to talk about her early life. Showed some regressive behavior and seemed to re-live childhood experiences.
- Patient 26: Relived traumatic episodes of childhood.
- Patient 27: Relived traumatic episodes of childhood. Previous amytal interviews had failed. This patient has 120 hours of therapy.
- Patient 28: Relived disturbing Navy experience. Previous attempts at narcosynthesis were only partially successful.

Again, this is suggestive, but the trial was clearly quite limited. The sample size was small, there was no control group, and all of the subjects were suffering from serious psychological distress, so we don't know how the supposed effect generalizes to healthy subjects.

It is also worth noting that there is some evidence against the hypothesis. Langs 1967 investigated the effect of LSD on the earliest memories subjects were able to recollect. At the beginning of the study, he asked subjects to describe their earliest memories, and then split the subjects into two groups: one receiving LSD and the other a placebo. Langs then asked subjects to describe their earliest memories again, and found that there was little difference between the two groups with respect to the number of subjects who reported new memories. Langs also found that subjects who had stronger reactions to the LSD were more likely to recollect a new earliest memory. Although there wasn't a corresponding correlation for placebo reactions, there was no statistical difference between those subjects who had a strong reaction to the LSD and placebo group.[24]

Another important question is how often the memories are of events that actually happened and how often they are false memories: fantasies that only *seem* like memories. As mentioned in Section 6.2, we know that false memories can occur even when psychedelic substances are not involved, so it is reasonable to expect that they will also occur during psychedelic-assisted psychotherapy sessions. There is also the concern that psychedelics may cause the frequency of such false memories to *increase*. Again, although Sandison and Grof report that some of the memories can be objectively verified, we don't know how many *other* cases involved memories that could not be verified—because they were

---

[24] To complicate matters further, LSD did have a significant effect on the *character* of the recollective experiences, which Langs characterized as an increase in regressive features and disorganized content.

fantasies of events that never happened. This concern is highlighted further by the fact that it is not uncommon for patients to report remembering being born or even remembering previous lives (Grof 1975). While one may wish to be open-minded about such reports, they certainly don't fit well with cognitive science, and so one might reasonably choose to be suspicious about them. For all we know, psychedelic-induced recollections of real memories may be the exception rather than the norm.

These concerns are especially important to address given the role that psychedelics are starting to play in psychotherapy. There is a worry, which goes back to at least Jung, that many of the traumatic memories uncovered during regular psychotherapy are actually false memories (Loftus 1993). It is worth noting that there is some evidence in support of this worry. For example, Clancy et al. 2000 found that subjects who reported recovered memories of childhood sexual abuse were more susceptible to DRM false memories. Geraerts et al. 2005 replicated this effect and found that the *fantasy-proneness* of subjects was more predictive of it than their self-reports of traumatization. However, consistent with these results is the possibility that increased susceptibility to DRM false memories and fantasy-proneness is a *consequence* of trauma. It is also not clear how, or even if, tendencies toward false memories under one paradigm generalize to other paradigms or to real-world memories (Patihis et al. 2018). So, this evidence is far from definitive.[25] Nevertheless, it is a distinct possibility that false memories are sometimes "uncovered" during regular psychotherapy, and the concern is that psychedelics may exacerbate this problem—for example, because of their tendency to increase suggestibility (Hartogsohn 2018).

In this regard, it should be noted that Speth et al. 2016 found that LSD resulted in fewer spontaneous mentations involving the past compared to placebos. This would seem to contradict the anecdotal evidence mentioned above. However, Speth et al. note that the conditions of their study design differ from those of typical psychedelic-therapy context, which may naturally prime subjects to orient their attention to the past. In short, we need randomized, double-blind, and active placebo-controlled experiments that objectively verify recollection frequencies and accuracies, before we can conclude that psychedelics have some tendency to reveal hidden memories.

Indeed, there is some evidence that psychedelics can make cued autobiographical memory recollections more psychedelic. Carhart-Harris et al. 2012 sought to examine whether psilocybin enhances autobiographical memory recollection. Ten subjects were given cues for memories of specific events in their lives and were given 16 seconds to bring those memories to mind. Afterwards, they were asked

---

[25] Also, even if the recovered memories of trauma are not of real events, they may nonetheless be real in the sense that they are active in the mind, causing real psychological suffering. This was a point that Jung was also aware of: even false traumatic memories may necessitate psychological intervention.

to subjectively rate their experiences with respect to the following properties: how vivid the memories were, how much mental imagery was involved, how emotionally charged they were, and how positive the emotions were. It was found that ratings of vividness and visual imagery were significantly higher under psilocybin than the placebo condition (of the within-subjects design). These increases suggest that psilocybin increased the scope and/or clarity of the recollective experiences. Notably, Carhart-Harris et al. also included a qualitative report that suggests that psilocybin may have also increased the *novelty* of recollections:

> I think my imagination had a lot to do with it last time [under psilocybin], but it seemed more vivid and real . . . I was more attached to the images and putting myself in the scenario than I was today. Today [in the placebo condition] it was like . . . I was thinking about it, it was nice, but it was nothing special—*nothing new came out of it*.
>
> Carhart-Harris et al. 2012, p. 242 (emphasis added)

Although this study moves us closer to having the kind of evidence we need, there are still several important limitations that future studies will need to address.

Another suggestive but indirect line of evidence comes from what we know about depression and memory. People with depression have been observed to have memories that are lower in specificity (Brown and Kulik 1977, Hermans et al. 2004), which is a way for the recollective experiences to lack clarity. Since psychedelics appear to be effective in treating depression, it's reasonable to expect that they may also thereby increase the specificity of memory recollections.

Finally, it should be noted that some other studies have examined the effects of psychedelics on memory, but they focused on the effects of the drug-induced state on encoding and retrieval together (Savage 1952, Sloane and Doust 1954, Jarvik et al. 1955, Doss et al. 2018). The problem with this is that while there is reason to expect that psychedelics will help with retrieval (at least, for certain kinds of memory), there is less reason to think that they will help with encoding (and they may even impair it). So, these studies don't quite target the hypothesis under consideration here—that is, whether psychedelics can improve access to memories that have been encoded *prior* to their administration.

Overall, the available evidence tentatively suggests that psychedelics reveal hidden memories and make memory recollections more psychedelic, but the research in this particular area is still nascent.[26] Also, based on what we know about attention and the accessibility of autobiographical memories, we have some theoretical reason to expect this—that is, if the Osmond-Grof hypothesis correct, and especially if the attentional-resource version is correct. With that said, it's

---

[26] Healy 2021 gives a review of the literature, including qualitative studies of follow-up interviews, and comes to a similar conclusion.

important to remember to keep these two issues—the effect and the process—distinct. Psychedelics may have the effect of revealing hidden memories but not do so via the process of amplifying unconscious currents of the mind or by freeing up the usual allocation of attentional resources. The most important issue, for the purposes of this book, is that of the *effect*, since it pertains to the hypothesis of whether psychedelics cause psychedelic experiences. The issue of the process by which they may deliver this effect is subsidiary in this respect.

While the case for the hypothesis that psychedelics reveal hidden memories looks promising, it is clear that more experimental work needs to be done before we can safely draw this conclusion. In particular, we need randomized double-blind controlled experiments that verify how frequently the memories that are allegedly revealed are real and not mere fantasies. This is especially important to establish given the role that psychedelics play in the psychotherapy. If it turns out that the alleged memories can rarely be verified—or significantly less so than the memories revealed by other methods—then this would be a sign that psychedelics do not reveal hidden memories, and are generating fantasies instead (which may nevertheless have psychotherapeutic value).[27]

6.5 Conclusion

A central idea of this chapter—and indeed of this book—is that the experience of remembering can be a *psychedelic* experience. This happens when the thing being remembered is *hidden*, such that it is difficult to retrieve, or is unlikely to appear in awareness involuntarily. The clearest examples of this are those occasions when a long-lost memory from childhood floods your conscious experience after being triggered by a rare taste or aroma in your environment. A famous example of this is Proust's flashback to his childhood times at Combray after tasting a tea-soaked madeleine. Such an experience is a *spontaneous* psychedelic experience, in which a hidden memory is revealed.

Another central idea is that the consumption of certain substances tends to make these experiences temporarily *more frequent* and/or *more psychedelic*. And if the consumption of a given substance tends to have this effect, then it earns some right to be called a 'psychedelic'. As we've seen, there is a lot of anecdotal evidence that substances such as LSD and psilocybin have this effect, especially within a psychotherapeutic context. These substances may also have other effects that could help them earn the right to be called 'psychedelic'—such as facilitating

---

[27] It's possible that people have hidden false memories and psychedelics reveal those more often than they reveal hidden true memories. Although this is a possibility that could be used to explain away a failure to objectively verify the supposed memories, we would need some independent evidence or reason in support of it.

emotional insights—but at least in this respect of revealing hidden memories, their name may be well-earned.

However, as we've seen, we should be careful in the conclusions we draw and how confidently we draw them. We do not yet have evidence that definitively shows that psychedelics reveal *real* hidden memories. It may be that many of the supposed memories being revealed are merely fantasies that seem like real memories. We know that people are susceptible to false memories during normal circumstances, and many of the strange reports from psychedelic-assisted psychotherapy—remembering previous lives, for example—suggest that psychedelics may exacerbate this tendency. Moreover, even when real memories are being revealed, they may nevertheless be laced with elements of fantasy. As such, although psychedelics may reveal deeply hidden memories, they may do so with *low clarity*—in the sense that errors of commission are present in the experience.

In contrast, we have seen that there is reason to think that the practice of meditation will tend to reveal hidden memories with high clarity. Roughly speaking, meditation cultivates *mindfulness*, which is the ability to bring things to mind, to hold them there, and to see them as they truly are. Remembering is one way of bringing something to mind, and we've seen empirical evidence that meditation helps people to do this. We've also seen that meditation helps people be less susceptible to false memory effects, which is one particular way of seeing things as they are. We didn't examine whether meditation helps people hold things in mind, since this effect is not essential to our main concern (of whether meditation reveals hidden memories). However, there is evidence that meditation has this effect as well. In terms of cognitive science, an improvement in the ability to hold things in mind would be an improvement in working memory, and there is evidence that meditation results in such improvements (Zeidan et al. 2010, Quach et al. 2016, Jha et al. 2019, Zanesco et al. 2019).[28] In short, while more research needs to be done, the empirical evidence that we have so far lines up neatly with the hypothesis that meditation reveals hidden memories—as well as the theory for why it does.

Our primary concern has been with the *effects* that psychedelics and meditation have on the mind since our focus is on the phenomenon of psychedelic experience and the circumstances under which it can happen. However, it also makes sense for us to consider the *processes or mechanisms* by which psychedelics and meditation may have these effects. In the case of meditation, it seems clear that many of its effects are achieved via an improvement in *attention*—by increasing the control one has over the allocation of attentional resource, or by increasing the efficiency

---

[28] One result that may point in the opposite direction is Baranski and Was 2018. However, see Jha et al. 2019 for discussion. Also, see Dreyfus 2011 who predicted, based on his understanding of mindfulness that goes beyond the bare attention definition, that cultivating mindfulness should improve working memory.

of its allocation. As I proposed in the previous chapter, new insights may be gained by thinking of the effects of psychedelics in similar terms. Briefly said, by "loosening up" the mind, psychedelics may free up attentional resources and make them more available for allocation to parts of the mind that would not normally receive them. If this is correct, the result would be more elements of the mind being sufficiently activated so that they appear in awareness and/or appear more vividly in awareness. In the specific case of hidden memories being thus revealed by psychedelics, this hypothesis fits well the research on attention and involuntary and autobiographical memories (for example, Barzykowski et al. 2019).[29]

To sum up, we can tentatively draw the following conclusions. Psychedelic experiences involving revelations of hidden memories can happen spontaneously, but they seem to be rare and typically not very psychedelic (experiences like those of Proust's are the exceptions that prove the rule). Psychedelics appear to temporarily make these experiences happen more frequently. They also seem to make these experiences *much more* psychedelic—in the sense that they are more revealing of our hidden memories. However, although psychedelics may bring about experiences with increased scope, novelty, and duration, there is an important concern that clarity is decreased. This concern is plausible given what we know about false memories, and it is not yet ruled out by the empirical evidence. Finally, meditation also appears to give us better access to our hidden memories. In the short term, this increase in access will manifest as psychedelic experiences. In the long term, the memories in question will no longer be hidden, and so the experience of them appearing in awareness will no longer count as being psychedelic. However, the individual in question will have become *more mindful*. In terms of the framework of psychedelic space, this means their default state will have moved deeper into psychedelic space, by moving out along each of the four dimensions of scope, novelty, duration, and clarity.

[29] It should be stressed, however, that there may also be *other* processes or mechanisms in operation. For example, MDMA, which is sometimes considered a psychedelic, appears to reveal traumatic hidden memories by blunting their emotional intensity, thus making it easier for people to engage with them. It's likely, therefore, that psychedelics in general achieve their mind-revealing effects by multiple processes and mechanisms. The same is probably also true for meditation, which is known to promote relaxation and improve the regulation of emotions.

7

Hallucinations

7.1 Introduction

In the previous chapter, we considered the evidence that psychedelics may reveal the mind by revealing hidden memories. In this chapter, we will examine some evidence that may initially appear to be *against* the hypothesis that psychedelics reveal the mind: namely, that psychedelics cause visual hallucinations.[1]

To many readers, the fact that psychedelics cause hallucinations suggests that psychedelics do something other than reveal the mind. One reason for this stems from the fact that the onset of hallucinations can be a sign of an underlying health problem. This can drive the intuition that psychedelic-induced hallucinations are the result of some *deleterious* effect on mind.

A second reason is that psychedelic-induced hallucinations appear to be *additions* to the mind rather than revelations of it. Consider the contrast with hidden memories: a long-lost memory from childhood is something that can be hidden in the mind and potentially revealed during a psychedelic trip.[2] Hallucinations don't appear to be like memories in this regard—they don't seem like the sort of things that are *already* in the mind. Instead, it seems they are *added* to the mind in some way. How those additions are understood will depend on one's general attitude towards psychedelics. To enthusiasts, psychedelic-induced hallucinations can seem as though they are new perceptions of previously hidden elements or aspects of reality. To sceptics, the hallucinations may seem more like delusional fantasies constructed by a disturbed mind. The enthusiasts therefore will be inclined to think that the hallucinations are *world*-revealing rather than mind-revealing.[3] And the sceptics might be inclined to say that the hallucinations are mind-*creating* or mind-*distorting* rather than mind-revealing. Either way, it would seem that the hallucinations involve something other than mind-revelation.

At first glance, these considerations appear to spell trouble for the hypothesis that psychedelics reveal the mind. However, there are ways to save the hypothesis. Recall from Chapter 3 that an experience can be more or less psychedelic by

---

[1] Hallucinations come in different forms (e.g. visual, auditory, and tactile), but in this chapter, I will focus on those that are visual in nature (and refer to them as hallucinations).

[2] Though it should be noted that the storage and retrieval mechanisms are more complex and nuanced than has been traditionally recognized—see Andonovski 2020 for a good discussion of this issue.

[3] For example, we can find this sort of view expressed in Huxley 1954.

varying in terms of its scope, clarity, novelty, and duration. It could be that psychedelics induce experiences that are low in clarity but are still revelatory because they score sufficiently high in terms of scope and novelty so as to compensate for the low clarity. From this perspective, experiences that involve hallucinations may be low in clarity, but nonetheless revelatory because they reveal large swaths of highly novel content. This could be because hallucinations are psychedelic *side effects*, or because there is some in-principle trade-off between clarity and the dimensions of scope and novelty (we will consider this second possibility in more detail in the next section). Whatever the reason may be, the point is that not all of the effects of psychedelics have to be psychedelic in order for the substances to be deserving of their name.

Although this point by itself is sufficient to block the concern, the fact that psychedelics induce hallucinations can actually be used to *support* the hypothesis that psychedelics reveal the mind. In the coming sections, I will argue that some hallucinations are themselves revelations of hidden elements of the mind. For some readers, this idea will seem counterintuitive and perhaps even conceptually impossible, since it would seem to entail that we have *unconscious hallucinations* during everyday experience. However, this is mostly due to an issue of conceptual imprecision—there's a sense in which it isn't true that psychedelics induce hallucinations. To appreciate this point, we need to sort out some basic conceptual issues about hallucinations and whether the visual effects that psychedelics induce are genuinely hallucinatory. This, in turn, will deflate some of the counterintuitiveness of the idea that psychedelic-induced "hallucinations" can themselves be psychedelic. That's the plan for Section 7.2. Then, in Sections 7.3 and 7.4, I will argue that the fact that psychedelics cause a particular kind of hallucination—namely, geometrical patterns of colourful light—is evidence in favour of the hypothesis that psychedelics induce psychedelic experiences.

7.2 Can Hallucinations Be Psychedelic?

It seems obvious that psychedelics induce hallucinations. Indeed, it is often thought that causing hallucinations is the *primary* effect of psychedelics—and for this reason they are frequently referred to as *hallucinogens*. However, such a simple statement only scratches the surface of the visual effects of psychedelics. When we consider them more carefully, we can see that the issue is more complex and nuanced than it may first appear.

For example, consider a common effect of psychedelics: they make the world appear brighter, clearer, more colourful, and more detailed. In short, they make the appearance of the world more *vivid*. Intuitively, such an effect is not a hallucination, and traditional definitions of hallucinations would agree. For example, one such definition says:

Hallucination: you have an experience of a worldly object but there is no corresponding object that you perceive in virtue of having that experience.[4]

Clearly, it is possible to experience the world more vividly than normal without also experiencing any non-existing objects. If anything, this effect may be better classified as an *illusion* rather than a hallucination:

Illusion: you perceive an object but you misperceive one or more of its properties.

However, even this classification is questionable, since it is not clear that experiencing the world more vividly counts as a *misperception* of any object's properties. This is further bolstered by the observation that colour detection (and low-level perception in general) can be left unaffected or potentially even *enhanced* by psychedelics (Chapter 5). The widespread anecdotal reports of psychedelics being used for performance enhancement in extreme sports (Oroc 2011) also suggest that these substances can be used to *enhance* one's perception of the world. Any conclusion from these early anecdotal reports should obviously be only tentative, but they are enough to warrant closer examination.[5]

To further complicate matters, there are visual effects that are not caused by psychedelics that are difficult to classify as hallucinations or illusions. To take an example that will be relevant later on, consider the Hermann grid illusion, depicted in Figure 7.1. The grey blobs you see at the intersections of horizontal and vertical white lines are not real. Seen as objects, they are hallucinatory. Seen as properties

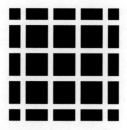

Figure 7.1 The Hermann grid illusion.

---

[4] This definition (and the one of illusion below) is adapted from Macpherson and Batty 2016, p. 265.

[5] One subtlety that I won't go into here but is worth mentioning concerns what we take the objective of the visual system to be. Traditionally (roughly speaking), the objective has been thought to be truth: to see the world as it truly is. However, it is increasingly recognized that the objective of the visual system more concerns enabling good action than it does truth. This view of perception may thus require further distinctions and refinements of our definitions of illusion and hallucination. To take a well-known case to illustrate: Doc Ellis famously pitched a no-hitter on 12 June 1970 while he was on LSD. Pitching a no-hitter is extremely difficult to do, and yet Ellis reported that while he was pitching, the ball appeared to change in size, the home plate umpire appeared as Richard Nixon, and the batter appeared as Jimi Hendrix batting with his guitar. It seems that the LSD may have enhanced his performance despite—or perhaps because of—the hallucinations.

projected into the white lines, they are illusory. This kind of example shows that we should be wary of expecting too much from our definitions of these concepts (Macpherson 2013, pp. 7–8).

Another common effect of psychedelics is that they cause people to experience geometric patterns of colourful light. Typically, these patterns appear during the early stages of a psychedelic trip, or during trips brought about by small doses, and they appear most clearly when one's eyes are closed. It is quite common for these patterns to be referred to as hallucinations. However, it is not clear that they meet the criteria of the above definition of hallucination (or illusion) since the patterns often don't appear as worldly objects. If we want to, we could consider other ways to define what a hallucination is; for example, there is the definition given by the American Psychological Association's *Dictionary of Psychology*:

> **hallucination** *n.* a false sensory perception that has a compelling sense of reality despite the absence of an external stimulus.[6]

However, it is also not clear whether this definition counts the geometric patterns as hallucinations. This is because the patterns may not appear as 'sensory perceptions', and they may also not have 'a compelling sense of reality' to them. Whether they do would seem to depend on the details of the experience—and, in particular, on its *phenomenal transparency/opacity* (Chapter 5). For example, a person may become so immersed in the geometric patterns that they take on a reality of their own. In that case, the experience would be high in phenomenal transparency, and so perhaps the patterns should count as hallucinations. However, another person may have a completely different kind of experience, one that is low in phenomenal transparency: the colourful patterns may be experienced from a detached perspective and have no sense of reality to them—that is, the person easily recognizes the patterns as just a form of mental imagery. For this reason, Metzinger 2003 calls these cases of phenomenally opaque images *pseudohallucinations* (p. 186) to signify the fact that they are not quite hallucinations—at least, according to a definition of hallucination that requires a commitment to the reality of the apparent perceptions. Shanon 2002 also makes a similar point about many of the visual effects of ayahuasca, and the distinction is made earlier in a conceptual analysis of hallucinatory experience by Horowitz 1975.

And so it goes. If we consider even more kinds of apparent hallucinations and even more definitions of hallucination, we arrive at similar results. The upshot is that is not clear whether the various effects caused by psychedelics are genuinely hallucinations. In many cases, the details of the specific experience matter, and it also matters what definition of hallucination we're working with. And so we see that it is a little too simple to say that psychedelics cause hallucinations. It

---

[6] VandenBos 2015, p. 480.

is perhaps better to say that psychedelics tend to increase *mental imagery*, and some cases of mental imagery may count as hallucinations if they meet certain criteria (Nanay 2016b). This general point, I think, deflates much of the counterintuitiveness of the idea that hallucinations could be instances of mind-revelation. Nevertheless, since it is commonplace to refer to these effects as hallucinations, I will continue to follow suit. Whether or not the visual effects are rightly classified as hallucinations is not really what is at stake. The important question is whether the effects are mind-revealing. So, now that we are clear on the terminology, let's turn to that issue.

There are two salient possibilities for how hallucinations may be psychedelic. The first is that the hallucinations may function as *vehicles* for content that is being revealed—similar to how psychoanalysts understand dreams as being revelatory of the inner mind. The second way is that the hallucinations may *themselves* be hidden elements of the mind that are being revealed.

Let's start with the thought that hallucinations function as vehicles for revealed content. This idea fits naturally with the view that all conscious content must be mediated by sensory data. For example, Carruthers 2011 has argued that conscious access to any mental content is always mediated by sensory representation.[7] For instance, if you know what you believe about a particular issue, it is because you have experienced a sensory manifestation of your belief. This sensory manifestation can take different forms. For example, you may find yourself voicing that belief in conversation, or expressing it in inner speech to yourself, or experiencing some mental imagery that represents the content of that belief. There are many ways in which you can come to be aware of your beliefs, but Carruthers argues that they are *always* bound to some kind of sensory representation. One may argue that there may be some exceptions to this claim, but on the whole, it does seem that our awareness of mental content is, at the very least, often mediated by sensory representation. So, if psychedelics expand awareness by revealing hidden mental content, then we should expect that there will be resulting changes in mental imagery. Moreover, if the mind has a limited bandwidth for sensory representations, then some of these changes will be rather strange. It would be a bit like trying to paint multiple pictures on a single canvas at the same time. Something has to give: the canvas has to get bigger, or the pictures are overlaid on each other, or they oscillate (like binocular rivalry) or they are distorted in strange ways so that they can fit together (like a dream), etc. In other words, the hallucinations that psychedelics induce may be the sensory manifestations of hidden contents being forced into a limited experiential space.

This sense in which hallucinations may be mind-revealing (i.e. as vehicles for content) is very similar to how the images produced by Google's *DeepDream* can be revealing of the hidden content of its "artificial mind". The DeepDream program

---

[7] Jung also held a similar view: that we can't directly experience the unconscious, but can only know it via images or ideas that represent unconscious instincts and archetypes.

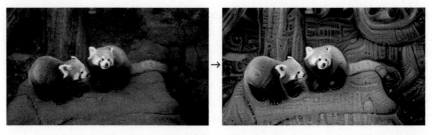

Figure 7.2 An example of the DeepDream algorithm applied to an input image (left).

(Mordvintsev et al. 2015) was developed in response to a problem that image classification engineers at Google were struggling with. The engineers were trying to figure out how to improve the classification performance but were running into the classic problem of not being able to see inside the "black box" of the neural network. A partial solution to the problem came from the idea of *inverting* the process that the network usually followed. The basic thought was: what would happen if instead of feeding the network an image—say, of a cat—and getting it to classify that image, the network was made to generate an image that would fit a pre-selected classification? Inverting the process in this way might facilitate an insight into how the network "thought" about the classification—and therefore how to improve it. What was immediately apparent from the resulting images was that they looked very similar to the visual experiences that people have under the influence of psychedelics. See Figure 7.2 for an example.

The neural network of DeepDream is known as a *convolutional neural network* and is based on the structure of human visual cortex: nodes of lower levels of the network are devoted to classifying low-level features of an image, such as edges, and nodes at higher levels are devoted to classifying higher-level features, such as whether the image contains a cat. The fact that DeepDream produces images that are so similar to hallucinations produced by psychedelics gives us some clues as to the neurocognitive processes by which they do so: it would seem that psychedelics are causing a strengthening of the top-down visual processes, relative to the bottom-up processes, that normally help us see the world.[8]

More importantly, though, DeepDream's images help us see how hallucinations can be mind-revealing by functioning as delivery vehicles for hidden content (that may require interpretative analysis). Take, for example, the dumbbell images that DeepDream produced from random noise, shown in Figure 7.3. As can be seen, all of the dumbbells have arms attached to them. This pattern across the images

---

[8] This point may seem in conflict with the REBUS model of the effects of psychedelics, which proposes that they are caused by a relaxation of high-level priors (Carhart-Harris and Friston 2019). However, a relaxation of high-level priors is compatible with a strengthening of top-down processes that start lower in the hierarchy. It has also been argued that the REBUS model should be expanded to include the strengthening of some priors (Safron 2020).

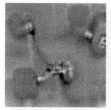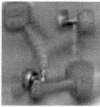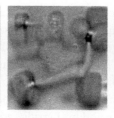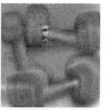

Figure 7.3 Dumbbell images produced by DeepDream from initial images of random noise.

affords us with a possible insight: because the training data typically contains images of people lifting dumbbells, DeepDream's network may not be good at distinguishing a dumbbell from a dumbbell with an arm attached to it. We can think of this as an artificial psychedelic experience: DeepDream's mind is being revealed. The thought, then, is that the same sort of thing could happen with real hallucinations: they may contain content generated by similar top-down processes that constitutes an immediate insight or provides source material that requires interpretative analysis.

It should be noted that this field is advancing rapidly and a new generation of image generation models has recently been developed (DALL-E 2, Imagen, Midjourney, Stable Diffusion, etc.) that create images that look less 'psychedelic' than DeepDream's images in that they are not as chaotic and involve less repetitiveness and fewer low-level distortions. However, although these new images don't appear as 'psychedelic' in this sense, they may in fact be more psychedelic in the sense of being better revelations of these artificial 'minds'. This is because these models are able to respond to more novel prompts and tend to produce images with greater clarity and richer and more cohesive contents (scope) than DeepDream's.[9] Presumably, as these models are further developed to produce videos and animations, we will also see improvements with respect to duration (e.g. in the form of compositional stability). Indeed, it may be that lessons can be learned from the development of these models that could inform the design of a new generation of psychedelics that are more psychedelic than classical psychedelics.[10] This doesn't mean that the models themselves are becoming more 'artificially psychedelic'; rather, it might be better to say that they are becoming more 'artificially mindful'.

Let's now consider the second way in which hallucinations may be psychedelic: the hallucinations *themselves* are hidden elements of the mind that are revealed. An initial reaction one may have is that this idea is conceptually impossible since

[9] These models also highlight how the distinction between mind-revelation and mind-generation can be tricky, especially when creativity is involved.

[10] More generally, the lessons could inform the development of more refined psychedelic methods (Chapter 11).

it is part of the concept of a hallucination that it be conscious—that is, there is no such thing as an unconscious hallucination. However, there is a growing trend in psychology to argue that elements of the conscious mind can also be elements of the unconscious. These extension arguments—also known as 'yes it can' arguments (Hassin 2013)—have targeted perception (Merikle et al. 2001), thought (Dijksterhuis and Strick 2016), bias (Baston and Vosgerau 2016), working memory (Hassin et al. 2009), emotion (Berridge and Winkielman 2003), attention (Prasad and Mishra 2019), mental imagery (Nanay 2021), and even insight (Siegler 2000). In particular, if we're ready to allow that there can be unconscious *perceptions* (Merikle et al. 2001), then it seems we should also be willing to admit that there can be unconscious hallucinations. And if these unconscious hallucinations can be hidden (hard to access), then perhaps they can also be revealed.

This gives us one way to argue for the mind-revealing hypothesis regarding psychedelic-induced hallucinations. However, we can sidestep some of this controversy and grant for the sake of argument that hallucinations must, by definition, always be conscious. Even with this assumption in place, it could still be that when we experience a hallucination, we are experiencing a hidden element of the mind being revealed. For example, we may have unconscious mental imagery, which, when made conscious, may sometimes appear to us in the form of a hallucination (Nanay 2021). This is a natural way for us to make sense of the idea that some hallucinations are themselves instances of mind-revelation—they are normally hidden in the mind as unconscious mental imagery and then manifest in conscious experience in the form of hallucinations.

This may seem like an unusual way of thinking about hallucinations, but there is a useful parallel with creative ideas that makes it more intuitive. As many authors have noted, the vast majority of our ideas aren't all that creative—while they may be novel, many of them aren't really good for anything (e.g. Eagleman and Brandt 2017). The ideas we have are often irrelevant to any problem we are concerned with, and even when relevant, they don't make for good solutions.[11] We have lots of problems and we have lots of ideas as potential solutions to those problems, but only a select few are any good. As a result, most of our ideas never see the light of consciousness, but the better ones make their way up and "pop into our minds". We'll come back to this in the next chapter, but the basic thought is that many of our creative ideas are hidden from us because they are not worthy of conscious processing. The parallel with hallucinations, then, is that many of our creative ideas are a bit like 'solution hallucinations': they pop into our minds as potential solutions to problems. To put it another way, hallucinations are like creative ideas in that they pop into our experience as apparent solutions to perceptual problems.

---

[11] The idea of a problem here is understood very broadly: from figuring out an engineering problem to writing a novel to composing a song that expresses a complex set of emotions.

There are, of course, some important differences between creative ideas and hallucinations. For example, we have far more cognitive control over the ideas we believe or choose to explore. And the creative ideas that make it into the conscious mind are a dime a dozen, whereas conscious hallucinations are quite rare. This latter difference can be explained by the fact that the problems that the perceptual system faces are fairly well defined and constant over time: each day you need to see where the food is, hear the people talking to you, and so on. In contrast, the problems that the epistemic system is confronted with are much more variegated and ambitious: people are figuring out how to solve global poverty, build space rockets, cure cancer, understand the fundamental nature of reality, etc. Given these differences between the epistemic and perceptual systems, it makes sense that the filter for our creative ideas might be more relaxed than the filter for our perceptions. The important point, though, is that both systems have a filter. The epistemic system keeps many of our ideas hidden from awareness, and the perceptual system keeps many of our mental images hidden from us.

In fact, we can see that a filter is at work when we challenge the perceptual system with problems it was not designed to solve. We have seen some of these already with examples of binocular rivalry and illusory motion. These are cases in which we can see the mind guessing as to what it is being presented with, as it usually does, but struggling to find a good guess because of the unusual situation. In the case of binocular rivalry, you can see the rival percepts moving in and out of awareness and sometimes fusing together, as the visual system struggles to make sense of the conflicting input. Under normal circumstances, the mind can quickly find a very good guess, and that is what you consciously perceive as a perception. However, there are still all the bad guesses that never make it to awareness. The thought, then, is that these bad guesses may be the hidden hallucinations that psychedelics can reveal.

This idea that the mind is constantly trying to guess what it is perceiving is becoming widely accepted in cognitive science. Perhaps the most popular theory, especially within the psychedelics literature, based on this idea is predictive processing (Friston 2002, Hohwy 2013, Carhart-Harris and Friston 2019). However, other Bayesian (Griffiths et al. 2008) and some non-Bayesian theories of perception (cf. Bowers and Davis 2012) share the same essential idea. Within the predictive processing framework, this idea has been expressed as the slogan *perception is controlled hallucination* (Clark 2015, Kirchhoff 2018). The thought is that the mind first constructs perceptions (as guesses) and *then* checks them against the sensory input that comes in from the external world.[12] The common sense view of perception has the story the other way around: sensory input comes in, and the brain processes it to construct perceptions and perceptual experiences. Hallucinations,

---

[12] The full story is more complicated than this, but this is a good first approximation.

on this common sense view, occur when the brain constructs a perception on its own instead of building one out of sensory input. According to predictive processing—as well as other modern theories of perception—hallucinations and perceptions are both constructed by the mind, with the difference being that perceptions are constructions that align with sensory stimuli. Another way to state the basic idea in slogan form is that *hallucination is uncontrolled perception*. The two slogans highlight the important point that perception and hallucination are fundamentally the same kind of thing and both are constructed by the same processes. Sensory input is used to decide which constructions are perceptions and are to be made available for conscious experience and which are hallucinatory and, therefore, should be kept hidden from awareness and eventually discarded.

The hypothesis we will examine in the following sections is whether psychedelics—as well as other interventions, such as meditation and sensory deprivation—can have the effect of revealing some of these hidden constructions. In particular, I will argue that the geometric patterns of colourful light often observed under the influence of psychedelics are instances of mental imagery that are normally hidden from conscious experience and which are revealed by psychedelics.

7.3 The Mathematics of Geometric Hallucinations

A visual effect that is frequently brought about by psychedelics is the appearance of vivid and intricate geometrical patterns of light. These tend to be most easily seen with the eyes closed, but they can also occur when the eyes are open, especially for stronger doses. In 1928, Heinrich Klüver began studying these geometric hallucinations by giving subjects doses of mescaline and asking them to describe their visual experiences. After studying their descriptions, Klüver concluded that these geometrical patterns came in four fundamental forms, which he called *form constants*: (i) tunnels, (ii) spirals, (iii) lattices, and (iv) cobwebs—see Figure 7.4.

Although these geometric hallucinations are often associated with psychedelics, they are known to occur under a wide variety of circumstances. Klüver 1942

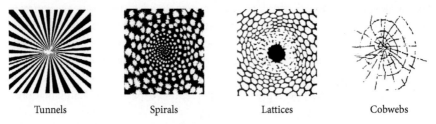

| Tunnels | Spirals | Lattices | Cobwebs |

Figure 7.4 The four form constants—four fundamental patterns of geometric hallucination: (i) tunnels, (ii) spirals, (iii) lattices, and (iv) cobwebs.

reported that they can occur during migraines, epileptic seizures, crystal gazing, when first waking up from sleep, and by putting pressure on one's eyes. It has also been noted that they can occur during meditation, especially for practices that involve (or resemble) sensory deprivation (Lindahl et al. 2014), which also has been documented to give rise to these hallucinations (Heron et al. 1956, Merabet et al. 2004, Mason and Brady 2009). They can also occur when flickering light is shone through closed eyelids. This wide variety of conditions lead Klüver, and others, to hypothesize that the hallucinations are the result of an underlying cortical mechanism.

Several decades later, we began to figure out what that mechanism could be. Ermentrout and Cowan 1979 were the first to put the major pieces of the puzzle together. In their seminal paper, they developed two major insights that help explain why the geometric hallucinations are so common. Their first insight was about the geometric relationship between our visual field and the primary visual cortex, V1, where low-level features of our visual experience are neurally encoded. Their second insight was about the dynamics of that neural activity: the field equations that govern this activity are very similar to the reaction-diffusion equations that Alan Turing used to explain the biological patterns we commonly observe in nature, such as leopard spots and zebra stripes (Turing 1952). Together, these two insights point to the hypothesis that the geometric hallucinations arise as a result of familiar mechanisms that generate structured patterns of neural activity in V1, which are then geometrically transformed into sensory representations in the visual field. This explanation requires unpacking, so we'll go through this step by step.

Let's start with the geometrical relationship between the visual field and V1. The geometry of V1 is relatively simple and, to a useful first approximation, can be modelled as a rectangular sheet. The geometry of our retinal fields is also fairly simple and can be modelled as circular discs.[13] When cells in the retina are stimulated by light, this activity is transmitted to neurons in V1. There's a special relationship between the location of a cell in the retina and its corresponding neurons in V1. Roughly speaking, this relationship allows the circular disc of the retina to be spread out efficiently over the rectangular sheet of neurons that is V1. This relationship is the retinal-cortical mapping, and Ermentrout and Cowan developed an equation to describe it. This mapping has several important features, but for our purposes, the most important feature is that it converts patterns of retinal stimulation into particular patterns of cortical activity: tunnels of stimulation are encoded as horizontal stripes of neural activity, concentric circles are encoded as vertical stripes, and spirals are encoded as diagonal stripes (Figure 7.5). This geometric transformation of retinal stimulation to cortical activity is also assumed

---

[13] With each eye containing left and right halves of the discs.

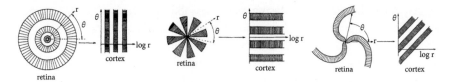

Figure 7.5 The retinal-cortical mapping.

to correspond to the transformation from cortical activity to visual experience, since what we perceive tends to line up with our retinal stimulation.

The retinal-cortical mapping goes some way to explain the geometric patterns. The tunnels and spirals correspond to stripes of activity in V1 oriented at different angles, the cobwebs are grids (horizontal and vertical stripes) of activity, and the lattices are hexagonal tilings of activity. So, if we can explain why psychedelics (and the other interventions/conditions mentioned earlier) cause V1 to produce these particular patterns of activity, then we'll have an explanation for why the geometrical hallucinations are so commonly observed.

This is where the second insight comes in: the neurons in V1 are connected to each other in such a way that, under the right conditions, they cause the structured patterns to arise spontaneously. Ermentrout and Cowan 1979 showed how the field equations that describe these neuronal connections can give rise to the patterns. It will be important for the discussion in the next section for us to understand these details, so I will present a simplified and slightly modified version of their mathematical model.

As I mentioned earlier, the geometry of V1 can be treated as a flat, two-dimensional surface of neurons. These neurons come in two kinds: *excitatory* and *inhibitory* neurons. When an excitatory neuron increases its firing rate (say, because of external stimulation), it influences nearby neurons by causing them to increase their firing rates (but to a lesser extent). When an inhibitory neuron increases its firing rate, it influences nearby neurons by causing them to *decrease* their firing rates. These excitatory and inhibitory neurons are interconnected: when the firing rate of excitatory neurons increases, it causes the firing rates of nearby inhibitory neurons to increase, which in turn causes the firing rates of nearby excitatory neurons to decrease. And so on. The overall influence of the neurons depends on the strengths of their connections and the reach of those connections. There is a particular configuration of these connections that gives rise to what is known as the *Mexican hat* effect: the influence of the excitatory neurons is stronger for nearby neurons than the influence of the inhibitory ones, and the influence of the inhibitory neurons is stronger for farther-away neurons than the influence of the excitatory neurons (Figure 7.6). This Mexican hat effect is the main driving force behind the spontaneous generation of the structured patterns of neuronal activity: the inhibitory neurons prevent an initial seed of

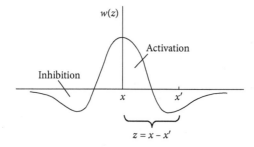

Figure 7.6 The Mexican hat effect: the function $w(z)$ represents the short-range excitation and long-range inhibition of neurons at position x.

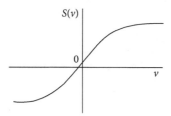

Figure 7.7 A typical neural response threshold function.

excitation from spreading uniformly over the entirety of V1, and the excitatory neurons "keep the party alive" in a local pocket of self-reinforcing activity around the initial seed.

There are two other facts about the neurons of V1 that we need in place before we can put everything together to build the model. The first fact is that the firing rates of the neurons are bounded in such a way that an input stimulation can only increase or decrease the firing of a neuron towards an asymptotic limit. A typical way of modelling this is with neural response threshold functions that have a sigmoidal shape (Figure 7.7). The second fact is that a neuron left to its own devices will gradually gravitate back to its baseline firing rate. So, if its firing rate is temporarily increased by an external stimulus, then it will slowly decrease back to where it started—and similarly if its firing rate is temporarily decreased.

We now have everything we need to present the Ermentrout and Cowan 1979 model. However, it will be useful for discussion in the next section if we work with a slightly modified version of the model. Following Billock and Tsou 2012, I'll incorporate the effect of *sensory input* and *mental imagery* into the model. I'll explain the model in plain English, but first let's see it written mathematically. In mathematical terms, the model is a pair of first-order nonlinear differential equations:

$$\frac{\partial E}{\partial t} = -E + S(aw_{EE} * E - bw_{IE} * I + \phi) \tag{7.1}$$

$$\frac{\partial I}{\partial t} = -I + S(cw_{EI} * E - dw_{II} * I + \phi) \tag{7.2}$$

Let's focus on the first equation. E represents the firing rate of the excitatory neurons, and the term on the left, $\partial E/\partial t$, describes how the firing rate of an excitatory neuron evolves over time. The terms on the right describe the influences on this evolution. The first term, the $-E$, describes dampening effect that brings the firing rate of a neuron back to its baseline—the higher the firing rate of the excitatory neurons, the stronger the force that brings them back to the resting state. The S function is a threshold function that ensures that the other effects on a neuron's firing rate don't cause it to increase or decrease beyond its bounds. These other effects are modelled by the three terms inside the S function. The simplest one is the ϕ term, which represents the effect of sensations caused by sensory input or mental imagery generated by other regions of the visual cortex. If ϕ is positive, it helps increase the neuron's firing rate. The $aw_{EE} * E$ term describes the positive effect that other excitatory neurons have on the neuron, and the $bw_{IE} * I$ term describes the negative effect that V1's inhibitory neurons have on the neuron. The w functions describe how the excitatory and inhibitory neurons influence each other, and the parameters a and b give us a convenient way of modelling the relative strengths of these influences. Roughly speaking, these parameters strengthen or weaken the Mexican hat effect described earlier. The second equation is very similar, except that it describes the evolution of *inhibitory* neuron firing rates, I.

These two equations describe the dynamical evolution of the firing rates of the excitatory and inhibitory neurons. To see how they work, it can help to examine a numerical simulation of how the firing rates evolve over time. Although V1 is a two-dimensional sheet of excitatory and inhibitory neurons, it will be easier to see this evolution if we look at a one-dimensional cross-section of the excitatory neurons. Figure 7.8 shows four time steps of the evolution. At $t = 0$, the neurons are all firing with a small amount of noise around their baseline firing rate of $E = 1$—this is the spatially homogenous state, where the firing rates are all uniform. At $t = 1$, we see the dynamics captured by the equations begin to take over and add shape to the noise: neurons near those that are excited also get excited, and those that are farther away get inhibited. At $t = 2$, we see a structured pattern of activity emerge from the noise, which begins to run into the physiological bounds on the firing rates, creating a pattern that is maximally differentiated between peaks of high activity and troughs of low activity.

It's important to note that this kind of evolution only happens for certain settings of the parameters (a, b, c, d). Ermentrout and Cowan focused on the strengths of a and c parameters, which can be understood as the *excitability* of V1. We can

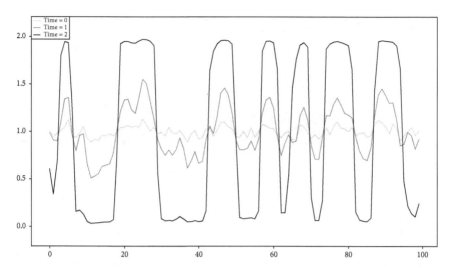

Figure 7.8 Three time steps of the evolution of the excitatory firing rates determined by the Ermentrout-Cowan dynamics.

parameterize excitability by introducing a new parameter, p: $a = pa'$ and $c = pc'$. Increasing p increases V1's excitability. Ermentrout and Cowan showed that p is a *bifurcation* parameter: when it is sufficiently high, above a critical value of p_c, the neural firing rates of V1 evolve in the way we just saw: small perturbations from the baseline grow and become structured to form the observed patterns. However, when p is below p_c, the dynamics are qualitatively different: perturbations are dampened back towards the baseline, and only the spatially homogenous pattern of activity is observed. Others have since demonstrated that other parameterizations also have these qualitative bifurcations of the model's dynamics. For example, motivated by hypothesis that epileptic seizures involve a weakening of the V1's inhibitory connections, Tass 1995 showed that weakening the parameters b and d below a critical value also results in the spontaneous emergence of structured patterns of neural activity.

There's one important point of clarification that needs to be made here. Numerical simulations of the Ermentrout-Cowan model typically don't lead to the patterns we are looking for—that is, the patterns of stripes, grids, and hexagonal lattices. Instead, what is far more typical is the kind of labyrinthine pattern shown in Figure 7.9. Because of this, the Ermentrout-Cowan model only gives us a *how-possibly* explanation for how the geometric patterns can spontaneously arise as a result of an intervention on V1 that increases its excitability. To complete the explanation, so that the patterns *inevitably* arise, additional assumptions need to be added to the model. One way to do this is to build more anatomical structure into the model, by incorporating the fact that neurons in V1 are organized into lattice structures that help with the detection of edges (Bressloff et al. 2002).

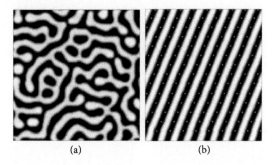

(a)   (b)

Figure 7.9 (a) An example of a labyrinthine pattern that spontaneously arises in the Ermentrout and Cowan 1979 model. (b) An example of a striped pattern emerging when long-range connections are pinned to neurons with similar orientation preferences (Baker and Cowan 2009).

Baker and Cowan 2009 show how this lattice structure combines with the Mexican hat effect to guarantee the emergence of the structured patterns that correspond to the Klüver's form constants, and Bressloff et al. 2002 show how the lattice structure allows for patterns that have even more realistic features, such as contours and depth. We don't need to go into the mathematical details here (see Cowan 2014 for a review of them). The crucial point for our purposes is that the models are improved as more details about the actual workings of V1 are included and, as a result, the hallucinatory patterns they generate become more realistic. In particular, the details about the neural mechanism that V1 uses to detect edges, contours, etc., are crucial to the explanatory power of the models. This will be an important point in the next section. It's also a good sign that the models are genuinely explaining how the appearance of hallucinatory patterns is brought about by the consumption of psychedelics (and other interventions).

7.4 Geometric Hallucinations Revealed?

Now that we have a rough idea of how these models of geometric hallucinations work, our next task is to figure out what they imply for our central question: do psychedelics *reveal* the geometric patterns, or do psychedelics *create* them (as side effects or as part of the necessary conditions for other psychedelic effects)?[14]

To answer this question, we must look at the models more carefully. In particular, we need to examine how the influence of a psychedelic substance is represented by the models and how this relates to the appearance of the geometric patterns. In

---

[14] In Section 7.2, we focused on the 'how possibly' question of whether psychedelics can reveal hidden hallucinations. In this section, we are focused on the 'how actually' question of whether the geometric patterns are, in fact, revelations of hidden hallucinations (or hidden mental imagery).

other words, we need to examine the interpretation of the models that allows them to explain the observed effect—that is, that psychedelics give rise to geometric hallucinations.

The standard interpretation of the models arises from a central aspect of their mathematical analysis, known as *bifurcation theory*. Recall from the previous section that a key component of the models is the existence of a bifurcation parameter: when the parameter p is above the critical value p_c, the baseline state becomes unstable, and patterns of neural activity emerge and grow towards their threshold limits. This invites the following natural interpretation: (i) the effect of the drug is to increase the bifurcation parameter past the critical value,[15] (ii) the consequence of that is that perturbations from the resting state are no longer dampened back to that state, and instead grow and evolve into the geometric patterns of cortical activity, and (iii) the appearance of hallucinations corresponds to the emergence of those patterns.

This interpretation was first expressed by Ermentrout and Cowan:

> [...S]imple formed hallucinations arise from an instability of the resting state leading to concomitant spatial patterns of activity in the cortex. This instability arises from a combination of enhanced excitatory modulation and decreased inhibition (disinhibition).
>
> Ermentrout and Cowan 1979, p. 138

And we find it in other discussions of the model:[16]

> The basic assumption in the model is that the effect of drugs, or any of the other causes of hallucinations, is to cause instabilities in the neural activity in the visual cortex and these instabilities result in the visual patterns experienced by the subject. [...] In the case of drug-induced hallucinations p [the bifurcation parameter] could be associated with drug dosage. [...] The mechanism for spatial pattern creation is then very like that with the other pattern formation mechanisms we have so far discussed. That is, the pattern is generated when a parameter passes through a bifurcation value, p_c [...].
>
> Murray 2003, pp. 629–33

---

[15] One potential problem with this aspect of the interpretation is that there isn't a *single* bifurcation parameter. Tass 1995, for example, showed that the patterns can emerge when the influence of the inhibitory neurons on the excitatory neurons is reduced—instead of the excitability of the excitatory and inhibitory neurons being increased. In other words, any given model can have several bifurcation parameters, each of which may correspond to a possible mechanism of action of a drug. However, for the sake of keeping the discussion as simple as possible, I will simply speak of *the* bifurcation parameter.

[16] The model discussed by Murray is almost the same as the model of Ermentrout and Cowan, except that the bifurcation parameters are slightly different. Ermentrout and Cowan examined a modulation of the excitatory connections (p. 141), whereas Murray examined the modulation of both the excitatory and inhibitory connections (p. 632).

And we also find a similar interpretation of the more complex models that have since been developed. For example:

> [T]he model is sensitive to the symmetries in the interaction patterns between neurons: the mathematics shows that it is these symmetries that drive the formation of periodic patterns of neural activity. [...] in other words [it is] the mechanisms that enable us to detect edges, contours, surfaces and textures in the visual world, that generate the hallucinations. [...] It is when these mechanisms become unstable, for example due to the influence of a drug, that patterns of neural activity arise, which in turn translate to the visual hallucinations.
>
> Freiberger 2009

Although the above quotes are referring to different models, each is applying the same interpretation: the effect of psychedelics is to increase the value of the relevant bifurcation parameter past its critical value, which corresponds to the resting state becoming unstable, thus allowing the geometric patterns to spontaneously form. As I mentioned earlier, this is an interpretation that naturally arises from the bifurcation analysis of the models.

On the face of it, this interpretation may seem to speak against the hypothesis that psychedelics reveal the geometric hallucinations. By causing the resting state to become unstable, it seems that psychedelics cause the *creation* of the patterns. If correct, this would be bad news for the hypothesis that the geometric hallucinations are psychedelic.

However, this simple argument is based on a mistake. The mistake is a conflation between the *creation* of the patterns and their *appearance in awareness*. These two things can come apart. It is true that, according to the models, the psychedelic-induced instability in the resting state allows the patterns of neural activity to grow in strength until the geometric hallucinations appear in awareness. However, this doesn't mean that the instability *creates* the patterns. In fact, we can see this by numerically simulating the models. For example, Figure 7.10 shows the output of a numerical simulation of a one-dimensional version of the Ermentrout-Cowan model (which I've adapted from the one-dimensional model presented in Murray 2003, pp. 614–22). The first graph shows what happens when the initial sensory input is random noise and the bifurcation parameter is *above* the critical value: the dynamics of the model smooth out the noise while also amplifying its accidental trends, turning them into structured oscillating patterns of neural activity. The second graph shows what happens when the bifurcation parameter is *below* the critical value: the initial noise is smoothed and dampened back to the uniform resting state. In this second graph, it looks like the pattern is not there. However, the third graph shows a zoomed-in version of the second graph: when we zoom in, we see that the pattern *is there*—it's just really small. So the difference between the first two graphs is not the *existence* of the pattern per se, but rather its *size*.

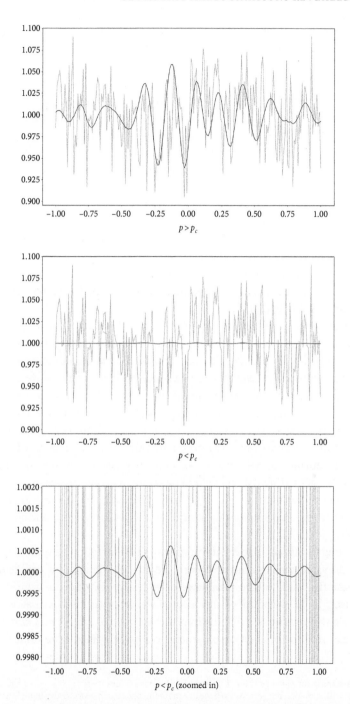

Figure 7.10 Top: The bifurcation parameter is greater than the critical value, and the structured patterns of neural activity can grow. Middle: The bifurcation parameter is less than the critical value, and the neural activity is dampened back to the resting state. Bottom: This is the middle image again, but zoomed in on the y-axis so that the small structured patterns can be seen.

If this is correct, then this would be good news for the hypothesis that the geometric hallucinations are psychedelic, since it is exactly the sort of thing we would expect to find. When the bifurcation parameter is below the critical value, the patterns of neural activity do exist, but they are so small that their corresponding representations/sensations—that is, the geometric hallucinations—are not sufficiently activated to appear in awareness and are easily dominated by sensory input and noise. Moreover, the reason why the patterns of neural activity are so small is because of the default tendency for the visual system to dampen neural activity back to the uniform resting state. So, there is a sense in which the patterns exist and are *hidden* from awareness.[17] When the bifurcation parameter is above the critical value, the patterns are allowed to grow away from the resting state and become strong enough so that their corresponding representations/sensations appear in awareness.[18] If all of this is correct, then we have a clear sense in which the appearance of geometric hallucinations constitutes a psychedelic experience. This explanation also fits well with the Osmond-Grof hypothesis that psychedelics reveal parts of the mind by amplifying them—and potentially its interpretation in terms of attention (Chapter 5).

Although this line of thought looks promising, we need to be careful in drawing conclusions. The reason is that there are now many different models of V1, and we don't know if they all have this property of the patterns existing when the bifurcation parameter is below the critical value. Moreover, even if we did know, we wouldn't be able to rule out the possibility that in the future, an even better model comes along that doesn't have this property. In other words, we need to be careful not to mistake a fact about a model for a fact about reality. So, it would be good if we had some other reason for thinking that the hallucinations exist subliminally during normal experience. There are some reasons for thinking this, but before we get to them, it will help to be aware of an alternative interpretation of the models that is just as plausible as the standard one. Doing so will help us appreciate the reasons for thinking that the patterns exist during normal experience.

According to this alternative interpretation, the bifurcation parameter is above the critical value during normal experience, and the effect of a psychedelic is to increase the value of the parameter *even further* beyond the critical value. One reason to be sceptical of this alternative interpretation is that we don't experience the geometric hallucinations during normal experience, and so that must mean that the bifurcation parameter is normally below the critical value.

---

[17] I'm assuming for now that there is no, or very little, visual sensory input (e.g. when the subject's eyes are closed) or mental imagery. As we'll see in a moment, the existence of sensory input functions as another dampening effect on the patterns and thus another way in which the hallucinations are hidden from awareness.

[18] Without going into the mathematical details of the models, Metzinger 2003 makes a similar proposal: that the geometric patterns are the appearance of early processing stages of the visual system.

However, although this reason may be intuitive, it is based on a confusion: the bifurcation parameter being above the critical value is a *necessary* condition for the emergence of the hallucinations, but it is not a *sufficient* condition. For example, if the sensation term consistently dominates the other terms inside the S function, then the patterns won't be able to grow, even when the bifurcation parameter is past the critical value. Therefore, it doesn't follow that because we don't see the geometric hallucinations during normal experience, the bifurcation parameter must therefore be below the critical value. It could be that the hallucinations do not emerge because they are dominated by other sensations. For example, we tend to have our eyes open during normal experience, and that provides a sensory input signal strong enough to dominate any other mental imagery. That's why it helps to close your eyes when you want to imagine something visual. So, this alternative interpretation has some plausibility to it.

We now have two ways in which the geometric hallucinations may be subliminal elements of our normal visual experience. This is an important point because it's tempting to think that the bifurcation parameter being above the critical value determines (i) the creation of the patterns and/or (ii) the appearance of the corresponding hallucinations in awareness. However, neither of these ideas is necessarily true. The hallucinations can exist subliminally when the parameter is below the critical value, and they can fail to appear in awareness even when it is above the critical value. To be clear, this is not to say that the value of the bifurcation parameter doesn't play an important role in the existence and appearance of the hallucinations. It's just that whether or not the parameter is above the critical value is not necessarily decisive for either point.

Let's now come back to the question of whether the hallucinations are subliminal during normal experience—either because they exist when the bifurcation parameter is below the critical value, or because they are usually hidden from awareness even when the parameter is past the critical value. Is there any reason to think the hallucinations are subliminal elements of normal experience?

One potential reason to think so is that we know that the geometric hallucinations also appear during meditation, sensory deprivation, and other ways of reducing the strength of other sensations associated with sensory input and mental imagery. For convenience, I will refer to all of these methods as 'sensory deprivation'. From the perspective of the mathematical models, sensory deprivation involves reducing the sensation term, ϕ, in the S function. By definition, this means that the other terms in the function, which are the terms responsible for the geometric hallucinations, dominate the total input to the S function, which then dominates the resulting neural activity. This suggests that the hallucinations are hidden during normal experience by our other sensations and that they are revealed when these sensations are reduced via sensory deprivation. Thus, these hallucinations may be like the stars in the sky, which are hidden during the day by the light of the sun and are revealed when the sun sets. The natural thought, then, is that the hallucinations are revealed by sensory deprivation because it clears the mind, and they are revealed by psychedelics because the substances amplify the underlying patterns of neural activity as a result of increasing the value of the bifurcation parameter.

This thought would also explain why closing the eyes, which is a mild form of sensory deprivation, makes it easier to see the hallucinations when one is under the influence of a psychedelic. Indeed, it is well known that people are normally unable to see the hallucinations unless they close their eyes. This suggests that the hallucinations appear in awareness because of two factors working together synergistically: closing the eyes reduces the sensation terms, and the psychedelic amplifies the terms responsible for the underlying patterns of neural activity. In many cases, either factor alone is not sufficient for the appearance of the hallucinations, but together they are more likely to be sufficient. This idea also fits well with the observation that it is *possible* for people to see the hallucinations with their eyes open when they are under the influence of a very strong dose or a particularly powerful psychedelic (such as DMT). In such cases, the psychedelic is able to sufficiently amplify the terms responsible for the patterns, so that the corresponding hallucinations come to dominate the sensation terms, even though they remain at their typical values.

Similarly, it has been observed that another way to generate the geometric hallucinations is to sit in front of a flickering light with one's eyes closed. The flickering has to be at the right intensity and frequency, and it can take a while for the hallucinations to appear. Smythies 1960 found that these flicker-induced hallucinations appeared more quickly and with more intensity and richness when subjects were given *sub*-hallucinatory doses of mescaline. At this dose level, the mescaline was not strong enough by itself to cause the hallucinations to appear in awareness. However, in combination with the flickering light, it was able to bring them into awareness faster and more vividly than they would have appeared otherwise. Again, this seems to speak in favour of the idea that the hallucinations are subliminal during normal experience and are amplified by the psychedelics.

Another line of evidence for this idea comes from a study by Kenet et al. 2003, which used high-resolution recordings of neural activity in the visual cortices of anaesthetized and unstimulated cats. Kenet et al. found that the cortical activity evolved into highly structured patterns resembling those of the Ermentrout-Cowan models. Goldberg et al. 2004 discussed how this effect could be explained in terms of different dynamical modelling assumptions about the attractor sets in cortical phase space. In other words, if you let a cat brain be unstimulated, the activity in its visual cortex naturally gravitates towards the patterns of neural activity that correspond to the geometric hallucinations. This suggests that this feature is not unique to the human mind. It also suggests that the patterns may not be curious accidental features of our visual systems and, instead, that they are somehow helping us see the world. We'll come back to this point in a moment.

There is one final line of evidence that we should consider, which stems from the Hermann grid illusion. As we saw earlier, the Hermann grid illusion involves the appearance of small grey patches at the intersection of vertical and horizontal white bands on a black background (Figure 7.1). The long-accepted explanation for this illusion is due to Baumgartner 1960 who proposed that the small grey patches arise because of edge-enhancing lateral connections between retinal ganglion cells. These lateral connections have the same excitatory and inhibitory Mexican hat effects that we saw in Section 7.3. Because of these lateral connections, a point at the intersection of two white bands receives four sources of inhibition (from the white regions above, below, and to its left and right), whereas other points in the white bands receive only two sources of inhibition (either from above and below or from the left and right). This creates a relative difference in apparent brightness that corresponds to the illusory grey patches. Although this is the long-accepted explanation for the illusion, Schiller and Carvey 2005 make a convincing argument that it is not quite correct: they argue that the illusory patches must be due to lateral connections in the visual cortex, rather than in the retina. That suggests that Hermann grid illusion is generated by the same mechanistic structure in the visual cortex that is responsible for the geometric hallucinations.

To put it in an overly simplistic but useful way: it seems that the grey patches of the Hermann grid illusion are fuzzy glimpses of the geometric patterns that exist subliminally during normal experience. This is because they are caused by the same neural mechanisms (and also bound to the same functional role of facilitating edge detection). This idea also suggests an empirical prediction: sub-hallucinatory doses of psychedelics should amplify the appearance of the grey patches. In other words, the experience of the grey patches is a *mildly* psychedelic experience, and so the consumption of a psychedelic should make it *more* psychedelic—so long as the dose is small enough to prevent other confounding effects. To my knowledge, this has not yet been examined empirically. However, there is evidence that alcohol has the *opposite* effect. Johnston and Timney 2013 report that the illusion appears less vividly for subjects under the influence of alcohol. Their explanation for this effect is that alcohol reduces the strength of lateral inhibitory connections. So, it seems reasonable to expect that a sub-hallucinatory dose of a psychedelic will cause the illusion to appear more vividly.

In summary, the case for the geometric hallucinations being subliminal elements of normal visual experience looks promising; however, it is by no means definitive. This is because it could be objected that in each of the situations just described, the intervention in question causes the bifurcation parameter to move past the critical value, and that this is necessary for the creation and appearance of the hallucinations. For example, it could be objected that sensory deprivation, which is an unusual situation to put the human mind in, causes the bifurcation parameter to move past the critical value. Similarly, exposure to flickering lights through the eyelids, anaesthetizing cats, and looking at the Hermann grid could all be ways of causing the bifurcation parameter to move past the critical value. Combined with the assumption that this is a necessary condition for the creation of the patterns, this would entail that the hallucinations are not subliminal elements of normal visual experience (and so this would cut against the hypothesis that they are revelations of the mind).

One potential way to decide the issue is to think about *why* the hallucinations would be subliminal elements of normal visual experience. This is the point we touched on earlier in connection with the results of Kenet et al. 2003 and Goldberg et al. 2004 involving the brains of anaesthetized and unstimulated cats. A natural thought here is that the subliminal hallucinations help the visual system to do its work of detecting features in the external environment. In particular, it would seem that they help the visual system to detect the *edges* of objects. This is because the Mexican hat effect that drives the hallucinations plays a role in the enhancement of edges in the visual scene. This can be seen in the Mach band illusion, which is closely related to the Hermann grid illusion, in which the local contrast surrounding edges is enhanced. In fact, a key assumption of some of the more advanced models (Baker and Cowan 2009 and Bressloff et al. 2002) is that neurons with similar orientation preferences have strong lateral connections between them. The idea, then, is that the brain is actively engaged in the creation of the experienced visual scene by making educated guesses as to the location and form of any existing edges and by automatically amplifying any signal that indicates the existence of an edge. In other words, the subliminal hallucinations are actively interacting with our sensory input to help us better see the edges of objects.[19] Normally, we don't notice this because the brain is doing a good job of finding the world's edges for us.[20] It is only in unusual visual circumstances, such as that of the Hermann grid illusion, or when we're under the influence of psychedelics, that we begin to see how the brain is actively constructing our visual experience in this way.

The hypothesis that the subliminal hallucinations are helping us see the world fits well with our modern understanding of cognition and perception, which says that there are top-down processing effects and/or predictive inferences that the brain is actively engaged in. This is a view that fits very naturally within the predictive processing framework, but it is also what we would expect from any Bayesian theory of cognition, as well as any other approach that posits anticipatory

---

[19] Ringach 2009 has suggested a very similar point for spontaneous cortical activity in general, hypothesizing that 'such patterns also emerge in the total absence of an external visual stimulus, as if the cortex were to be spontaneously hallucinating a physical stimulus with a particular orientation' (p. 2).

[20] It is worth noting that in some situations that the human brain clearly did not evolve to handle, these educated guesses can result in substantial errors. For example, the Mexican hat effect is an important factor behind common misinterpretations of dental radiographs (Nielsen 2001).

top-down effects on cognition and perception. For example, here is a recent explanation of the effects of sensory deprivation in these terms:

> Within the framework of the Bayesian model, we suggest that a healthy individual under sensory deprivation experiences a lack of bottom-up sensory stimulation. Since sensory stimulation is normally much greater, the predictions of higher brain regions are violated. In addition, sensory deprivation by physical means is never complete and there are baseline, noisy, fluctuations of firing in the brain. In other words, the sensorially deprived state involves low-level noisy bottom-up signals combined with strong priors that are accustomed to acting upon stronger signals.
>
> Corlett et al. 2009, p. 524

To put it in other words, and in terms of predictive processing (which we need not be committed to), having the bifurcation parameter above the critical value is a way for the brain to encode a prior that expects edges in the world to appear and for them to appear in particular ways (to form shapes of objects with depth, for instance). The work of this prior is normally hidden from us because it generally does its job well, but it can be revealed to us in experience via the effects of psychedelics, sensory deprivation, and the other interventions we have discussed.[21]

In conclusion, a good (but not definitive) case can be made that the geometric hallucinations are psychedelic in the sense that we have been focused on. It seems that these hallucinations exist during normal experience as subliminal elements of our visual experience that actively help us see the world. If this is correct, then it raises the question of whether we really should be classifying the geometric patterns of colourful light as *hallucinations*. At the very least, it may be better to say that they are cases of unconscious mental imagery that become hallucinations only when they appear in conscious experience. However, as discussed in Section 7.2, this definitional point is probably not something we should worry too much about—so long as it is clear what is meant. Nevertheless, it is useful to think about the basic idea using different terminology: roughly speaking, the experiences of geometric patterns *seem* hallucinatory, but they are actually the revelation of the visual system's building blocks—or raw ingredients—that it uses to construct our visual experience of the world. We are not aware of them under normal circumstances, as that would interfere with their purpose, but, under the right conditions, and especially with the help of psychedelics, they can be revealed to us in experience.

---

[21] Smythies 1960 considered a similar hypothesis put forward by H. Barlow (in personal communication, 1956) to explain stroboscopic-induced hallucinations (p. 252).

7.5 Conclusion

The bulk of this chapter has been devoted to arguing that some psychedelic-induced hallucinations are psychedelic because they are hidden elements of normal experience and are revealed as a result of the consumption of a psychedelic substance. As I pointed out in Section 7.2, this may seem like a counterintuitive idea, but it can be made less counterintuitive once we appreciate the sense in which these hallucinations are not genuine hallucinations and that all perception may be viewed as a kind of controlled or limited form of hallucination. As Corlett et al. 2018 put it, 'hallucinations [are] an exaggeration of normal non-hallucinatory perception, to which we are all sometimes prone' (p. 124).

It should be emphasized that we need to be cautious in concluding that *all* hallucinations are psychedelic. As I mentioned in the introduction, it is entirely possible that some hallucinations should be considered as non-psychedelic side-effects. That is, they could be the byproducts of a dramatic disturbance to the normal functioning of the brain that allows *other* effects that are psychedelic—such as emotional insights, long-lost memories being relived, etc. It could therefore be the case that the vast bulk of psychedelic-induced hallucinations are not psychedelic. Therefore, the conclusion here is just that there is a good case to be made that *some* hallucinations are psychedelic—in the sense that they directly involve the revelation of a hidden part or aspect of the mind.

Although this conclusion is somewhat modest, it is enough to mitigate the general concern raised at the beginning of this chapter that psychedelics are not psychedelic because they cause hallucinations. This concern is based on the assumption that hallucinations must always involve some kind of *addition* to the mind rather than a revelation of it. I've argued that at least in some cases, psychedelic-induced hallucinations are revelations of the mind, and not mere additions to it.

8
Creativity

8.1 Introduction

In the previous two chapters, we've seen how the recovery of lost memories and the appearance of certain kinds of hallucinations may be psychedelic—in the sense that they are revelations of hidden elements of the mind. In this chapter, we will turn to another potential kind of psychedelic experience: experiences that involve increases in creativity.

This choice of focus is motivated by the fact that psychedelics and meditation are widely believed to enhance creativity. The anecdotal evidence for this claim is compelling and, as we'll see in the coming sections, the scientific evidence for it is also slowly accumulating. This naturally gives rise to a question for us: if psychedelics and meditation enhance creativity, is it because they induce psychedelic experiences? In other words, can these alleged enhancements in creativity be explained in terms of the mind being revealed?

In his seminal book, *The Antipodes of the Mind*, Benny Shanon presents an argument that they cannot. While his primary focus is on ayahuasca and on a particular version of our hypothesis that psychedelics reveal the mind, which he calls the *informational account*, his objection is applicable here:

> [T]he informational account ignores the creative aspect of the Ayahuasca experience. Its main theoretical conceptualization is information processing. Under the intoxication, much more than information processing seems to take place. Rather than reveal what has hitherto been hidden, Ayahuasca seems to induce creativity and the generation of novelty.
>
> Shanon 2002, p. 368

The structure to Shanon's objection is similar to the concern that we saw in the previous chapter: the fact that psychedelics cause hallucinations can be taken as a sign that psychedelics do *not* reveal the mind. In both cases, the underlying thought is that psychedelics are mind-*creating* rather than mind-*revealing*: somehow psychedelics add hallucinations and creativity to the mind rather than reveal these things. So, just as we considered whether hallucinations can be hidden in the mind and revealed, we will pursue a similar line of thought here: can our creativity be hidden in the mind and potentially revealed? By exploring this idea, we will get a better sense of how psychedelics and meditation may enhance creativity by revealing the mind—and thus develop a response to Shanon's objection.

In order to explore this idea, we first need to make it more precise and address some foundational concepts and questions. There are several immediate questions we need to address. How can creativity be hidden in the mind? What does it mean to reveal creativity? And what is creativity, anyway? The first three sections of this chapter will be focused on sorting out these issues. In Section 8.2, we will lay out some basic details about the nature of creativity. In Section 8.3, we will consider what it could mean for creativity to be hidden in the mind and whether there is any reason to think this may be the case. In Section 8.4, we will then consider what it would mean for this creativity to be revealed.

Having sorted out these details, we will then consider, in Sections 8.5 and 8.6, what reasons we may have to think that meditation and psychedelics enhance creativity by revealing it. In Section 8.7, we will then examine another conceptual issue: if psychedelic experiences can enhance one's creativity by revealing it, does that mean there is some kind of relationship between creativity and the dimensions of psychedelic space? I'll argue that there is a surprisingly neat correspondence between the key factors contributing to one's creativity and the degree to which an experience is psychedelic. This will give us a general framework for analysing how different ways of inducing psychedelic experiences might enhance creativity.

8.2 What Is Creativity?

The notion of creativity is notoriously difficult to define. In part, this is because we attribute creativity to so many different kinds of things, such as ideas, objects, processes, people, and organizations. Since the underlying motivation for this chapter is the thought that psychedelics and meditation can help people become more creative, our starting point is, therefore, what it takes for a *person* to be creative.

A common way of understanding what it takes for a person to be creative is that they produce lots of *creative objects*, such as paintings, books, songs, theorems, technologies, clothes, recipes, etc. And an object is generally considered to be creative if it has a high degree of *novelty* and *quality*. That means that the creativity of an individual is related to the novelty, quality, and quantity of the objects that they produce.[1] Some trade-offs between these three factors are possible. For example, if you sacrifice some quantity to get a large increase in novelty and quality, then you will probably increase your creativity. Nevertheless, generally speaking, all three factors need to be in place for a person to be considered creative.

However, when it comes to *measuring* creativity, cognitive psychologists sometimes define creativity slightly differently. The production of objects is often impractical in a laboratory setting, which makes creativity difficult to measure if we focus on this particular output.

---

[1] For example, see Boden 1990, Runco and Jaeger 2012, Simonton 2013, and Fox and Beaty 2019.

Thus, there tends to be a focus on *creative ideas*, which can be thought of as precursors to creative objects. So, if a person has lots of ideas that are novel and good, then that can be taken as an indicator of their creativity. Moreover, in many creative domains, you often need an idea for an object before you can make it, which further justifies the focus on creative ideas. To be sure, there are cases in which creative objects are produced without the ideas preceding them. For example, a piece of jazz improvisation may occur spontaneously without being preceded by an idea for it (Johnson-Laird 2002). Nevertheless, it seems safe to say that many of our creative objects are preceded by corresponding ideas for them. So, the thought is that focusing on creative ideas is a good first step in the study of human creativity.

Focusing on creative ideas also leads us to consider the *creative processes* that generate those ideas. By intervening on the brain/mind in certain ways, we may be able to intervene on the processes that produce creative ideas, and measure the effects of these interventions by the resulting changes in the creative ideas. For many people, the creative processes behind our creative ideas can seem mysterious, even magical. Artists and writers, for example, often speak of ideas appearing out of nowhere, or the muses descending, or divine inspiration striking, and so on. However, a fairly common view in cognitive science is that a creative process is just a process that transforms old ideas into new ones. For example, Eagleman and Brandt 2017 argue that all creativity can be accounted for in terms of old ideas being blended, bended, or broken into new ones. Kounios and Beeman 2015 also describe creative processes as the breaking up of old ideas into their elements and then recombining those elements into new ideas. Similarly, Boden 1990 offers a computational view of creativity that involves the exploration and transformation of conceptual spaces. These sorts of views take the apparent magic out of the creative process by making it a purely mechanical process. In what follows, I'll assume that this kind of view gets something right about the creative processes that generate our creative ideas. To be clear, this assumption doesn't entail that all of our creative processes fit this mould. Perhaps there is some genuine magic to creativity, and perhaps divine inspiration is a real thing. However, in what follows, I will rely only on the assumption that many of our creative processes involve the transformation of old ideas into new ones.[2]

To summarize, we have something of a conceptual chain of creativity: our interest in creative *people* entails an interest in the production of creative *objects*, which leads to an interest in the creative *ideas* for those objects, which leads to an interest in the creative *processes* that produce those ideas. With this in place, it will also help to have on the table two basic distinctions from the cognitive science literature on creativity.

---

[2] This is also compatible with Nanay's 2014 proposal that what is distinctive about a creative process is that it produces an idea that is *experienced* as something that one would have not thought to be possible before.

The first is the distinction between convergent and divergent thinking tasks. A convergent thinking task is a puzzle that has only one solution to it (or at least a very narrow range of solutions). One common convergent thinking task is the *remote associates task*, which involves finding a word that relates three other seemingly unrelated words. For example, what word is related to each of these three words: shoe, French, car? The answer is *horn*: shoehorn, French horn, car horn. In contrast, a divergent thinking task is a puzzle that has a potentially infinite number of solutions to it. One common divergent thinking task is the *alternative uses task*, which involves coming up with as many different uses of a common object as possible. For example, what are all the possible uses of a brick? Answers include: the building of a house, the breaking of windows, a door stop, a paperweight, a bird feeder, a prop in a play, a symbol for Protestant work ethic, and so on. Both convergent and divergent thinking tasks are used to measure creativity and, arguably, both are necessary to properly measure it.

The second distinction is between analytic and insight solutions to creative problem-solving (Bowden et al. 2005). Analytic thinking consists in the employment of conscious, step-by-step reasoning to solve a problem. In contrast, an insight is a solution to a problem that suddenly appears in awareness—it's sometimes known as an "aha!" or "eureka!" moment. Creativity often involves different mixtures of these two styles of thinking (Jung-Beeman et al. 2004, Hommel 2012). For example, solutions to remote associates tasks often come via insight: you look at the three words, mull over them for a bit, and, at some point, if you're lucky, the word 'horn' may pop into your awareness. However, solutions to remote associates tasks can also come via analytic thinking. For example, you might first break a remote associates task into three divergent thinking tasks: come up with as many associated words for each of the three words. Then, as a logical next step, you could search those three lists for any point of overlap. If the word 'horn' appears on each of the three lists, then you know you have found a solution to the remote associates task. So, we see how a creative problem might be solved using different combinations of these two styles of thinking.

A lot more could be said about creativity. However, we now have enough for our purposes. So, as our next step, let's consider what it could mean for one's creativity to be hidden in the mind.

8.3 Hidden Creativity

What could it mean for creativity to be hidden in the mind? Given our definition of creativity, there are two things it could mean: (i) some creative *ideas* are hidden from awareness, and (ii) some creative *processes* are hidden from awareness. So, let's unpack each of these possibilities, starting with the possibility that creative processes are hidden from awareness.

One thing that we can be certain of right away is that not *all* creative processes are hidden from awareness. Analytic thinking is clearly something that can be creative, and it is a process that we are aware of. Indeed, in many cases, our creative processes can be analytically encapsulated in the form of *creativity heuristics* (Hájek 2014, 2016). For example, one such heuristic consists in writing down some ideas or concepts that you are already familiar with and then considering novel combinations of them. To see how this works, let's suppose I wanted to come up with a new idea for this chapter. Following the heuristic, I would first write down some of the ideas and concepts that we have already covered in this book:

mind-revelation, hallucinations, opium, creative ideas, mindfulness, memory, convolutional neural networks, optical illusions, . . .

And then I would start trying out various novel combinations of these ideas. Of course, most combinations of the above ideas will seem like dead ends—for example, opium & convolutional neural networks. However, other combinations show more promise. For example, hallucinations & creative ideas: maybe they are the same kind of thing? As I suggested in the previous chapter, some hallucinations and ideas may be understood as potential solutions to problems that challenge the perceptual and epistemic systems respectively. That seems like a potentially useful idea to develop. And so on. By systematically trying out different combinations, one can potentially discover all sorts of creative ideas.

Such creativity heuristics clearly have some value to them. If you're struggling to be creative, the heuristics can be a useful way to get some new ideas. However, it is also clear that using these heuristics can be a tedious, time-consuming process and that the heuristics will often lead you to dead ends. Moreover, it's not clear that heuristics can lead to creative ideas all by themselves. For example, it's one thing to analytically identify the combination of hallucinations & creative ideas, and it's quite another to come up with the insight that these two things may be the same. That insight doesn't just fall out of the combination of the ideas.

As Hájek puts it, a creative idea is like a spark that leaps across two electrically charged wires, and while the heuristics don't cause the spark, they bring the two wires together, and thus make it *easier* for the spark to occur. In this sense, the heuristics capture an important part of the creative process. However, they also miss an important part of it: the spark. Indeed, some have argued for a stronger claim: that what is distinctive about creative processes is that they are *not* analytic or mechanical (Gaut 2003). Following the heuristics is clearly an analytic and mechanical procedure, and so this point reflects the intuition that it is not a process of "real" creativity. However, we needn't accept such a strong conclusion. If we're serious that creative processes involve transformations of old ideas into new ones, then we can accept that the heuristics capture part of our creative processes, while accepting that they also miss something important.

The question, then, is: what is it about our creative processes that the heuristics are missing? Part of the intuition that creative processes cannot be analytic and mechanical is that "real" creativity is somehow outside of our control. The intuitions we often have about "real" creativity is that it is something mysterious and organic: the opposite of analytic thought. Creativity is something that happens *to* us rather than something that we do (Nanay 2014). It's the spark that seemingly comes from nowhere. Artists and poets speak of muses and divine inspiration, and of ideas suddenly appearing from nowhere. Even mathematicians and scientists often speak of creativity working in similarly mysterious ways. However, a big part of the mystery stems from our tendency to identify with our conscious mind— or, at least, the part of the conscious mind that we typically conceive of as the self (or as involving it). We tend to say things like 'the idea just popped into my mind', because we don't habitually think of our minds as mostly operating outside of our awareness. However, just as a real spark doesn't come from nowhere and is a product of unseen processes, so are our creative ideas. Ideas don't pop into our *minds*. Rather, they pop into our *awareness* after having been generated by unconscious processes. The mathematician Henri Poincaré once described how this works for his mathematical creativity:

> Most striking at first is this appearance of sudden illumination, a manifest sign of long, unconscious prior work. The role of this unconscious work in mathematical invention appears to me incontestable, and traces of it would be found in other cases where it is less evident. Often when one works at a hard question, nothing good is accomplished at the first attack. Then one takes a rest, longer or shorter, and sits down anew to the work. During the first half-hour, as before, nothing is found, and then all of a sudden the decisive idea presents itself to the mind.
>
> Poincaré 1910, p. 328

And Arthur Koestler, following Poincaré, had a similar reflection about the creative process:

> The moment of truth, the sudden emergence of a new insight, is an act of intuition. Such intuitions give the appearance of miraculous flashes, or short-circuits of reasoning. In fact they may be likened to an immersed chain, of which only the beginning and the end are visible above the surface of consciousness. The diver vanishes at one end of the chain and comes up at the other end, guided by invisible links.
>
> Koestler 1964, p. 211

This quote highlights the respect in which the heuristics miss something important about our creative processes. A crucial aspect to creative processes is that they operate largely outside of our awareness. This is also why it can seem like creativity is something that happens to us rather than something we do: it emerges out of parts of the mind with which we normally don't identify.

It makes sense for the human mind to be built this way. Conscious, analytic thinking is considered to be slow, serial, and expensive. It is a precious and limited cognitive resource that should be used only for high-value tasks. In contrast, unconscious thinking is often considered to be fast, massively parallel, and relatively inexpensive. And that is exactly what you want in a procedure that has to search an incredibly vast space of possibilities (remember how the heuristics can lead you down many dead ends). The thought, then, is that our creative processes are operating outside of conscious experience because this is an efficient way for the human mind to operate.

This shows that creative processes can be hidden from us (in fact, most of them are). What about their outputs—creative ideas? Could they also be hidden from us? That doesn't follow automatically, but it wouldn't make much sense for them to be otherwise. Part of the reason why the processes are hidden is so that the conscious mind doesn't have to execute them. However, another important reason is that the conscious mind doesn't have to *evaluate* every one of their outputs. It would make sense for the ideas (the outputs) to pass some kind of initial assessment before they flow into conscious experience. Otherwise, the conscious mind would be burdened with having to assess every "creative" idea that the unconscious mind comes up with. So, it makes sense that many of the ideas produced by the unconscious processes remain hidden from awareness and that only a select few—hopefully, the *better* ideas—make their way into our conscious experience.

This view of creative processing is not just one that can be arrived at through introspection and philosophical reflection. It has become a fairly mainstream view in cognitive science. For example, Eagleman and Brandt describe part of the view in *The Runaway Species*:

> Just like the massive computer programs running silently in the circuitry of our laptops, our inventiveness typically runs in the background, outside of our direct awareness.
>
> Eagleman and Brandt 2017, p. 6

And Eagleman states the idea even more explicitly in *Incognito*:

> You gleefully say, 'I just thought of something!', when in fact your brain performed an enormous amount of work before your moment of genius struck. When an idea is served up from behind the scenes, the neural circuitry has been working on the problems for hours or days or years, consolidating information and trying out new combinations. But you take credit without further wonderment at the vast, hidden machinery behind the scenes.
>
> Eagleman 2011, p. 7

And in *The Eureka Factor*, Kounios and Beeman write of insights, which they understand as a particular kind of creative thought:

> Insights have two key features. The first one is that they pop into your awareness, seemingly out of nowhere. They don't feel like a product of your ongoing thoughts. In fact, you can't control them in the way you can control your deliberate, conscious thought. Insights are like cats. They can be coaxed but don't usually come when called.
>
> Kounios and Beeman 2015, p. 23

> This is how insight is supposed to work. Your brain is processing the problem, but you don't have any sense of how it's going because this processing occurs outside of your awareness. At some point, the solution pops into awareness. You are surprised and may experience an emotional rush.
>
> Kounios and Beeman 2015, p. 120

Eagleman and Brandt also go on to articulate the thought that many of our ideas remain hidden from awareness:

> In the active brain, ideas multiply furiously and compete. A few get promoted into conscious awareness, but most don't reach the necessary threshold and they peter out.
>
> Eagleman and Brandt 2017, p. 211

These quotes represent a fairly consensus view that creative processes operate unconsciously, and we can find similar views expressed in the research literature as well. For example:

> We propose that unconscious thought may indeed be better at associative search than conscious thought (Dijksterhuis and Meurs 2006, Dijksterhuis and Nordgren 2006), but the products of unconscious thought may not always be immediately entered into consciousness. Instead, they may remain unconscious, only later emerging into consciousness as insight (Maier 1931) or eventually dissipating. Alternatively they may surface as tacit cognitive or affective recognition of patterns, coherences, or themes. For example, when presented with coherent stimuli such as an incomplete drawing of a camel, participants were able to recognize better than by chance the existence of some coherence in the incomplete drawings but could not always articulate what it was (Bowers et al. 1990). *We suggest that this feeling of 'something is there' may be a partial manifestation of unconscious generation.*
>
> Zhong et al. 2008, p. 913 (emphasis added)

I've highlighted the last sentence of this passage because it nicely anticipates the coming sections: that a partial manifestation is a partial revelation. That is, it is a psychedelic experience that could potentially be made *more* psychedelic by a suitable intervention—say, the consumption of a psychedelic or the practice of meditation. At any rate, the point for now is just that this has become a fairly standard view of creativity: a lot of what we associate with creativity is hidden from our awareness.

On the one hand, this theory of human creativity is quite straightforward. It's hard to see how it *can't* be true, at least in its broad outlines. It also takes a lot of the mystery and "magic" out of creativity, while also explaining why creativity seems so mysterious to us. On the other hand, this theory may also seem counterintuitive—or even creepy. It makes our creativity more like an alien intelligence living inside our minds that sometimes decides to speak to us. Right now, as you read these words, this alien intelligence is in your mind, churning away, melding old ideas into new ones through interlacing eddies of thought. And at any point, it may decide to speak up and share with you one of its latest creations. We don't normally conceive of our minds in this way, and that can make the theory counterintuitive. Nevertheless, once you get used to the basic idea, this view of creativity makes a lot of sense.[3]

8.4 Revealed Creativity

Now that we've established that creativity can be hidden, let's think about what it would be like if some of this hidden creativity were revealed. Remember, there are two things hidden from us: our creative ideas and the creative processes that produce those ideas. So, let's consider what it would be like for each of these to be revealed.

It's easy to imagine what it might be like to have some of your hidden ideas revealed to you in awareness: from your perspective, it could seem, for example, like you are having more ideas than usual. Or, it may seem like one idea that has been frustratingly difficult to come up with finally occurs to you. For example, we see this in Poincaré's description of his mathematical creativity:

I turned my attention to the study of some arithmetical questions apparently without much success and without a suspicion of any connection with my preceding researches. Disgusted with my failure, I went to spend a few days at the seaside and thought of something else. One morning, walking on the bluff, the idea came to me, with just the same characteristics of brevity, suddenness and

---

[3] To be clear, this view of creativity is not committed to these unconscious processes as having, or belonging to, some kind of unconscious *persona* or *agency*.

immediate certainty, that the arithmetic transformations of indefinite ternary quadratic forms were identical with those of non-Euclidian geometry.

Poincaré 1910, p. 327

Such breakthrough insights are not uncommon, and most of us know what it is like to have days when ideas come to us more freely. So, the experience of having hidden ideas revealed could be quite familiar.

However, what if such experiences were more psychedelic? If they were more psychedelic, then they would be more remarkable. For example, if the ideas being revealed are very strange (high in novelty), then you might be unsettled by the experience of suddenly having them in your conscious mind. Similarly, if your experience is *flooded* with ideas (high in scope), then you may become overwhelmed by them. Moreover, suddenly experiencing an overwhelming number of very strange ideas may even lead you to become concerned about your mental health—especially if this change is inexplicable and long-lasting or frequently occurring. These two examples correspond to the scope and novelty dimensions of psychedelic space. We'll come back to the relationship between creativity and the rest of psychedelic space in Section 8.7. For now, these two examples suffice to illustrate what the phenomenology of having creative ideas revealed in experience can be like. If just a few relatively normal ideas are revealed in experience, then this will count as an experience that is only mildly psychedelic, and it won't stand out to us. In contrast, if lots of very strange ideas are revealed, then the experience will be much more psychedelic (all else being equal), and it will feel much more remarkable to us.

Let's now consider what it would be like to have your hidden creative *processes* revealed in experience. This is a bit more difficult to imagine, but we can make it easier by first thinking about how these processes normally behave. As we know, they are operating outside of our awareness. However, they are also operating outside of what we take to be our *control*. To be sure, there are some things we can do to influence these processes. For example, we may deliberately feed them material that we would like them to work on. Or, we may train ourselves to become more finely attuned to what would make for a high-quality product. However, for the most part, we don't control these processes. This lack of control entails that the experience of having these processes revealed would involve one's experience evolving in an uncontrollable way. Recall from the previous section that the processes are constantly morphing old ideas—by bending, blending, and breaking them—into new ones. The processes are also operating in parallel, and likely interacting with one another, cross-pollinating with each other's intermediary outputs. Thus, having a psychedelic experience in which hidden creative processes are revealed would be remarkable to us, even if it were only mildly psychedelic. For example, Poincaré describes having had such an experience after having drunk some coffee:

One evening, contrary to my custom, I drank black coffee and could not sleep. Ideas rose in crowds; I felt them collide until pairs interlocked, so to speak, making a stable combination. [...] It seems, in such cases, that one is present at his own unconscious work, made partially perceptible to the over-excited consciousness, yet without having changed its nature. Then we vaguely comprehend what distinguishes the two mechanisms or, if you wish, the working methods of the two egos.

Poincaré 1910, pp. 326–35

Even though the experience was triggered by coffee, which is not usually considered a psychedelic substance, it nonetheless counts as a psychedelic experience since it involves Poincaré's unconscious processes being made partially perceptible (assuming he was right about this). However, the experience was, arguably, only a *mildly* psychedelic experience. An experience that was much more psychedelic, and much more revelatory of one's hidden creative processes, would be even more noticeable, and likely have a phenomenological profile that is similar to that of dreaming. We'll come back to this point later in Section 8.6, when we discuss the effects that psychedelics may have on creativity.

To summarize, from the previous two sections, we have reasons to think that at least some of our creative ideas and processes are hidden from our awareness, and from this section, we have a sense of what it would be like for these ideas and processes to be revealed in experience. Let's now consider whether there is reason to think that the practice of meditation can reveal our hidden creativity.

8.5 Meditation and Creativity

We have three kinds of reason for thinking that meditation reveals hidden creativity: (i) anecdotal evidence, (ii) a theoretical connection, and (iii) scientific evidence. Let's consider each of these in turn, starting with the anecdotal evidence.

Perhaps no one else has been more vocal about how meditation can increase creativity than David Lynch. In his book, *Catching the Big Fish: Meditation, Consciousness, and Creativity*, Lynch explains how meditation enhances his creativity:

Ideas are like fish.

If you want to catch little fish, you can stay in the shallow water. But if you want to catch the big fish, you've got to go deeper. Down deep, the fish are more powerful and more pure. They're huge and abstract. And they're very beautiful.

I look for a certain kind of fish that is important to me, one that can translate to cinema. But there are all kinds of fish swimming down there. There are fish for business, fish for sports. There are fish for everything.

Everything, anything that is a thing, comes up from the deepest level. [...] The more your consciousness—your awareness—is expanded, the deeper you go toward this source, and the bigger the fish you can catch.

My thirty-three-year practice of [meditation] has been central to my work in film and painting and to all areas of my life. For me it has been the way to dive deeper in search of the big fish.

Lynch 2007, p. 11[4]

It's clear from Lynch's description and, in particular, his metaphor of catching fish, that meditation enhances his creativity by making hidden parts of his mind available to consciousness.

Jumping fields, from cinema to investment decision-making, Ray Dalio, founder of Bridgewater (currently one of the most successful hedge funds), describes the effect of meditation on creativity similarly in his book, *Principles*:

Our greatest moments of inspiration often 'pop' up from our unconscious. We experience these creative breakthroughs when we are relaxed and not trying to access the part of the brain in which they reside, which is generally the neocortex. When you say, 'I just thought of something,' you noticed your unconscious mind telling your conscious mind something. With training [which includes meditation], it's possible to open this stream of communication.

Dalio 2017, p. 309[5]

Again, we see the same idea: meditation may increase creativity by enhancing the access one has to the unconscious.

Let's now consider the theoretical connection. As we saw in Chapter 5, both focused-attention meditation and open-monitoring meditation can be defined as interventions on the distribution of attention, and there is good scientific evidence that these interventions have measurable effects on attention. We also know, from the scientific research on creativity, that attention interacts with creativity in various ways (see Zabelina 2018 for an overview). For example, Kounios et al. 2008 found that diffused states of attention are associated with *insight* solutions to a convergent thinking task. And Carruthers et al. 2018 found that the concentration of attention was positively associated with performance on a divergent thinking task. Therefore, it stands to reason that meditation probably influences creativity via its effects on attention. Indeed, Horan 2009 has given a detailed argument

[4] The particular form of meditation that Lynch practises is known as Transcendental Meditation (TM), which is a mantra-based form of meditation and can be thought of as occupying a middle ground between focused-attention and open-monitoring meditation. I have omitted some details from Lynch's description that involve his views about fundamental physics since they are not essential to the core point that meditation can reveal hidden creative ideas.

[5] Incidentally, like Lynch, Dalio practises Transcendental Meditation.

along these lines. Vervaeke and Ferraro 2016 have also argued that meditation (and mindfulness more generally) facilitates creative insights by developing one's ability to scale attention up and down.[6]

In particular, there are three effects that meditation has on attention that are likely to have a positive impact on creativity: (i) it enhances the focusing of attentional resources, (ii) it enhances the diffusing of attentional resources, and (iii) it enhances the flexibility of how attentional resources are allocated and reallocated. The connection with creativity that is perhaps easiest to understand concerns the diffusing of attention. In a diffused state of attention, more attentional resources are available for allocation to unusual ideas, and these ideas are more likely to be promoted into awareness. In Lynch's metaphor of catching fish, a diffused state of attention corresponds to you surveying a larger, and deeper, region of the water. Now, once you see a potentially good fish, in order to catch it, it helps to flexibly switch from a diffused state of attention to a focused one. Then, the ability to focus attentional resources allows you to hold the idea in mind and reveal more of its details and connections with other ideas. If it turns out that the idea is not a good one, then you also need the flexibility to let it go, and shift back either to a diffused state of attention or to an alternative, focused one—for example, perhaps one that focuses on another idea that has appeared in awareness.

There's also a fourth effect that meditation has on attention that benefits creativity. Recall, from Chapter 5, that open-monitoring meditation involves the observing and non-reacting to sensations (both internal and external). The skill of non-reactivity is very important for creativity. We can see this by considering how the creativity-revealing process can go awry. By expanding awareness, a novel idea can get closer to consciousness and yet still remain outside of it. Let's assume, however, that it is a misleading idea—that is, it looks like it is a good idea but actually isn't. Because it is misleading in this way, your attention may be drawn towards it, causing it to suddenly appear in your mind in a vivid and captivating fashion. The result, then, would be a case of a *false insight*, and it can be problematic since it has the phenomenology of a true insight and thus feels more convincing than it should (Laukkonen et al. 2020). This can lead to precious time and resources being devoted to the idea (either exploring it in more detail or, worse, converting it into some real-world action). This sort of outcome can be prevented, to some extent, by reducing one's reactivity to one's ideas through the practice of meditation.

Once we see this connection between meditation and creativity, it's hard to unsee it. It explains not only the typical anecdotal reports that meditation enhances

---

[6] Scaling attention up corresponds to increasing the phenomenal transparency of experience (Chapter 5) while also expanding the scope of one's attention to include global or gestalt properties. Scaling down corresponds to increasing phenomenal opacity while decreasing the scope of one's attention to focus on local or featural properties.

creativity, but also the multifaceted connection between attention and creativity.[7] It also makes sense that if ideas really are created in the unconscious, then allocating additional attention to them will make them more likely to appear in awareness. To the extent that meditation can facilitate this (for example, by helping the ego to 'get out of the way'), then meditation will facilitate creativity. Moreover, to the extent that meditation can facilitate *good* ideas being promoted into awareness, it will further facilitate creativity.

We've now seen some of the anecdotal evidence and the theoretical reasons for believing that meditation enhances creativity by facilitating the revelation of hidden creativity. There is also some scientific evidence for this view. However, there is one caveat: many of the early studies into meditation and creativity did not clearly define the meditative techniques they used, and the choices of creativity measures were somewhat haphazard. For this reason, I'll focus on research that more clearly specifies the kind of meditative technique studied and the reasons for expecting it to enhance performance on the chosen measures of creativity. I'll also focus on the research that explores this connection directly.[8]

It makes sense to begin with the study of Strick et al. 2012 (from Chapter 5) since they set out to test specifically the hypothesis that a form of focused-attention—*susokukan*, or counting breaths—meditation provides greater access to the unconscious mind. They did this in two experiments. In the first experiment, they found that 20 minutes of meditation improved performance on a remote associates task, which is a common measure of creativity. In the second experiment, they found that subjects in the meditation condition were more likely to make use of subliminal primes when solving another task. Together, the two experiments suggest that meditation improves performance on remote associates tasks by increasing access to unconscious solutions.

On the one hand, the results of Strick et al. are somewhat in tension with the results that associate diffused attentional states with insight solutions to convergent thinking tasks (for example, Kounios et al. 2008). On the other hand, the results fit well with the thought that directing attentional resources to internal phenomena, and away from external stimuli, makes it easier to notice creative ideas. The tension may also be partly resolved by the results of Colzato et al. 2014 who studied the comparative effects of focused-attention and open-monitoring meditation on creativity. In particular, they found that for experienced meditators, 20 minutes of open-monitoring meditation increased insight-based solutions to remote associates tasks, relative to a session of focused-attention meditation of the same duration. This fits well with the natural thought that directing attention to internal phenomena *while also* diffusing attention would be most conducive

---

[7] For example, see Zabelina 2018, Kounios et al. 2008, Vervaeke and Ferraro 2016, Carruthers et al. 2018, and Wronska et al. 2018.

[8] See Horan 2009 for a nice review of the indirect evidence.

to having creative insights. Colzato et al. also found that 20 minutes of open-monitoring meditation improved performance on the alternative uses task in comparison with a session of focused-attention meditation of the same duration (for both experienced and inexperienced meditators). In general, these results seem to indicate that open-monitoring meditation may be more conducive to creative insight than focused-attention meditation.

Greenberg et al. 2012 conducted two experiments to investigate whether mindfulness and meditation would reduce the Einstellung effect, whereby preexisting knowledge impedes one's ability to reach an optimal solution to a problem task. The Einstellung effect can be thought of as the opposite of *shoshin* (beginner's mind). Their hypothesis was that mindfulness and meditative practices should help subjects be less blinded by previous experience and be more aware of the details of the present problem, which would then facilitate a more optimal solution. In the first experiment, they found that experienced meditators had a reduced Einstellung effect, and in the second, they found that participation in a 6-week mindfulness meditation programme also reduced the Einstellung effect (in comparison to controls who had not participated in the programme).

In another study, Müller et al. 2016 found that for experienced meditators, both kinds of meditation[9] led to increases in creativity as measured by performance on alternative uses tasks (which involve divergent thinking), relative to a within-subject non-meditation control condition. One important feature of this study to note is that subjects only performed the kind of meditation that they were experienced in. This makes the results of the study less comparable to those of other studies. For example, Müller et al. also found that focused-attention meditation increased cognitive flexibility, whereas open-monitoring meditation had no statistically significant effect on it. This could, however, have been due to initial differences between the two groups.

Ren et al. 2011 examined whether a particular form of focused-attention meditation would result in an improvement on a set of insight problems. The particular form of meditation they studied was *susokukan* meditation (similar to that of the study by Strick et al. 2012), which involves focusing attention on the breath and counting on each exhale. In order to control for possible effects from relaxation and a reduction in vigilance, Ren et al. divided subjects into three groups: a relaxation control, a meditation group that raised their hand every 10 exhales (M10), and a second meditation group that raised their hand every 100 exhales (M100). Subjects attempted to solve 10 insight problems for 30 minutes, then they either relaxed or meditated for 20 minutes, and then they attempted to solve any remaining insight problems. Meditators of both groups solved more remaining problems than the controls. Moreover, the M10 meditators solved more remaining problems than

---

[9] Müller et al. use the terms 'concentrative meditation' and 'mindfulness meditation' to refer to focused-attention meditation and open-monitoring meditation, respectively.

the M100 meditators did (although this effect only approached significance, with p = 0.051). Ren et al. interpret this result as indicating that the effects were due to maintaining a state of *watchfulness* rather than one of relaxation. This supports the idea that meditation can enhance creativity by expanding one's awareness and promoting an active, watchful state that is alert to new ideas produced by the unconscious.[10]

In summary, these effects of meditation on creativity are what we should expect to see if meditation enhances creativity by revealing hidden ideas. It is worth noting that Haase et al. 2022 conducted meta-analyses for 12 different methods of creativity enhancement and found that meditation interventions to be among the most effective. However, the research is still nascent, and so we should be cautious in drawing strong conclusions from these results. Nevertheless, the anecdotal evidence, the theory, and these initial scientific results all point in the same direction.

Before moving on, it's worth mentioning another interesting line of evidence that comes from a potential connection between mindfulness and creativity. Ostafin and Kassman 2012 found that mindfulness correlated with better insight problem-solving and not with non-insight problem-solving. They also found that 10 minutes of mindfulness meditation (following audio instructions) improved performance on insight problem-solving and not on non-insight problem-solving, in comparison to a control group (listening to a natural history text). Lebuda et al. 2016 conducted a meta-analysis of mindfulness and creativity studies and found a weak, but significant positive relationship between mindfulness and creativity. They also found that the effect was stronger when creativity was measured with tasks that required insight-based solutions, and that creativity tended to improve when mindfulness was manipulated with a meditation intervention (indicating a causal link between mindfulness and creativity). Again, this fits well with our hypothesis that meditation enhances creativity by improving access to the ideas produced in the unconscious mind.

Finally, Baas et al. 2014 broke the concept of mindfulness into four specific skills:

1. Observation: the ability to observe internal phenomena and external stimuli.
2. Acting with awareness: engaging in activities with undivided attention.
3. Description: being able to describe phenomena without analysing conceptually.
4. Accepting without judgment: being non-evaluative about present-moment experience.

They then sought to establish which of these specific skills were most associated with creativity. They found that the skill of observation was the only skill that

---

[10] This form of meditation is often used to develop attentional stability, so the effect could also be seen in terms of a shift in psychedelic space along the dimension of duration.

was a consistently reliable predictor of creativity and, moreover, that an increase in observation skills, due to intensive open-monitoring meditation training, was positively associated with an increase in creative behaviour. Baas et al. conclude:

> To be creative, you need to have, or be trained in, the ability to observe, notice, and attend to phenomena that pass your mind's eye.
>
> Baas et al. 2014, p. 1104

This result also fits well with the view that meditation can enhance creativity by making one more observant of the ideas created by one's unconscious processes.

To summarize, the anecdotal evidence, theory, and scientific evidence all appear to point in the same direction: meditation can enhance creativity by making it easier to notice ideas created by the unconscious mind. Again, to be clear, this does not entail that this is the *only* way by which meditation may enhance creativity. Instead, the point is that inducing psychedelic experiences (and/or increasing mindfulness) that reveal hidden ideas is *one* way that meditation may enhance creativity.

8.6 Psychedelics and Creativity

Let's now consider whether there is reason to think that the consumption of psychedelic substances can also reveal our hidden creativity. A natural place to begin is with the objection, inspired by Shanon 2002, that the hypothesis that psychedelics cause mind-revealing experiences cannot account for their supposed enhancements of creativity. The basic thought behind the objection is that since creativity involves the generation of novel ideas, then if psychedelics enhance creativity, it follows that they don't do so by revealing ideas that already exist in the mind.

We're now in a position to see why this objection is mistaken. Although creativity involves the generation of novel ideas, it doesn't follow that those novel ideas necessarily appear in awareness (most do not). Moreover, just because a novel idea suddenly appears in awareness, it doesn't follow that the idea was generated in that very moment. New ideas are constantly being generated by unconscious processes, and although some of them may appear in awareness right way, many may remain hidden in the unconscious mind. Therefore, it is entirely possible that psychedelics may enhance creativity by revealing ideas that are concealed from awareness.

There is also an important point about the *counterfactual* effects that psychedelics may have in this regard. Imagine a person who suddenly has a creative idea during a psychedelic trip, and let's suppose that this idea appeared in awareness in the very moment that it was generated. Since it appeared as soon as it was generated, it follows that the idea was never hidden from awareness. Does this mean that the appearance of the idea counts as an increase in creativity that doesn't involve mind-revelation? Not necessarily. It could be the case that if the person hadn't been under the influence of the psychedelic, then the idea would have been generated but kept hidden from awareness. For conditions when such a counterfactual is true, it is reasonable to say that the trip increases the individual's creativity by revealing their mind. In this case, the experience didn't reveal the particular idea, but it did reveal the "space" where the idea was generated.[11]

We therefore have two distinct ways in which a psychedelic trip may enhance creativity by revealing the mind. First, the trip may reveal ideas that are already in the unconscious—that is, before the trip has begun. Second, the trip may reveal newly generated ideas which would otherwise have remained hidden from awareness. Therefore, we have at least two ways in which psychedelics may enhance creativity by revealing the mind, and both are entirely consistent with Shanon's point that creativity involves the generation of novel ideas.

That gives us a response to the objection that psychedelics do not enhance creativity by revealing hidden information. However, we do not yet have any *positive* reason for thinking that they do this. So, let us now to turn to that issue. From a theoretical perspective, we can draw one line of argument from the Osmond-Grof hypothesis. This argument proceeds in two steps.

First, let's think about why a creative idea may fail to appear in awareness: it doesn't pass the initial filtering process that is checking ideas for quality and relevance. The mechanisms responsible for this filtering process are likely similar to those that prevent most of our memories from appearing in awareness at any given moment (Chapter 6). In both cases, the filter is imperfect, but the imperfections are more obvious when it comes to memory. This is because there are situations in which it can be quite clear that we have something in memory but are unable to access it temporarily—such as when a word is stuck on the tip of one's tongue. In contrast, it is often unclear as to whether we already have a creative idea and are unable to access it.

Nevertheless, it appears that there are situations in which this occurs. For example, recall from Section 8.3 the result observed by Bowers et al. 1990 that people could tell that an incomplete drawing of a camel had some coherence to it, even though they couldn't identify what it was a drawing of. As Zhong et al. 2008 propose, this feeling of coherence may be a *partial* manifestation of an unconscious idea as to what the drawing is meant to represent. Indeed, Boden 1990 described the phenomenon in more absolute terms:

> Up to a point, tacit knowledge can be made explicit [. . .] and doing so 'immensely expands the powers of the mind, by creating a machinery of precise thought'. But

---

[11] A similar point also holds true for meditation.

some unformalized knowledge always remains, and the new insights arising from it cannot be immediately captured by conscious thought. As the mathematician Carl Gauss put it: 'I have had my solutions for a long time, but I do not yet know how I am to arrive at them'.

Boden 1990, p. 35

So, it looks like there can be cases in which, just as we know we can't call to mind a memory, we are also unable to call to mind a creative idea that we already have. The point, then, is that not only do we have hidden ideas, but that we sometimes have hidden creative ideas, marked by novelty and quality.

Let's now move to the second step of the argument. Recall that, according to the Osmond-Grof hypothesis, psychedelics indiscriminately amplify elements of the unconscious, so that they are more likely to appear in awareness (or more vividly in awareness). In terms of attentional resources, this is the hypothesis that psychedelics disrupt the attention system and create a surplus of attentional resources that can flow somewhat freely throughout the mind. When some of this surplus is allocated to an element of the unconscious, then that element is more likely to appear in awareness. In Chapter 6, we considered what could happen when this element is an autobiographical memory: the memory is more likely to pass the threshold of activation and thus appear in awareness as an involuntary autobiographical memory (Barzykowski et al. 2019). The thought here is that essentially the same thing can happen for an unconscious idea: if an idea receives more attentional resources than it otherwise would, then it might be sufficiently activated to appear in awareness.

However, this doesn't yet entail that psychedelics *enhance* creativity. Remember, our interest is in the hypothesis that psychedelics enhance the creativity of an individual by revealing their hidden creativity. The revelation of an idea doesn't entail that one's creativity is enhanced, because an untold number of *uncreative* ideas could be revealed. As far as the Osmond-Grof hypothesis goes, there's no reason to expect that psychedelics will somehow selectively target only the good ideas that have been mistakenly prevented from making their way into their awareness. If psychedelics are non-specific amplifiers of the unconscious mind, then they will amplify *all* ideas—the good and the bad. Moreover, since there are, presumably, many more bad ideas than good ones, it seems that we should expect the opposite of an enhancement of creativity from psychedelics: the conscious mind will be inundated by junk. To make matters worse, if the experiences are lacking in clarity, then it will be difficult to accurately assess the quality of each idea. As Laukkonen et al. 2020 have observed, people can mistake the phenomenological profile of a creative insight for a sign that the insight is true. Putting all this together, we arrive at an unexpected conclusion: psychedelics may *diminish* creativity by revealing one's hidden ideas.

Indeed, there is some evidence in support of this. For example, indiscriminate amplification is a natural interpretation of the increased spread of semantic activation that has been observed to be brought about by psilocybin (Spitzer et al. 1996) and LSD (Family et al. 2016). More generally, as Baggott 2015 has pointed out, it was not uncommon for the early research on psychedelics and creativity to find a discrepancy between *perceived* enhancements of creativity and *actual* enhancements. This also lines up with a common anecdotal report: new ideas can seem to be of profound importance during a psychedelic trip and then recognized to be banal or nonsense once the trip is over.

There is another line of evidence that psychedelics indiscriminately amplify ideas into awareness. A common description of psychedelic trips is that they are like waking dreams (Jacobs 1978, Fischman 1983). Indeed, after analysing a large database of descriptions of trip and dream experiences, Sanz et al. 2018 found that there was a strong similarity between the two. Kraehenmann et al. 2017 also report that LSD produces mental imagery similar to that of dreaming, and Kraehenmann 2017 argued that psychedelic-induced experiences are most similar to those of lucid dreams.[12] This phenomenological similarity between dreams and psychedelics therefore suggests that psychedelics may also amplify our unconscious *creative processes* into awareness (Section 8.4). This entails that psychedelics are indiscriminately amplifying all (or at least many) of the ideas that these processes generate and which would normally be kept out of awareness due to their lack of quality or relevance.

Does this mean that psychedelic enhancements of creativity are illusory? Not necessarily. There is growing evidence that psychedelics can, in some circumstances, enhance creativity.[13] There is also indirect evidence: psychedelics have been observed to increase openness,[14] which is strongly associated with creativity (Silvia et al. 2009). However, there are also results that are mixed or against the hypothesis.[15] In general, there appears to be weak support for the claim that psychedelics can enhance creativity, but it is too early to draw conclusions at this stage.[16]

Part of the challenge in obtaining clear results with respect to this issue involves designing experiments that tap into the relevant mechanisms that psychedelics are likely to enhance. For example, while psychedelics may enhance divergent thinking, tasks that measure divergent thinking are unlikely to be personally relevant to the subjects. Thus, if psychedelics enhance creativity by revealing

---

[12] See also Carhart-Harris 2007 for a review of the literature on dream and psychedelic states and the discussion in Carhart-Harris and Nutt 2014.

[13] Harman et al. 1966, Zegans et al. 1967, Rios and Janiger 2003, Kuypers et al. 2016, Sweat et al. 2016, Mason et al. 2019, Mason et al. 2021.

[14] MacLean et al. 2011, Lebedev et al. 2016, Nour et al. 2017, Bouso et al. 2018, Erritzoe et al. 2018, Erritzoe et al. 2019, Madsen et al. 2020.

[15] McGlothlin et al. 1967, Uthaug et al. 2018, Mason et al. 2021, Kiraga et al. 2021.

[16] For reviews, see Sessa 2008, Baggott 2015, Iszáj et al. 2016, Girn et al. 2020, and Prochazkova and Hommel 2020.

hidden creative ideas, experiments designed using such tasks are likely to miss actual enhancements of creativity. This is because it appears that in order for a psychedelic to enhance one's creativity, one must already be working on a problem that requires a creative solution (Narby 2001, Shanon 2002). As Poincaré pointed out, insights that pop into awareness from the unconscious do not come for free: intense and disciplined conscious effort must be deployed on both sides of the insight's occurrence. Such conscious work must be conducted in order to sufficiently encode the problem, and the criteria for solving it, in the unconscious. Only then could it be reasonable to expect that the problem might be solved via creative insight. So, it may be that psychedelics enhance creativity only under these circumstances. They may do so by revealing our creative ideas and facilitating such insights. Alternatively, they may do so by revealing our creative processes and making them more available for conscious guidance. As Kounios and Beeman 2015 put it: 'Insights are like cats. They can be coaxed but don't usually come when called' (p. 23). It could be that by revealing one's unconscious creative processes, psychedelics enhance one's ability to coax them in the right direction. At any rate, each possibility (the revelation of ideas and the revelation of processes) requires that disciplined conscious work has already been done.

The experimental design of Harman et al. 1966 study is important to highlight in this regard. As Baggott 2015 points out, this study suffered from several problems: it had no placebo controls, it allowed for group work, and it involved the administration of stimulants in addition to LSD. It was also a pilot study that was meant to be the start of a subsequent line of research, but this was interrupted when psychedelics research was banned by the government. Nevertheless, this study was unique in an important respect. Instead of having subjects perform arbitrary divergent and convergent thinking tasks, the researchers required that subjects try to solve problems they had already been struggling with in their professional careers. This design choice helped ensure that the materials for LSD-induced insights were already in the unconscious minds of the subjects and that genuine solutions could be accurately recognized and externally validated. From the perspective of the Osmond-Grof hypothesis, it would be interesting to see what the results would be if this experimental design was developed appropriately to control for confounding factors (such as placebo effects).

To summarize, we now have a better idea of how psychedelics may enhance creativity by revealing hidden creative ideas and processes. The above discussion is primarily theoretical in nature because we currently have limited empirical evidence that psychedelics can, in fact, enhance creativity—let alone evidence that psychedelics do this specifically by revealing hidden ideas and creative processes. Nevertheless, there is reason to expect that this is at least one way in which psychedelics may enhance creativity.

8.7 Creativity and Psychedelic Space

The main point of this chapter was to explore how psychedelics and meditation may enhance one's creativity by revealing hidden creative ideas and processes, and we now have an idea for how this may happen. In this section, we'll briefly look at how we may develop a deeper understanding of the relationship between creativity and psychedelic experience using the conceptual framework of psychedelic space. The reason for thinking that this may be a worthwhile pursuit is that there are some suggestive similarities between what it takes for an experience to be more or less psychedelic and what it takes for someone to be more or less creative. For example, one way an experience can be more psychedelic is if it involves the revelation of more *novel* content, and one way that someone can be more creative is if they have more *novel* ideas. Is this similarity just a coincidence, or is there something deeper going? Let's take a closer look.

Recall what it takes for someone to be creative. The standard definition says that a creative person tends to produce many novel objects of high quality, where the notion of 'object' is understood broadly to include things such as poems, movies, theorems, hypotheses, furniture, technology, and so on. Although it's common to speak of someone as either being a creative person or not, creativity is clearly something that comes in degrees. You can become more creative by producing *more* objects, or by producing objects with *higher quality*, or by producing products with *greater novelty*. Some trade-offs are possible, but generally speaking, the higher you score on each of these dimensions, the more creative you are. So let's examine how having psychedelic experiences that score higher on the four dimensions of psychedelic space may facilitate one scoring higher with respect to these three dimensions of creativity.

Let's start with the dimension of novelty since that is the most obvious point of contact between creativity and psychedelic space. All else being equal, if an idea revealed in an experience is more novel than one revealed in another experience, then the former experience will be more psychedelic than the latter. So there is clearly a connection between an idea being more creative in this respect and an experience being more psychedelic by being more novel. What about the other direction? Can we say that if a psychedelic experience is more novel, then the idea it reveals is more novel? Not quite. This is because the source of novelty of the experience may not lie in the revelation of a novel idea but in the revelation of a novel memory, or a novel emotional insight, etc. (which could, of course, spark the generation of a novel idea). However, to the extent that an experience can be directed towards the revelation of ideas, we can say that the more novel the experience is, the more novel are its revealed ideas. This raises the question of whether and how psychedelic experiences can be directed, which we'll come back to in the next chapter. For now, we can rely on the observation that it is well recognized that the content and nature of a psychedelic trip can be shaped to some degree by appropriately choosing its set and setting.

Next, let's consider the dimension of scope. The dimension of creativity that scope appears to line up with is the number of one's creative ideas. All else being equal, if an experience reveals more ideas than another experience does, then the first experience will be more psychedelic than the second. This makes sense, but there is a subtlety regarding how we count ideas, which depends on how we individuate them. For example, is an idea for an entire film just one idea, or is it a collection of ideas—for example, for the set, cast, location, music, cinematography, etc.? It seems that we should say that an experience that reveals an idea for an entire film has greater scope than an experience that reveals only an idea for the cast. Or, rather than counting ideas, it may make more sense to treat *idea* as a mass noun and instead to speak of the total "amount of idea" revealed in an experience (or instead just speak of revealed content or revealed information). So, all else being equal, if an experience reveals "more idea" than another, then it has larger scope to it and is thus more psychedelic. We obviously lack a fully general way of measuring how much idea (content) an experience contains, but it does seem to be a sensible notion and one that we can use at least to a rough approximation. For example, compare Lynch's description of how his ideas for films come to him with Dostoyevsky's claim about creative ideas:

It would be great if the entire film came all at once. But it comes, for me, in fragments. That first fragment is like the Rosetta Stone. It's the piece of the puzzle that indicates the rest. It's a hopeful puzzle piece.

In Blue Velvet, it was red lips, green lawns, and the song—Bobby Vinton's version of 'Blue Velvet'. The next thing was an ear lying in a field. And that was it.

You fall in love with the first idea, that little tiny piece. And once you've got it, the rest will come in time.

Lynch 2007, p. 23

And:

[...] certainly a creative work comes suddenly, as a complete whole, finished and ready, out of the soul of a poet.

Dostoyevsky, as quoted in Miller 1981, p. 49[17]

Another famous example of a large creative idea coming all at once is Coleridge's *Kubla Khan*. Here is Coleridge's description of his experience (written in the third person):

In the summer of the year 1797, the Author, then in ill health, had retired to a lonely farm house between Porlock and Linton, on the Exmoor confines of

[17] It should be noted that there is some reason to think Dostoyevsky might have been taking some poetic license with this description (Weisberg 1993, pp. 230–1).

Somerset and Devonshire. In consequence of a slight indisposition, an anodyne [a dose of opium] had been prescribed, from the effects of which he fell asleep in his chair at the moment that he was reading the following sentence, or words of the same substance, in 'Purchas's Pilgrimes': 'Here the Khan Kubla commanded a palace to be built, and a stately garden thereunto: and thus ten miles of fertile ground were inclosed with a wall'.

The Author continued for about three hours in a profound sleep, at least of the external senses, during which time he has the most vivid confidence, that he could not have composed less than from two to three hundred lines; if that indeed can be called composition in which all the images rose up before him as things, with a parallel production of the correspondent expressions, without any sensation or consciousness of effort. On awakening he appeared to himself to have a distinct recollection of the whole, and taking his pen, ink, and paper, instantly and eagerly wrote down the lines that are here preserved. At this moment he was unfortunately called out by a person on business from Porlock, and detained by him above an hour, and on his return to his room, found, to his no small surprise and mortification, that though he still retained some vague and dim recollection of the general purport of the vision, yet, with the exception of some eight or ten scattered lines and images, all the rest had passed away like the images on the surface of a stream into which a stone had been cast, but alas! without the after-restoration of the latter [...]

Coleridge 1816, pp. 51–3

While opium isn't typically considered a psychedelic, the above example demonstrates how it's possible for a large idea to come to someone in an experience. Consider, also, the following anecdotal report from the Harman et al. pilot study on the effects of psychedelics on creativity:

I looked at the paper I was to draw on. I was completely blank. I knew that I would work with a property 300 square feet. I drew the property lines [...] *Suddenly I saw the finished project.* I did some quick calculations. [...] it would fit on the property and not only that [...] it would meet the cost and income requirements [...] it would park enough cars [...] it met all the requirements.

Harman et al. 1966, p. 224 (emphasis added)

Again, we see the same phenomenon of an idea appearing in its entirety. It's conceivable that, say, only half of the idea for the project could have appeared instead. If that had happened, then the experience would have had less scope to it and therefore been less psychedelic.

As is the case with novelty, the direction of the connection between the scope of an experience and the amount of idea revealed isn't guaranteed to go in the other direction. That is, if one psychedelic experience has more scope to it than another, then it doesn't follow that more idea is revealed in the experience. Again, the reason is that other things besides ideas could be revealed in the experience that could increase its scope. However, to the extent that the experience is guided towards revealing ideas—as was attemped by Harman et al. 1966—then this direction of the connection would be established.

Let's now consider clarity. All else being equal, if an idea is revealed more clearly in one experience than another, then the experience is clearer and therefore more psychedelic. That much seems straightforward. However, what is the connection between the psychedelic dimension of clarity and the dimensions of creativity? To see this connection, we need to remember that our focus on the generation of creative ideas is in service of something else: the production of creative *objects*. For each idea that is revealed in experience, one is faced with the decision of whether or not to convert it into an object. The clarity of the experience will help with these decisions. If the clarity is high, then it will be easier to see the ideas for what they are and whether they are *good* or not. Moreover, clarity will also help with the execution that is necessary for producing the object. For example, it may be difficult to paint a painting if the idea of it can only be seen vaguely in the mind— it's much easier if the painting can be visualized clearly and vividly.[18] As before, increasing the clarity of a psychedelic experience won't necessarily increase the quality of the ideas being revealed or the number of ideas executed. However, to the extent that the experience can be guided towards the revelation of ideas, then increasing its clarity will increase the creativity associated with the experience in these respects.

Finally, let's consider duration. It's clear that duration is also closely tied to execution. For example, another participant of the Harman et al. 1966 pilot study gave the following description of their experience:

> Looking at the same problem with the materials, I was able to consider it in a much more basic way, because I could form and keep in mind a much broader picture.
>
> Harman et al. 1966, p. 220

Here we see both a reference to scope—'a broader picture'—but also to duration: *keeping* the broader picture in mind. The execution in this case, though, is a further consideration and evaluation of the idea. It's possible that the further consideration could have led the participant to judge the idea as a bad one. Duration can, therefore, also help ensure that more *good* ideas are eventually executed (this will depend also on their scope, novelty, and clarity). Krippner 1968 (pp. 57–60) also describes some initial empirical work (done between 1950

---

[18] Of course, this is not the only way to paint—one can, for example, paint to find an idea.

and 1970) that investigated how the hypnotic induction of time dilation could enhance creative output. The general thought behind this work was similar to the one here: an increase in subjective duration will permit a more efficient processing and more complete comprehension of the creative idea, leading to an increase in creative output. Finally, as before, extending the duration of a psychedelic experience doesn't necessarily enhance the associated creativity, but to the extent that experience is directed towards that purpose—as it was in the experiments described by Krippner, for instance—it will.

We now have a clear set of connections between the dimensions of psychedelic space and the key factors that contribute to one's creativity. It's important to note, though, that many simplifying assumptions have been made in order to tease out these connections. For example, it's possible that getting a fragment of an idea rather than the entire idea all at once may ultimately lead to more creativity. By only getting the fragment, one may have to work much harder and longer than one otherwise would. And perhaps by doing so, one ends up meeting new people, who introduce all sorts of new ideas that one wouldn't have had otherwise. Nevertheless, I think we can sensibly keep such external factors fixed and analyse a person's creativity during some period of time. That is, all else being equal, it's better to get the idea all at once rather than in fragments. As we saw in the quote from Lynch earlier: it would be great if the entire film came all at once.

Bringing everything together, I think we have a surprisingly fruitful theoretical connection between psychedelic experience and creativity via the conceptual framework of psychedelic space. This is because the dimensions of psychedelic space—scope, novelty, clarity, and duration—coincide with, or contribute to, the three dimensions of creativity: quantity, novelty, and quality. In short, being more creative is closely aligned with being more psychedelic (and more mindful; see Chapters 6 and 9).

8.8 Conclusion

The jury is still out on whether psychedelics actually increase creativity, but the evidence looks promising. At first glance, it would seem that if psychedelics do enhance creativity, then this would be a problem for the hypothesis that psychedelics reveal the mind. The apparent problem is that an increase in creativity looks like it is mind-*creating* rather than mind-*revealing*. However, in this chapter, I have argued that increases in creativity may arise because much of our creativity is often hidden from awareness and some of this hidden creativity is revealed in psychedelic experience.

9
Well-Being

9.1 Introduction

A central thesis of this book is that a psychedelic experience is a *mind-revealing* experience and that this concept can be successfully explicated in terms of psychedelic space, with its four dimensions of scope, novelty, clarity, and duration. In the previous chapters, we have seen how this explication can be used to unify and illuminate a range of phenomena relating to the consumption of psychedelics and the practice of meditation. In this chapter, we will consider how the explication may also help us understand the psychotherapeutic benefits of these interventions.

There is a rapidly growing body of scientific evidence indicating that meditation and psychedelics, when used appropriately, can alleviate a wide range of psychological conditions, including depression, anxiety, obsessive-compulsive disorder, substance use disorder, and post-traumatic stress disorder (Wielgosz et al. 2019, Nutt and Carhart-Harris 2020). There is also accumulating evidence that meditation and psychedelics may be used in combination to produce synergistic improvements in well-being (Heuschkel and Kuypers 2020, Payne et al. 2021, Simonsson and Goldberg 2022).

Naturally, these results give rise to a question about the fruitfulness of our account of psychedelic experience: can it be used to explain the therapeutic benefits of psychedelics and meditation? It seems so. Indeed, the explanation would appear to be rather simple: many psychological conditions are psychecryptic in nature—that, or their treatment is often thwarted by some psychecryptic part or aspect of the mind—and so a psychedelic experience can help unlock the mind and allow it to heal into a healthier state. The classic example is that of a traumatic memory that is hidden from awareness but nevertheless drives unhealthy behaviour and experiences of depression or anxiety. However, the general idea may be applied to other parts or aspects of the mind that are hidden from awareness and yet manage to influence conscious experience and behaviour with undesirable effects (coping mechanisms that have become maladaptive would be another example).

This simple explanation has been around since the early days of psychedelic research. For example:

> There is now an increasingly firm body of opinion that the psychological basis of LSD treatment lies in its peculiar property of releasing unconscious material. Earlier discussions and symposia (1955-1957) hinted at this possibility. In 1959

a Macy Foundation Conference considered that there was abundant evidence for this view, whilst the participants at the first European Symposium on LSD therapy held last November in Göttingen were unanimous that this theory was the only satisfactory explanation for the quality of the LSD subjective experience and thus of its healing effects on the individual.

Sandison 1963, p. 34

It has also been suggested that this feature of psychedelics may lead to a scientifically credible revival of psychoanalytic theory and therapy (Carhart-Harris et al. 2014), which tend to focus on bringing unconscious material into awareness. A number of recent studies also suggest that the ability of psychedelics to reveal the mind and facilitate psychological insight may be a key component of their therapeutic efficacy.[1]

While there is something to this simple explanation, it is not entirely satisfactory. This is borne out by the fact that new promising explanations have been put forward that do not involve the revelation of the mind—at least, not apparently so. For example, it has been proposed that the therapeutic power of psychedelics may lie in their tendency to promote experiences of connectedness (Carhart-Harris et al. 2018), psychological flexibility (Davis et al. 2021), the dissolving of self-representations (Lebedev et al. 2015, Letheby and Gerrans 2017), neuroplasticity and neurogenesis (see Rieser et al. 2021 for a review), and even placebo effects (Hartogsohn 2016, 2018). These proposals are fascinating and clearly have merit. Some may also be viewed as compatible with each other and as targeting the same phenomenon at different levels of analysis (e.g. as may be the case for psychological flexibility and some forms of neuroplasticity). Some of the proposals may also be specific cases of mind-revelation. For example, experiences of connectedness likely arise due to increases in phenomenal transparency, which in turn likely arise via the release of attentional resources, allowing them to flow more easily through some mental representations to others that wouldn't have received those resources otherwise (Chapter 5, Lyon and Farennikova 2022). However, some of the proposals are less obviously related to mind-revelation—for example, those involving psychological flexibility. Therefore, in this chapter, I will develop another explanation—one that generalizes the simple explanation involving mind-revelation and subsumes many of those just mentioned. This explanation stems from the growing evidence that the therapeutic power of psychedelics may lie in their tendency to enhance *mindfulness* (and mindfulness-related capacities).[2]

---

[1] For example, see Roseman et al. 2018, Carhart-Harris 2018, Roseman et al. 2019, Garcia-Romeu et al. 2019, Agin-Liebes et al. 2021, Davis et al. 2021, and Peill et al. 2022.

[2] For example, see Thomas et al. 2013, Soler et al. 2016, 2018, Sampedro et al. 2017, Domínguez-Clavé et al. 2019, Smigielski et al. 2019, Uthaug et al. 2019, 2020, Mian et al. 2020, Davis et al. 2020, Madsen et al. 2020, Murphy-Beiner and Soar 2020, Oorsouw et al. 2022, and Søndergaard et al. 2022; and see Radakovic et al. 2022 for a meta-analysis.

There are four key motivations for this choice of focus. First, as I argued in Chapter 6, the concepts of mindfulness and psychedelic experience are closely interrelated. Second, mindfulness has a special relationship to well-being. In fact, many Buddhist teachers refer to it as a *direct path* to liberation from suffering (*duhkha*). Therefore, we should be able to deepen our understanding of the therapeutic potential of psychedelic experiences by combining these two connections (psychedelic experience and mindfulness, and mindfulness and well-being). Third, the empirical result that psychedelics can enhance mindfulness may seem like good news in this respect. Indeed, I believe it is, but we should also pause on this point. For some readers, the effects of psychedelics may look nothing like mindfulness or the effects of meditation—indeed, they may even seem like opposites. Therefore, this empirical result requires an explanation, and the relationship between psychedelic experience and mindfulness can provide one. Fourth, a related puzzling result is that psychedelics can induce mystical-type experiences, and these appear to be associated with the therapeutic and other beneficial outcomes of psychedelics.[3] Part of the puzzling nature of this result is that these experiences have typically been associated with spiritual practices such as meditation, and some spiritual teachers and scholars have rejected the idea that the consumption of psychedelic drugs could induce these experiences (e.g. Suzuki 1971). There is definitely some wisdom in this rejection, but it is also increasingly difficult to deny that there is at least *something* in common to the mystical-type experiences induced by psychedelics and those induced by meditation. I propose that focusing on a mindfulness-based explanation of the therapeutic effects of psychedelics will help us understand the nuances involved and thus resolve this philosophical tension.

The plan for this chapter is as follows. In Section 9.2, we will return to the relationship between psychedelic experience and mindfulness and how both concepts can be explicated in terms of psychedelic space. In Section 9.3, we will consider the deep connection between mindfulness and psychological well-being. The results of these two sections will then allow us, in Section 9.4, to establish a relationship between psychedelic experience and well-being, which, in turn, will allow us to establish a novel theoretical relationship between psychedelics and well-being that is mediated by mindfulness. In Sections 9.5 and 9.6, we will then examine how this explanation can account for the well-being benefits that appear to be conferred by the mystical-type experiences induced by psychedelics.

[3] For example, see O'Reilly and Funk 1964, Klavetter and Mogar 1967, Griffiths et al. 2006, 2008, 2011, 2016, Maclean et al. 2011, Bogenschutz et al. 2015, Johnson et al. 2016, Ross et al. 2016, Roseman et al. 2018, Schmid and Liechti, 2018, Garcia-Romeu et al. 2019, Davis et al. 2020, McCulloch et al. 2022, Søndergaard et al. 2022, and Qiu and Minda 2022.

9.2 Mindfulness and Psychedelic Experience

Let's begin with the relationship between psychedelic experience and mindfulness. We've already discussed this relationship in Chapter 6, but it will help to review it so that it is fresh in our minds.

Perhaps the most common definition used in psychology is that mindfulness consists in paying non-judgemental attention to the present moment (Kabat-Zinn 1994). Another common and closely related definition says that mindfulness is an awareness that arises from paying non-judgemental attention to the present moment (Kabat-Zinn 2005). Such definitions are sometimes known as *bare-attention* definitions of mindfulness. As we saw in Chapter 6, while these definitions can be useful as instructions for the *practice and cultivation* of mindfulness, they don't quite fully capture mindfulness itself. The second definition is better than the first in this regard since it captures the fact that mindfulness involves a kind of awareness that arises from the practice circumscribed by the first definition. However, this second definition doesn't tell us about the nature of this awareness or what it is an awareness of. To be fair, Kabat-Zinn was well aware of these issues (for example, see Kabat-Zinn 2011); however, the resulting literature has not always appreciated the necessary subtleties in defining mindfulness, as several authors have pointed out.[4] The upshot is that, while they are good for informing the practice and cultivation of mindfulness, the above definitions lack sufficient detail for us to do any serious analytical work with them. So, we need a definition of mindfulness with more flesh on the bone.

Several authors have highlighted particular aspects of mindfulness that are missing from the above definitions. One aspect that is important for our purposes is that mindfulness is closely related to *memory* (Dreyfus 2011, Levman 2017). In Chapter 6, I used this relation to motivate the hypothesis that meditative practices (that are thought to cultivate mindfulness) should have positive effects on memory—particularly on the recollection of memories that are otherwise difficult to retrieve. However, this memory aspect of mindfulness isn't just about remembering learned facts or life experiences. It also involves a kind of *prospective* memory that makes it easier to remember one's values and intentions (Wallace 2006, Thānissaro 2012). There is, thus, also a relationship between the memory and present-moment aspects of mindfulness. As Bhikkhu Anālayo put it:

> [...] it is due to the presence of *sati* [mindfulness] that one is able to remember what is otherwise only too easily forgotten: the present moment.
>
> Anālayo 2004, p. 64

---

[4] For example, see Dreyfus 2011, Bodhi 2011, Purser and Milillo 2015, and Vervaeke and Ferraro 2016.

Another important aspect of mindfulness is that it involves *lucid* awareness of the mind's objects (Bodhi 2011). In other words, mindfulness is an awareness of mental objects—broadly defined so as to include thoughts, perceptions, the body, and even awareness itself (awareness of awareness)—that is clear and uncontaminated by distorting factors. This gives us reason to expect that mindfulness is at odds with failures to maintain lucid awareness, and there is some evidence in support of this—for example, the introspection illusion (Fox et al. 2012), change blindness (Hodgins and Adair 2010), inattentional blindness (Schofield et al. 2015, Pandit et al. 2022), and choice-blindness (Lachaud et al. 2022).

A better definition of mindfulness should therefore capture these various aspects of mindfulness (Shulman 2010, Bodhi 2011). As a way to do this, I proposed in Chapter 6 that we define mindfulness as the ability to call anything in the mind (broadly construed) into awareness and to hold it there indefinitely with perfect clarity. For example, if a memory of a past event is in the mind, then it can be called into awareness at will, experienced in its completeness with no erroneous details added, and for as long as needed. Or, if one has a complex plan for the future, then this plan can be held clearly in awareness in its full detail, and for as long as one wishes. One could also see with perfect clarity the value of the plan and how much time should be spent developing it. As another example, if one is looking at a painting, one sees the painting in all of its detail and all that the mind may associate with it (and the fact that the mind has those associations). As a consequence of this definition, mindfulness also involves a kind of cognitive dexterity: the more mindful someone is, the more easily they can shift from one object of thought to another, or from one mental state to another. They can also more easily adopt different attentional states. In particular, they can more easily maintain a diffused and stable allocation of attention, resulting in a form of open awareness or breadth of mind (Anālayo 2004, pp. 65–6).

With this definition of mindfulness, we can see that there is a substantial overlap between the different aspects of mindfulness and the dimensions of psychedelic space. For example, the dimension of scope corresponds to the breadth of mind just mentioned, including the meta-cognitive objects and aspects of the mind—awareness of awareness, awareness of the mind's associations, etc. The dimension of clarity corresponds to the lucid awareness aspect of mindfulness and what the bare-attention definitions of mindfulness focus on—particularly, the removal of distortions that arise through judgement and conceptualization (or at least the awareness of those distortions). The dimension of novelty corresponds to, among other things, the memory aspect of mindfulness and its associated cognitive dexterity: no part or aspect of the mind counts as forgotten and thus too difficult to bring into awareness.[5] Finally, duration corresponds to the stability and

---

[5] To be sure, there is more to novelty than this. Novelty can also be in the present moment—for example, in the form of somatic and energetic phenomena that are often hidden from awareness.

equanimity of mindfulness—the absence of "wobbling" and reflexively reacting—as well as the working-memory aspect of mindfulness (Dreyfus 2011), which I briefly discussed in Chapter 6.[6] In a way, these connections shouldn't be surprising: the framework of psychedelic space was designed to capture how an experience can be more or less revelatory of the mind, and mindfulness involves being able to be aware of the mind. (Recall that 'mind' is understood broadly here. It is common to mistake mindfulness as not including embodiment, somatic awareness, etc.)

This doesn't mean that psychedelic experience and mindfulness are identical, but it does entail that they are closely related. The relationship between them is somewhat like the relationship between having finally found your keys after losing them (a key-revealing experience) and never having lost your keys in the first place (being mindful of your keys). Given these parallels, the framework of psychedelic space is also useful for understanding mindfulness, and it provides us with new conceptual resources for understanding the relationship between psychedelic experience and mindfulness. In particular, the framework of psychedelic space provides us with a common language for analysing psychedelic experiences, mindfulness, and the interventions that are hypothesized to bring them about.

One example of this that will be relevant later on, when we discuss mystical-type experiences, is the effects that psychedelics and meditation may typically have on one's location in psychedelic space. Recall in Chapter 4 that I proposed, as a rough hypothesis, that psychedelics will tend to shift an individual temporarily deeper into psychedelic space before returning them to normal consciousness and that, in contrast, meditation tends to move one deeper into psychedelic space in a more enduring fashion—corresponding to a shift in one's coordinate system (one's default state of consciousness). Said another way, this hypothesis amounts to the following: psychedelics tend to produce psychedelic experiences, and meditation tends to enhance mindfulness. This is by no means a necessary difference between psychedelics and meditation, but if one had to guess what these interventions do to a randomly selected human being, this rough hypothesis would be a good guide. However, this rough hypothesis can easily be false. For example, if the psychedelic is consumed in a well-designed context with appropriate preparation and integration, the effect of the psychedelic can be more like that of meditation.[7] The analogy with finding your keys helps illustrate this point: finding your keys makes it easier for you be to more mindful of them in the future, especially if you take the time to learn from your experience of losing and subsequently finding them.

One may wonder, then, about the opposite direction: does all of this imply that as you become more mindful, you also become more psychedelic? After all,

---

[6] As I also mentioned in Chapter 6, the dimension of duration can be seen not as an aspect of mindfulness (*sati*) but as one of concentration (*samādhi*).

[7] Indeed, the effect can result in more mindfulness than from meditation alone. For example, in some ayahuasca ceremonies, the set and setting are so well designed that the ceremony is effectively a meditation retreat during which one's meditation practice is enhanced by a psychedelic.

as you become more mindful, your default state of consciousness moves deeper into psychedelic space. Perhaps somewhat counterintuitively, the answer is no. In fact, there is a sense in which the opposite is true. As you become more mindful, various experiences that were originally psychedelic for you become *less* psychedelic—the items that were once hidden either become less hidden or not hidden at all. This means that the nature of one's psychedelic experiences changes as one's mindfulness develops over time. However, we can also recognize a sense in which becoming more mindful entails becoming more psychedelic. This is because mindfulness is a *movable launchpad* for psychedelic experiences: all else being equal, the more mindful one is, the deeper in psychedelic space one's psychedelic experiences will tend to be. In other words, becoming more mindful makes it easier to access experiences that are deeper in psychedelic space (for example, one can use one's meditative skills to bring more stability and clarity to a psychedelic trip that is otherwise chaotic and overwhelming). Thus, we see that while mindfulness and psychedelic experience are interrelated concepts, there is still an important difference between the awareness afforded by mindfulness and the revelation of a psychedelic experience. This will be relevant later when we consider the nuances of entering mystical-type experiences via meditation and psychedelics.

Another important point of clarification is that for a shift in one's coordinate system to count as an increase in mindfulness, it should be *robust* and *enduring*. If the shift is fragile and can be immediately undone, then there's a sense in which this is not genuine mindfulness. This corresponds to a distinction made in the literature between *state mindfulness* and *trait mindfulness* (Kiken et al. 2015). An increase in state mindfulness is what we may expect to occur during, and soon after, a session of meditation. If an increase in mindfulness is enduring and robust, then this would count as an increase in trait mindfulness. Trait mindfulness is what we would expect expert meditators to have. This is important because, plausibly, a key part of mindfulness is that it also involves the skill of *developing more* mindfulness and *protecting against decreases* in mindfulness. It also reflects the difference between practising being non-judgementally aware of the present moment and not being *stuck* in judgemental awareness or awareness of one's past and future.[8] Therefore, it is probably best to reserve the term 'mindfulness' to refer to trait mindfulness, and view state mindfulness as a closely related and important concept.[9] Similarly, whereas the revelation of some specific part or aspect of the mind counts as a psychedelic experience, mindfulness is probably better understood as a general capacity that is not specific to any particular part or aspect of the mind. To be sure, practising being mindful of specific mental contents (e.g. the sensation of one's breath) can result in improved mindfulness (as a general capacity), but these are still different attributes.

---

[8] As I argued in Chapter 6, one can, for instance, mindfully think about the future.
[9] Moreover, a case could be made that increases in state mindfulness are, in fact, psychedelic experiences.

The definition of mindfulness given above is somewhat clunky—it says that mindfulness involves being able to call parts or aspects of the mind into awareness, hold them there indefinitely, and see them as they truly are. The reason for this formulation was to highlight the connections to psychedelic space. However, a simpler definition can be given in terms of the concept of a psychecryptic state. Recall, from Chapter 3, that a psychecryptic *experience* is the opposite of a psychedelic experience: it is a mind-concealing experience (a ship sailing into the fog). Accordingly, psychecryptic *state* is a mental state in which some parts or aspects of the mind are hidden from awareness (a ship already hidden in the fog). Although our mental states are always psychecryptic to some degree, we can recognize that some mental states are more psychecryptic than others. Moreover, just as psychedelic experiences can be more or less psychedelic with respect to the dimensions of psychedelic space, experiences and states can be more or less psychecryptic in these ways as well. We can thus define mindfulness simply as the inverse of a psychecryptic state: the more mindful you are, the less psychecryptic your default mental state is.

In summary, the framework of psychedelic space provides us with a clearer understanding of how psychedelic experience and mindfulness are related to each other. Indeed, as I've been arguing in the previous chapters, psychedelic space gives us an elegant framework for understanding many of the key concepts and ideas we have come across so far. It allows us to see how experiences can be more or less psychedelic, how meditation and psychedelics can both give rise to psychedelic experiences (but of different kinds), how psychedelic experiences are related to mindfulness, and how psychedelics and meditation may contribute to developing mindfulness in their different ways.

To be sure, a lot more can and should be said about mindfulness, and we should be wary of concluding that the definition of it in terms of psychedelic space captures all there is to mindfulness. Nevertheless, the definition does a better job of capturing mindfulness compared to the standard, bare-attention definitions, and it provides enough detail for us to connect the concept with other important concepts we care about, such as psychedelic experience. With this definition in hand, let us now turn to the connection between mindfulness and well-being.

9.3 Mindfulness and Well-Being

There are three ways we can approach the relationship between mindfulness and well-being. The first is to see how Buddhists understand the relationship. This is an appropriate place to start because the concept of mindfulness is, after all, originally a Buddhist one (although various precursors can be found in Hinduism). The second way we can approach it is scientifically: there is a growing body of evidence in support of a positive relationship between mindfulness and well-being. The third way is a first-principles approach: using our understanding of mindfulness and well-being, we can discover a positive relationship between them. Let's examine these three approaches in turn.

The claim that mindfulness and well-being are positively related to each other is perhaps one of the most basic and fundamental ideas of Buddhism. As I mentioned earlier, there is no one thing that is Buddhism: there are many schools of thought, and multiple perspectives can be taken on any given issue. However, as a broad brushstroke, it is fair to say that there are four fundamental ideas to Buddhism:

(i) Being in the world, *samsara*, necessarily involves *duhkha*—which is often translated as *suffering*, but more broadly construed so as to include dissatisfaction and also understood more narrowly so as to potentially exclude some forms of physical pain.

(ii) We are trapped in *samsara*, and the experience of *duhkha* that comes along with it, by our mental habits of attachment (desire, craving, etc.), many of which are difficult for us to recognize or change.

(iii) Nevertheless, it is possible to be released from *samsara* and to attain *nirvana*.

(iv) *Marga*, often referred to as the Noble Eightfold Path, is a way to achieve this release.

These four ideas correspond, roughly speaking, to the Four Noble Truths. The Noble Eightfold Path referred to in the fourth noble truth involves developing: (i) right view, (ii) right intention, (iii) right speech, (iv) right action, (v) right livelihood, (vi) right effort, (vii) right mindfulness, and (viii) right concentration. Explaining how this works will take us too far afield, and there is some debate among Buddhists as to how to understand the "folds" and their relationship to each other. For our purposes, we can make do with the observation that mindfulness often receives special emphasis, with it also occasionally being treated as necessary for release from *samsara*, and even sufficient, as the direct path to *nirvana* (Anālayo 2004). (Since the goal of this book is not to explicate Buddhist philosophy, nor to defend any particular school of Buddhist thought, I will leave the discussion here.)

Let's now turn to the scientific evidence concerning the relationship between mindfulness and well-being. We immediately run into a problem: how can we define and measure mindfulness? As I mentioned earlier, there are different definitions of mindfulness in the literature, and they don't always quite line up with traditional understandings of the concept. Nevertheless, there is a growing literature on using interventions that are thought to enhance mindfulness and therefore promote well-being by treating a wide array of psychological ailments (Wielgosz et al. 2019). Two interventions stand out in the literature: mindfulness-based stress reduction (Kabat-Zinn 1990) and mindfulness-based cognitive therapy (Teasdale et al. 1995). There are also different measures of mindfulness used in the literature, such as the Mindful Attention Awareness Scale (MAAS), the Freiburg Mindfulness Inventory (FMI), the Five Factor Mindfulness Questionnaire (FFMQ), and the Toronto Mindfulness Scale (TMS).

Not surprisingly, it can be difficult to interpret the results of this literature. On the one hand, the evidence that the cultivation of mindfulness promotes well-being appears clear-cut. For example, MacDonald and Olsen 2020 state that mindfulness 'has been robustly associated with psychological health, predicting greater well-being, and lower levels of anxiety, depression, and stress across samples'. On the other hand, it has been argued that current empirical results are mixed, and because of various methodological problems that arise from the issues with defining and measuring mindfulness, as well as defining consistently what mindfulness-based interventions amount to, it is difficult to draw conclusions about the effectiveness of mindfulness, let alone its clinical significance (Dam et al. 2018a). It has also been pointed out that techniques that are thought to cultivate mindfulness, such as various meditative practices, were never designed to treat mental health problems, and were instead designed to promote flourishing, self-actualization or self-transcendence, and enlightenment (Davidson and Dahl 2018). So, while the scientific evidence certainly looks promising, we need to be cautious when drawing conclusions from it.

The third, and final, approach we can consider is to examine the relationship between mindfulness and well-being from first principles. The idea is to take the most basic things we know about the two concepts and see if we can establish a theoretical connection between them. The advantage of this kind of approach is that it may allow us to sidestep many of the issues just discussed. That is, it may be possible to avoid many of the debates within Buddhism and not get caught up in the various definitional and methodological issues that have arisen in the scientific literature.

In order to begin, we need to lay out our basic definitions of mindfulness and well-being. We have a definition of mindfulness already, which is one half of the equation. The other half requires a definition of well-being, which we don't yet have. As usual, different definitions can be given, and there is a large literature on the analysis of well-being. In general, though, the concept of well-being is rooted in the idea that health is more than the absence of disease. Common definitions say that well-being involves an overall combination of physical health, positive relationships with others, positive emotions, personal mastery and autonomy, finding purpose and meaning in life, and personal growth and development (Ryff 1989, Seligman 2011). Some trade-offs between these components may be possible, but generally speaking, the better you are doing on each of them, the greater your well-being.[10]

---

[10] This definition is admittedly vague, but I think it is precise enough for our purposes while also being abstract enough to allow specific theories of well-being to be plugged into the main argument.

It wouldn't be an overstatement to say that the connections between mindfulness and well-being are many and nuanced, and a full discussion of them requires the space of another book. Nevertheless, we can make do with a limited discussion for our present purposes. I'll first discuss some of the fairly straightforward and practical ways in which mindfulness is conducive to well-being and then briefly consider one of the connections that is less straightforward and more spiritual in nature.

One straightforward connection between mindfulness and well-being is one we have touched upon already: we often learn all sorts of lessons for how to live well but then *forget* them. Becoming more mindful helps us to retain these critical insights so that we can apply them to our lives. Consider whatever lessons you have learned from life. These could be anything: good sleep is vital, it's better to be kind than right, you should exercise regularly, fear isn't conducive to good decision-making, comparison is the thief of joy, and so on. You don't have to agree with these examples. Think of your own list of lessons. And now think of all the times you forgot them, and all the reasons why. That, too, is a variegated list: you became tired, angry, distracted, sick, an emergency happened, you were manipulated by someone careless or malevolent, you allowed bad habits to form, etc. In short, you could read all of the self-help books in the world, and yet none of this knowledge will amount to anything if you forget it. Cultivating mindfulness makes it easier to remember this knowledge and convert it into action—*good* action—which, in turn, will typically lead to improved well-being.

A second connection draws upon the lucid awareness aspect of mindfulness. Many hindrances to well-being are fairly obvious and even easy to remove, but they often lurk just outside of awareness (in its hazy fringes), and we fail to notice them. The list is endless—bad posture, shallow breathing, poor eating habits, lies that we unknowingly tell ourselves, etc. These sorts of things can easily occur without us noticing, even though we know they are detrimental to our well-being. Cultivating mindfulness makes it easier to remove these hindrances to our well-being by bringing them into lucid awareness.[11]

A third connection between mindfulness and well-being stems from the psychological flexibility aspect of mindfulness. As noted earlier, many definitions of mindfulness often focus on the idea of paying non-judgemental attention to the present moment. Although paying attention in this way is certainly an important component of mindfulness, it is also a method for developing psychological flexibility. For example, our minds tend to gravitate towards certain styles of thought that involve judgemental attitudes and fixations, such as worrying about the future

---

[11] It should be noted that many of these examples are examples of the other folds of the Noble Eightfold Path—not lying (right speech), avoiding bad eating (right action), etc. To a certain extent, we're reinventing the dharma wheel here, but the difference—and the advantage—is that by doing so, we're not bound to any particular Buddhist school of thought or interpretation of classic texts.

or ruminating about the past. By practising the skill of focusing non-judgementally on the present moment, one develops the ability to not get trapped in these patterns of thinking. One can *choose* to think about the future, but one doesn't *have* to—one doesn't have to get caught up in such thoughts involuntarily. This aspect of mindfulness gives us another important connection to well-being, since psychological flexibility has been identified as a crucial element of psychological health (Kashdan and Rottenberg 2010).[12]

This brief discussion gives us a sense of some of the more straightforward connections between mindfulness and well-being. Based on these connections, we see that mindfulness is, at the very least, *necessary* for well-being. It is part of the nature of being human that we have to learn from the world while balancing the need to remember what we have learned with the need to adapt to changing circumstances. Learning, remembering, and adapting all require mindfulness. There is also a case to be made that mindfulness may be sufficient for (or at least highly conducive to) greater well-being (in Chapter 11, we will see that mindfulness is related to *phronēsis*, or practical wisdom). That is, the more mindful we are, the greater our well-being will tend to be. This stems from the fact that most (if not all) people want to live better, and that human civilization already has an abundance of unused, or inefficiently used, knowledge and resources that could be put to better use. By remembering more of life's lessons, becoming more aware of the situations we find ourselves in, and increasing our flexibility in how we respond to those situations, we're almost guaranteed to end up doing better in life (on average).[13]

We've just examined some of the more straightforward connections from different aspects of mindfulness to well-being. Let's now turn to the deeper connection between mindfulness and well-being I alluded to earlier. Recall the various aspects of mindfulness that we have come across. Mindfulness involves being able to call anything to mind, see it as it is, and hold it in awareness indefinitely. It also involves psychological flexibility and a kind of stability to the mind. A feature that emerges from all of these aspects of mindfulness is a kind of unification or integration of the mind—a certain *oneness* or *wholeness* to the quality of one's mind. One way to see this point is to consider mindfulness as the inverse of how psychecryptic one's default state of mind is. If one is more mindful, one's overall mental state is less psychecryptic, and thus less fragmented and less siloed. There's a resulting integration of mind that makes it easy to flexibly call things into awareness, see them as they truly are, and hold them there indefinitely.[14]

---

[12] It is also worth noting here that increased psychological flexibility has been proposed as one of the mechanisms by which psychedelics may improve well-being (e.g. Davis et al. 2021).

[13] It is important to emphasize that this point is about the *outcome* of being more mindful and not the *process of cultivating* mindfulness, which may involve travelling along a very bumpy road.

[14] Remember that we're using the term 'mind' rather broadly, so as to include bodily sensations, feelings, perspectives, etc.

Many psychologists have noticed a connection between well-being and having this unified, integrated state of wholeness. Perhaps the most noteworthy in this respect are Carl Jung and Abraham Maslow.[15] For example, Maslow wrote:

> In the healthy person and especially the healthy person who creates, I find that he has somehow managed a fusion and a synthesis of both primary and secondary processes; both conscious and unconscious; both of deeper self and of conscious self. And he manages to do this gracefully and fruitfully.
>
> Maslow 1963, p. 85

And:

> We are learning that complete health means being available to yourself at all levels.
>
> Maslow 1963, p. 88

Similarly, in a commentary by Jung on the relationship between Zen Buddhism and psychotherapy, we find:

> If the fragments offered by, or forced up from, the unconscious are successfully built into the life of the conscious, a psychic essence form results, which corresponds better to the whole of the individual personality, and therefore abolishes fruitless conflict between the conscious and the unconscious personality. Modern psycotherapy rests upon this principle, inasmuch as it was able to break away from the historic prejudice that the unconscious harbors only infantile and morally inferior contents.
>
> Jung 1949, p. 23

As we'll see in the next section, the larger context of this passage from Jung concerns the *psychedelic experience* that can be brought about by Zen practice— hence the reference to fragments being 'forced up' from the unconscious. Despite this difference (between psychedelic experience and mindfulness), the essential idea concerning the connection between the integrated state of mindfulness and well-being is clearly present. Indeed, it is at the core of Jung's notion of the *individuation process*, whereby the individual's personal and collective unconscious are

---

[15] In the rest of the chapter, I include several quotes from Jung and Maslow. This isn't because of an implicit commitment to their particular views on psychology and psychotherapy. Instead, it is simply to recognize that the ideas presented here are not entirely new. Also, the works of Jung and Maslow were seminal in the development of psychology and psychotherapy—particularly person-centred therapy, transpersonal psychology, and most recently, positive psychology and non-directional therapy. See also Kaufman 2020 for a comprehensive discussion of how many of these ideas—particularly those of Maslow—have found scientific support in recent decades.

assimilated with the conscious mind to form an integrated whole.[16] It also has sub-stantial overlap with Maslow's notions of *self-actualization* and *self-transcendence*, and similar concepts can be found in other works of humanistic psychology (such as Rogers' *fully functioning person* and Fromm's *autonomous person*). It also contains Ernst Kris' 1936 notion of *voluntary regression in service of the ego* as one particular way of being able to call a part or aspect of the unconscious to awareness (see also Knafo 2002).[17]

The idea that mindfulness is essential to well-being in this holistic way has been around for quite some time, and it gets expressed in different ways by those coming from different perspectives and schools of thought. The basic idea is that psychological suffering is caused by hidden mental elements that drive behaviour and decision-making in undesirable ways. All else being equal, by developing the ability to bring them into awareness at will, the individual begins to break free from the grip of these hidden elements. This idea is at the heart of many psychodynamic, humanistic, and transpersonal theories of psychotherapy, but it is also central to other approaches, such as cognitive-behavioural therapy—from which mindfulness-based cognitive therapy has emerged (Teasdale et al. 1995). To be sure, these approaches tend to differ in how they understand the human mind. For example, psychodynamic approaches tend to postulate complex structures in the unconscious, and cognitive-behavioural approaches tend to take a more parsimonious view of the unconscious mind. They also tend to differ with respect to the kinds of interventions they focus on. Taking our two examples again, psychodynamic approaches can involve years of talk-based therapy, tending to focus on extracting and analysing content from the early stages of life, whereas cognitive-behavioural interventions can be much shorter (weeks, days, and even hours) and tend to focus on improving the patient's strategies for dealing with the present. Nevertheless, they both often involve increases in mindfulness (perhaps via revelatory experiences). The only approach to psychotherapy that may not have mindfulness at its heart in some form or other is behavioural therapy. However, it has been argued that even radical behaviourism is compatible with, and even complementary to, a Buddhist understanding of the mind (Diller and Lattal 2008). In any case, the point here is not that the connection between mindfulness and well-being is at the heart of every school of psychotherapy. Rather, it is just that the idea of their connection has been around for some time, exists in different forms, and is congenial to many schools of psychotherapy.

We now have a fairly clear connection between mindfulness and well-being. It's worth emphasizing, again, that nothing that has been said so far entails anything about the effectiveness of specific mindfulness-based *interventions* (such

---

[16] For a similar commentary on psychoanalysis and Zen, see Fromm 1959.

[17] See also the discussion of Fabbro et al. 2017 concerning the relationship between mindfulness and Freud's concept of *free-floating* or *evenly-suspended* attention.

as meditative practices). All that has been established is that the more mindful one is, the greater one's well-being will likely be (all else being equal). This says nothing about the *process* of becoming more mindful. It could easily be the case, for example, that certain meditative practices may worsen various psychological conditions. Indeed, there is growing evidence that adverse effects from mindfulness-based interventions are not uncommon.[18] For instance, it's conceivable that the last thing someone suffering from suicidal ideation should do is go on a five-day silent meditation retreat. We'll address the issue of intervention at the end of the next section. For now, we just have a plausible conceptual relationship between established mindfulness and well-being. With that in place, we can now turn to the final step of the argument: the relationship between psychedelic experience and well-being.

9.4 Psychedelic Experience and Well-Being

To summarize where we are so far, we have established two connections: (i) between psychedelic experience and mindfulness (Section 9.2) and (ii) between mindfulness and well-being (Section 9.3). The task of this section is to use these two connections to establish a connection between psychedelic experience and well-being.

There are two key ideas that will help us arrive at this third connection. The first is that a psychedelic experience is a kind of "downgraded" form of an increase in mindfulness. Or, to put the idea more positively, a psychedelic experience can *approximate* an increase in mindfulness.[19] The second key idea is an inheritance principle: to the extent that a psychedelic experience approximates an increase in mindfulness, it inherits the benefits to well-being that that increase in mindfulness would bring. Putting these two ideas together gives us a way to extend the simple answer to our question we considered in Section 9.1: the more a psychedelic experience approximates an increase in mindfulness, and the greater that increase in mindfulness is, the more the experience will have a positive impact on one's well-being. This answer will help us understand why psychedelics and meditation tend to produce psychotherapeutic benefits. It will also highlight some ways in which we may improve upon them as therapeutic interventions.

To get to that conclusion, we need to unpack the two key ideas. We can do this by "peeling off" some of the features that constitute mindfulness and seeing how what is left inherits many of the mindfulness' benefits to well-being. This peeling

---

[18] For example, see Cebolla et al. 2017, Lindahl et al. 2017, Baer et al. 2019, Schlosser et al. 2019, and Farias et al. 2020, but also see Anālayo 2019 for a nuanced discussion of this issue.

[19] Recall that we are using the dispositional form of mindfulness here. In contrast, increases in state mindfulness may be understood as psychedelic experiences. This helps us see why practising state mindfulness cultivates mindfulness, since the former can approximate the latter.

off process comes in two stages. First, we peel off the features that *distinguish* increases in mindfulness from psychedelic experiences: (i) the robustness, or enduring nature of mindfulness, (ii) the generality, or lack of content specificity of mindfulness, and (iii) the volitional quality of mindfulness. Second, we peel off the features that constitute an *increase* in mindfulness, which correspond to the four dimensions of psychedelic space. As we do all this peeling, we can see how many of the benefits of increases in mindfulness may still be inherited and also how there are things we can do to patch up the difference.

The first feature to peel off is the enduring nature of mindfulness. Recall, from Section 9.2, that an increase in mindfulness corresponds to a shift of one's coordinate system deeper into psychedelic space, which is understood as change in one's default mental state. We can imagine how a similar change that is less robust and enduring would still bring about many of the same benefits. Suppose one's newfound mindfulness tends to fluctuate throughout the day—for example, it deteriorates in the evening but returns in the morning after a good night's sleep. It would be better to have one's newfound mindfulness consistently throughout the day, but many of the same benefits can still be acquired. For instance, one can have insights in the morning about how to protect one's self in the evening from self-undermining behaviours (e.g. by locking away the cookies). One can also make changes to one's daily schedule to take advantage of the mindful mornings.[20] The details will vary depending on one's situation, and how one's mindfulness fluctuates, but the general idea will hold: if the mind is appropriately scaffolded, a fluctuating mindfulness can have many of the same benefits as a mindfulness that is more robust and enduring.

The second feature to peel off is the generality, or lack of content specificity, of mindfulness. It seems that a genuine increase in mindfulness must have a generality to it that psychedelic experiences often lack but can, nonetheless, approximate. For example, by revealing a hidden memory, a psychedelic experience may cause a long-term increase in the accessibility of associated memories without those memories appearing in awareness during the experience. This improvement in accessibility could be considered an increase in mindfulness. However, it could also be argued that the improvement may be too specific to count as a genuine increase in mindfulness. It's not clear where to draw the line between being too specific and sufficiently general, and it probably makes sense to say that it is a matter of degree: the more general the new accessibility is, the more it will count as an increase in mindfulness. Thus, this generality can be approximated by a psychedelic experience, and the better it is approximated, the more of mindfulness' benefits will be inherited by the experience.

---

[20] Of course, to the extent this can be done will depend on one's life circumstances. Thus, these examples should be understood with implied *ceteris paribus* qualifications and are simply meant to help illustrate the general idea.

The third feature to peel off is the volitional quality of mindfulness. This is the idea that when something is brought into awareness using mindfulness, it is done with voluntary control, and as such, it is not *revelatory* in nature. This volitional quality is a key difference maker between mindfulness and psychedelic experience. There is a sense in which psychedelic experiences happen *to* you: things are hidden in your mind, and then they are shown to you. Mindfulness is the opposite of that: things are not hidden, and so you can call them to awareness at will.[21] However, as with the peeling off of the previous two features, many of the benefits of an increase in mindfulness can also be inherited by involuntary revelations. For example, you may have enough mindfulness to be aware that you are now in an agitated state, but not enough to remember how to resolve this. Nevertheless, your mindfulness may *also* enable you to remember that a session of meditation will likely reveal a way for resolving your agitation. For instance, it may reveal some nugget of wisdom that you've temporarily forgotten (e.g. that comparison is the thief of joy). It would be better to be able to call upon that nugget as needed, but remembering that there's something like it that meditation can help one recollect is almost as good.[22]

We've now completed the first stage of our analysis. We've considered how even if the features of robustness, generality, and volition are lost, many of the mindfulness' benefits can remain.[23] This first stage is about how a change in mental trait can approximate an increase in mindfulness to varying degrees and proportionally inherit benefits of that increase. The second stage involves peeling back the dimensions of psychedelic space. As we peel back these features, we make the resulting experiences less psychedelic and the associated increases in mindfulness less substantial. This should be familiar territory by now but reviewing it will help us see, from a philosophical perspective, the sorts of things we can do to enhance psychedelics and meditation as therapeutic interventions.

Let's pick a hypothetical example to help fix our ideas: suppose you have the problem (by your own lights) of eating too much cheesecake (or pick your favourite indulgence) and that a psychedelic experience may help you solve this problem. Consider how this experience can vary with respect to the four dimensions. First, if the experience is lacking in clarity, you may erroneously guess that your desire to eat cheesecake is driven by, say, the stress of checking your bank account when, in fact, it is driven by any kind of stress. Second, if the experience is lacking in scope, you may only get a fragmentary insight concerning your desire to eat cheesecake. For instance, you may notice that the desire arises when you check your bank

---

[21] I'm bracketing here the debate over the existence of genuine free will and its relation to mindfulness.

[22] The nugget of wisdom also needn't be propositional. It could also be, for instance, a shift in perspective, an increase in embodiment, an enhanced awareness of one's breath, etc.

[23] While these features can be peeled off independently, they can also be peeled off in conjunction. For example, your newfound mindfulness may only occur in the morning and be limited to the retention of the insight that practising meditation will somehow mitigate your morning stress.

account and also when you have to give a presentation at work, but fail to notice other occasions and so fail to connect the dots. Third, if the experience is lacking in novelty, you may see that you reach for the cheesecake after stressful events (or in anticipation of them), but fail to notice that this is a coping mechanism you acquired as a child. Fourth, if the experience is lacking in duration, you may have the above novel insight about coping but only be able to hold it in mind briefly, thus precluding it from being consolidated into long-term memory—which, in turn, would make it difficult for you to integrate the insight into your daily life.

While it may be desirable to have an experience that is psychedelic in each of these four respects, many of the benefits may still be acquired by an experience that is only partially psychedelic, especially if we supplement it with *surrogates* for the respects in which it is lacking. For example, knowing that one's experience may be lacking in clarity and scope, one could adopt the mindset that Wilson 2002 advocates: treat yourself as though you were another person and carefully piece together the clues and test hypotheses about them (like a detective or scientist). In the case of lacking novelty, while it may be better to know the origins of the coping mechanism, there are still cognitive-behavioural modifications you can make based on the shallower insight that cheesecake-eating is triggered by stress. Finally, having some way of recording the experience can help mitigate the problems presented by limited duration. This could be a notebook, an audio recorder, a reliable friend, a therapist, etc. Thus, we see how an experience that isn't very psychedelic in various respects, and is a poor approximation to mindfulness, may still be able to inherit many of the benefits of mindfulness with appropriate surrogates in place. To put it another way, simply by being mindful of the fact that one may undergo imperfect psychedelic experiences, one can extract benefits from those experiences that would otherwise be easily lost.

That completes the second stage of our analysis, and we can now put everything together. First, there is a continuum from messy and chaotic psychedelic experiences all the way up to pristine and enduring increases in mindfulness. The more one's mental state approximates an increase in mindfulness, and the greater that increase in mindfulness, the more the benefits of mindfulness will be inherited. Second, as we just saw, for the sake of acquiring these benefits, we needn't be limited to psychedelic experiences alone: we can make use of psychedelic experiences combined with surrogates for mindfulness. For example, supplementing a messy and chaotic psychedelic experience with a careful and critical mindset afterwards can help one acquire the same benefits as those of a psychedelic experience that is clear and stable. Similarly, the features of the first stage of analysis can have surrogates as well. For example, a lack of volitional control can be made up for by setting an intention and carefully deploying one's psychological resources during a psychedelic experience. In short, there is a positive feedback loop between psychedelic experiences and increases in mindfulness. A mindfulness of a psychedelic experience even at a high level can help one either make the experience more like an increase in mindfulness or supplement it with a surrogate (e.g. a pen and paper) with the same effect.

With all of that in place, we can now address the issue of *interventions*—the consumption of psychedelics and the practice of meditation. The argument I've presented implies that these interventions are going to be beneficial to the extent that they give rise to psychedelic experiences that approximate substantial increases in mindfulness. Moreover, the interventions can be enhanced—and safeguarded against deleterious effects—by ensuring that appropriate surrogates for mindfulness are in place.

This is essentially what happens—to varying degrees—in psychedelic research and therapeutic practice. For instance, extensive preparatory discussions between patient and therapist may be conducted before the patient undergoes a psychedelic session (Grof 1975). Such discussions lead to the appropriate setting of intentions, which naturally guide the experiences to certain kinds of mental contents (e.g. the patient's difficulties with substance addiction). Patients and subjects are also often advised to surrender to the psychedelic session: to accept what comes up and avoid resisting the experience. This, effectively, is a strategy for enhancing the mindfulness of the subject's mental state during the session—in particular, by reducing their reactivity and increasing their psychological flexibility. Similarly, integration sessions after the psychedelic session help ensure any insights (or other kinds of experiences) are processed appropriately and healthily integrated into the subject's daily life and subsequent therapeutic work. There are many more examples that could be given. Notably, Griffiths et al. 2018 and Smigielski et al. 2019 found that mindfulness training appeared to enhance the positive effects of psychedelic-induced experiences (and mitigate their negative qualities). The upshot is that much of the therapeutic practice surrounding the psychedelic state can be justified in terms of the effectiveness of causing the state to approximate an increase in mindfulness, or by playing a surrogate role for mindfulness.[24]

Understanding the therapeutic techniques from this particular theoretical perspective may also help practitioners make further improvements to their practices. For example, this perspective of viewing psychedelic experiences in terms of their ability to approximate increases in mindfulness can help us address a practical question that can come up during psychedelic sessions. It is quite common for one to have an insight that is especially profound and valuable—e.g. a change of perspective on one's life—that would be desirable to take into regular life. However, such insights often fade once the trip is over, leaving behind only a vague trace, if anything at all, as one returns to everyday life. This common phenomenon raises the practical question: can anything be done to bring such insights back into

---

[24] In other contexts, the external source of mindfulness may come from a shaman, meditation teacher, ritual, or a team of people focused on different aspects of the session. See, for example, Metzner and Leary 1967 for a discussion of the various ways a psychedelic session may be "programmed".

regular life from the depths of a psychedelic trip? The above picture suggests that the answer is yes. By immediately applying one's mindfulness skills to the insight during the trip, one may begin the consolidation process while the insight is still active and thus increase the continuity of experience between the psychedelic trip and regular life. The result would be to make the insight more readily available to one's default state of consciousness and thus better integrated into one's life.

Finally, with respect to mindfulness-based interventions, the above analysis can help practitioners appreciate that meditation is not a panacea. As mentioned earlier, there is growing evidence that adverse effects from mindfulness-based interventions are not uncommon. Part of the explanation for this is that a practice of cultivating mindfulness is not the same thing as having mindfulness. The psychedelic experiences that occur as a result of meditative practice can be just as chaotic and terrifying as those that arise during "bad" trips, and such experiences may do more harm than good, especially if preparations are not in place to manage them appropriately. Moreover, it is also possible that *psychecryptic* experiences may occur, and the degree to which one's usual state of mind is psychecryptic may even increase. That is, it is entirely possible for mindfulness to *decrease* as a result of meditative practice. Moreover, even when it does increase, it doesn't always do so in a linear or predictable fashion.[25]

Before concluding this section, it is worth noting that this difference between therapy and traditional mindfulness practice was highlighted by Jung. In the lead-up to the quote we saw in the previous section, he writes:

> The unconscious is an unglimpsable completeness of all subliminal psychic factors, a 'total exhibition' of potential nature. It constitutes the entire disposition from which consciousness takes fragments from time to time. Now if the consciousness is emptied as far as possible of its contents, the latter will fall into a state (at least a transitory state) of unconsciousness. This displacement ensures as a rule in Zen through the fact of the energy of the conscious being withdrawn from the contents and transferred either to the conception of emptiness or to the *koan*. As the two last-named must be stable, the succession of images is also abolished, and with it the energy which maintains the kinetic of the conscious. The amount of the energy [which we may understand as attentional resource] that is saved goes over to the unconscious, and reinforces its natural supply up to a certain maximum. This increases the readiness of the unconscious contents to break through to the conscious. Since the emptying and the closing down of the conscious is no easy matter, a special training and an indefinitely long period of time is necessary to produce that maximum of tension which leads to the final break-through of unconscious contents into the conscious [a psychedelic experience].

---

[25] It is also important to emphasize that these considerations are only part of the explanation. One's physical health and general life circumstances are also major factors in one's well-being.

The contents which break through are by no means completely unspecified. As psychiatric experience with insanity shows, peculiar relations exist between the contents of the conscious and the delusions and deliria that break in upon it. They are the same relations that exist between the dreams and the working conscious of normal men. The connection is in substance a *compensatory relationship*: the contents of the unconscious bring to the surface everything necessary in the boards sense for the completion, i.e., *the completeness, of conscious orientation*.

Jung 1949, pp. 22–3

Jung then continues with the passage cited earlier, expressing the connection between this breakthrough of the unconscious into the conscious and the goals of psychotherapy. And a little later, he writes:

[...] psychotherapy is by no means dealing with men who, like Zen monks, are ready to make any sacrifice for the sake of truth, but very often with the most stubborn of all Europeans. Thus the tasks of psychotherapy are of course much more varied, and the individual phases of the long process meet with far more opposition than in Zen.

Jung 1949, pp. 23–4

Although Jung has in mind his particular approach to psychotherapy and the practices of Zen Buddhism, we can see that what he is highlighting is a specific form of the connection between psychedelic experience and well-being discussed in this section. In Jung's opinion, the "stubborn Europeans" need the therapist to resolve the discrepancy between their psychological dispositions and those of the monks.

In this regard, it is also worth noting that Jung was wary of psychedelics. In a letter to Father Victor White in 1954, Jung wrote:

Is the LSD-drug mescalin? It has indeed very curious effects—*vide* Aldous Huxley—which I know far too little. I don't know either what its psychotherapeutic value with neurotic or psychotic patients is. I only know there is no point in wishing to know more of the collective unconscious than one gets through dreams and intuition. The more you know of it, the greater and heavier becomes your moral burden, because the unconscious contents transform themselves into your individual tasks and duties as soon as they begin to become conscious. Do you want to increase loneliness and misunderstanding? Do you want to find more and more complications and increasing responsibilities? You get enough of it. If I once could say that I had done everything I know I had to do, then perhaps I should realize a legitimate need to take mescalin. [...] There are some poor impoverished creatures, perhaps, for whom mescalin would be a heavensent gift without a counterpoison, but I am profoundly mistrustful of the 'pure gifts of the Gods'. You pay very dearly for them. [...]

[...] If you are too unconscious it is a great relief to know a bit of the collective unconscious. But it soon becomes dangerous to know more, because one does not learn at the same time how to balance it through a conscious equivalent. That is the mistake Aldous Huxley makes: he does not know that he is in the role of the 'Zauberlehrling' [the Magician's apprentice], who learned from his master how to call the ghosts but did not know how to get rid of them again [...]

[...] It is quite awful that the alienists have caught hold of a new poison to play with, without the faintest knowledge or feeling of responsibility. It is just as if a surgeon had never learned further than to cut open his patient's belly and to leave things there. When one gets to know unconscious contents one should know how to deal with them. I can only hope that the doctors will feed themselves thoroughly with mescalin, the *alkaloid of divine grace*, so that they learn for themselves its marvellous effect. You have not finished with the conscious side yet. Why should you expect more from the unconscious? For 35 years I have known enough of the collective unconscious and my whole effort is concentrated upon preparing the ways and means to deal with it.

Jung 1954, pp. 172–3

Again, we see the same sentiment expressed. Psychedelic experience by itself is a potentially dangerous thing, and Jung aptly highlights the knowledge, structure, discipline, and respect required in order for the experience to be managed in a beneficial way. Maslow also expressed essentially the same idea with respect to psychotherapy in general:

Perhaps I can now say something more about this openness to the unconscious. This whole business of psychotherapy, of self-therapy, of self-knowledge is a difficult process because, as things stand now for most of us, the conscious and the unconscious are walled off from each other. How do you get these two worlds, the psychic world and the world of reality, to be comfortable with each other? In general, the process of psychotherapy is a matter of slow confrontation, bit by bit, with the help of a technician, with the uppermost layers of the unconscious. They are exposed and tolerated and assimilated and turn out to be not so dangerous after all, not so horrible. Then comes the next layer, and then the next, in this same process of getting a person to face something which he is terribly afraid of, and then find in, when he does face it, that there was nothing to be afraid of in the first place. He has been afraid of it because he has been looking at it through the eyes of the child that he used to be. This is childish misinterpretation. What the child was afraid of and therefore repressed, was pushed beyond the reach of common-sense learning and experience and growing up, and it has to stay there

until it's dragged out by some special process. The conscious must become strong
enough to dare friendliness with the enemy.

Maslow 1963, pp. 86–7

We see here again the importance of an external surrogate of mindfulness ('the technician'), and the process of ensuring that certain qualities of the subject's mental state are maintained throughout the process (such as clarity and duration, at the cost of novelty and scope).

To summarize the main line of thought of this section, perfect mindfulness is a holy grail of well-being, but it is far from easy to achieve, and the path towards that goal can be long and littered with obstacles. Psychedelic experiences—induced by psychedelics, meditation, or by other means—can play an extremely valuable role in moving along that path, but they can also easily take one off the path. It is for this reason that any *treatment* involving these experiences must be handled with great care and implemented within a robust therapeutic framework and supportive environment. It is also for this reason that it is crucial that we do not conflate psychedelic experiences with the experiences produced by psychedelics and meditation. Those may sometimes amount to the same thing, but they can also come apart. So, it is essential that we establish the degree to which these interventions reliably produce psychedelic experiences. In other words, while we have established a connection between psychedelic experience and well-being, we only have a resulting connection between experiences induced by psychedelics and meditation and well-being to the degree that we can establish that these interventions induce psychedelic experiences that approximate increases in mindfulness (perhaps with the help of mindfulness surrogates).

We now have a clearer understanding of the connection between psychedelic experience and well-being. The connection is nuanced, so we can't simply say that a psychedelic experience is guaranteed to improve well-being. Moreover, we certainly can't say that any particular intervention that induces psychedelic experience, such as meditating or consuming a psychedelic substance, is a universal cure for psychological suffering. However, we can say that there is a generally positive relationship between psychedelic experiences and well-being and that this relationship becomes stronger the more the psychedelic experiences approximate increases in mindfulness.

9.5 From Mystical to Mystical-Type Experience

As I mentioned in the introduction to this chapter, there is growing evidence that psychedelics induce mystical experiences and the degree to which they do so appears to correlate with their therapeutic outcomes.[26] Can the account developed in this chapter explain this observed connection between mystical experience and well-being?

In order to address this question, we first need to say what a mystical experience is—to pinpoint the phenomenon in question. However, it is commonly reported that these experiences are *ineffable*: as we'll see in the next chapter, there's a deep and important sense in which mystical experiences are indescribable. Paradoxically, it could even be said that ineffability is a *defining* feature of a mystical experience. That, obviously, creates a problem: how can we assess the relationship between mystical experiences and well-being if we can't say what mystical experiences are? We will explore this issue in much greater detail in the next chapter, but for now, there's an easy solution to this problem: we can focus instead on a close cousin of mystical experience, known as mystical-*type* experience.

We can shift our focus in this way because we need not be committed to the claim that the experiences induced by psychedelics are genuinely mystical. Instead, we can make do with the weaker claim that these experiences appear to have *interesting similarities* with mystical experiences, and so they can be said to be mystical-like, or of a mystical-type. The reason we can do that is because, despite their ineffability, mystics have had plenty to say about their experiences— throughout the ages and across many cultures. These different descriptions were given a systematic analysis by Stace 1960, who argued that mystical experiences have common characteristics. Stace's analysis then allowed for the development of questionnaires and psychometric scores that could be used to ascertain the degree to which someone has had a mystical experience. These include the Pahnke-Richards Mystical Experience Questionnaire (Pahnke 1969, Richards 1975) and the Hood Mysticism Scale (Hood 1975, Hood et al. 2001, Spilka et al. 2005). A common assumption in this work is that experiences are mystical to the extent that they involve the following characteristics: (i) a sense of oneness, unity, and interconnectedness, (ii) a noetic quality, in which profound knowledge of a metaphysical or spiritual nature is revealed with great clarity and certainty, (iii) a transcendence of time and space, (iv) an indescribability or ineffability, (v) a paradoxical character, (vi) a sense of sacredness, and (vii) positive feelings of bliss, joy, wonder, and awe.

While these measures of mystical-type experiences appear to be measuring something real—in the sense that they have been validated and shown to be predictive—they are not uncontroversial. As mentioned, they are based on Stace's

---

[26] For example, see O'Reilly and Funk 1964, Klavetter and Mogar 1967, Griffiths et al. 2006, 2008, 2011, 2016, Maclean et al. 2011, Bogenschutz et al. 2015, Johnson et al. 2016, Ross et al. 2016, Roseman et al. 2018, Schmid and Liechti, 2018, Garcia-Romeu et al. 2019, Davis et al. 2020, McCulloch et al. 2022, Søndergaard et al. 2022, and Qiu and Minda 2022.

analysis, which has been criticized for advancing a perennialist view of religion without appropriate justification (Katz 1978). More recently, the measures have come under fire for methodological issues and for potentially biasing how subjects report their experiences (Taves 2020, Sanders and Zijlmans 2021, but also see Breeksema and Elk 2021). The scores have also been suggested to be too generous in classifying an experience as being mystical in nature (Pollan 2018, pp. 283–4), and there has long been a debate as to whether psychedelics really can induce the experiences that have historically been engendered through religious and spiritual practices (Zaehner 1957, Smith 1964, Suzuki 1971, Zaehner 1972, Smith et al. 2004). Nevertheless, it is clear that psychedelics can induce experiences that appear to be of a different category or magnitude than those we have been focusing on so far. That is, they appear to induce experiences that are not merely memory recollections, hallucinations, creative ideas, psychological insights, etc. For lack of a better term, we will refer to these distinctive experiences as being of a mystical-type, and save the discussion of genuine mystical experiences for the next chapter.

Another issue that needs to be flagged is that while mystical-type experiences appear to correlate with observed improvements in well-being, they may not play any *causal* role in bringing about those improvements. For example, it's possible that some mystical-type experiences are simply *blow-out* experiences, whereby all the usual structures of cognition and perception are temporarily dissolved. Such experiences may not be therapeutically efficacious in themselves, but they may nevertheless correlate with other aspects of a psychedelic trip that are therapeutic. For instance, it could be that immediately before (or after) a mystical-type experience, people tend to have experiences that are very psychedelic and which thereby tend to afford unusually deep and clear psychological insights that are of tremendous therapeutic value. If so, then this would explain why mystical-type experiences are predictive of therapeutic benefits, even though they themselves are not therapeutically beneficial.

Alternatively, if we examine the common characteristics of mystical-type experiences, they appear to be what one would expect from experiences that are *very* psychedelic—that is, they appear to be located *deep* in psychedelic space.[27] If an experience is extremely *novel*, then it will tend to be difficult to describe—feature (iv) in the above list. It will also tend to appear paradoxical in nature (v), for it will likely surpass one's present conceptual schemes. If the experience also has extreme *clarity* to it, then it will likely also engender a feeling of certainty, which, when combined with novelty, is likely to give rise to a noetic quality and a sense of ultimate reality (ii) to the experience. Combined with extreme *scope*, this is

---

[27] There is also some evidence indicating mystical-type experiences are not predictive of psychological insights and that psychological insight does not significantly mediate the benefits of mystical-type experiences (Peill et al. 2022). It is also important to note that their measure of psychological insight focused on personal insight and not the transpersonal or philosophical-spiritual insights that may be associated with mystical-type experiences.

also likely to lead to feelings of wonder and awe as well as bliss and joy (vii), because of the lack of constraints and the enjoyable nature of clarity. An experience that is extreme in scope is also likely to give rise to a feeling that everything is interconnected (i), since many things would be in awareness simultaneously, along with the mind's associations between them. If an experience is extremely high in *duration*, then there will be a sense in which the experience transcends time (iii)—it may even seem as though time stands still. Finally, it is easy to imagine that all of these factors, combined, can lead to a feeling of sacredness of the experience (vi). In summary, the seven core characteristics of mystical experience appear to be somewhat explainable in terms of high scores with respect to the four dimensions of psychedelic space. This suggests, then, that mystical-type experiences are very psychedelic and so they may be particularly therapeutic.

Another reason to think that mystical-type experiences are very psychedelic stems from the observed interactions between psychedelics and mindfulness practices. If mystical-type experiences are deep in psychedelic space, and if being more mindful places one's coordinate system deeper in psychedelic space, then we should expect that people who are more mindful are more likely to have mystical-type experiences during psychedelic trips. As I mentioned in Section 9.2, mindfulness can be thought of as a moveable launchpad for psychedelic trips. The more mindful you are, the deeper into psychedelic space a given psychedelic trip will take you, and so the more likely you are to land in a region of psychedelic space that corresponds to mystical-type experiences. Interestingly, there is some evidence in support of this. Griffiths et al. 2018 found that the psilocybin-induced experiences of subjects who received more support during a programme of meditation (and spiritual) practice scored higher on the Hood Mysticism Scale, and Smigielski et al. 2019 found that mindfulness training appears to deepen psychedelic-induced experiences and enhance psilocybin's positive effects while counteracting possible dysphoric responses.[28] These sorts of observations are what we would expect to see if mindfulness functions as a launchpad for psychedelic trips. Therefore, this gives us additional reason to think that mystical-type experiences are deep in psychedelic space—and therefore are very psychedelic—and for this reason can be especially therapeutic.

That said, this reason also introduces a new complexity that we need to account for. Recall, from Section 9.2, that as you become more mindful, some psychedelic experiences tend to become *less psychedelic*. This is because the experiences become *less revelatory* as you become more mindful: their contents are less hidden and therefore easier to call into awareness. This introduces an important subtlety concerning the degree to which mystical-type experiences are

---

[28] Simonsson and Goldberg 2022 also found that meditators are more likely to have experienced psychedelic-induced ego dissolution than non-meditators. However, the study design doesn't determine whether this is a causal effect of meditative practice.

psychedelic. Consider a given mystical-type experience and suppose that it is deep in psychedelic space. If you get to it because you've increased your overall mindfulness (say, by practising meditation), then it would be barely psychedelic (if at all). However, if you are low in mindfulness but succeed in getting to the experience anyway—say, via a high-dose psychedelic trip—then the experience will count as being very psychedelic. Therefore, the degree to which a given mystical-type experience is psychedelic is a relative matter, dependent on your starting point.

Thus, we may wish to distinguish between those mystical-type experiences that are revelatory and those that are not. Indeed, we can find a similar, if not identical, distinction drawn in Zen Buddhism using the concepts of *kensho*, *satori*, and *daigo*. These terms are often used interchangeably, and their meaning can depend on the context and discussion, but they can be used to distinguish three stages of enlightenment (Kapleau 1965). Roughly speaking, *kensho* is sometimes understood to be an initial and partial glimpse of enlightenment, whereas *satori* typically arises after additional training that deepens this initial insight. *Satori* is also said to be more enduring and brought about with some degree of control (and is thus less revelatory). *Daigo* is then said to be a complete and final transition into enlightenment. Although these stages are different from one another, they still involve the same "content".[29] A key difference between these stages is that whereas *kensho* is an initial and revelatory insight, *daigo* is an enduring and final understanding that is no longer revelatory (in part, because it is enduring). *Satori* sits somewhere between the two, being more revelatory than *kensho* in that it is more complete, pure, and deep (scoring higher on scope, clarity, and novelty), but also not more revelatory in that it can be more easily brought about at will (as a consequence of increased mindfulness). Whether any of these experiences can be said to be of a mystical-type (or akin to any of the experiences induced by psychedelics) is a matter of some debate (Suzuki 1971). Nevertheless, we can at least take inspiration from these distinctions and similarly distinguish between mystical-type experiences that are revelatory and those that are not. Irrespective of their revelatory nature, there is a clear sense in which mystical-type experiences are deep in psychedelic space.

To summarize, we have two reasons to think that mystical-type experiences are not only psychedelic, but are *very* psychedelic. With that established, we can now consider why they may be beneficial to well-being.

---

[29] I use scare quotes to indicate that we should be careful in thinking of these experiences in terms of content. Indeed, some say that what is distinctive of these experiences is that they are empty of all possible content. It is also worth noting that the term 'experience' can be similarly inappropriate, and 'insight' or 'understanding' may be better alternatives, depending on context.

9.6 Mystical-Type Experience, Well-Being, and the Self

Our central question is whether the observed improvements in well-being that correlate with mystical-type experiences can be explained in terms of the latter being psychedelic. Based on the arguments in Sections 9.2–5, we already have an answer. The more an experience approximates an increase in mindfulness, the more it will inherit the benefits of mindfulness; and the more psychedelic the experience is, the greater the increase in mindfulness it can approximate. A mystical-type experience is either very psychedelic or afforded by a substantial increase in mindfulness. If the latter, then the individual will simply enjoy the benefits of the cultivated mindfulness. If the former, then since the supporting therapeutic context (or mindfulness training) either helps ensure the experience approximates mindfulness or plays a surrogate role for mindfulness, it is likely that the experience in question is indeed a good approximation of a substantial increase in mindfulness.

Despite the complexity involved in getting to this answer, the answer itself is fairly straightforward: mystical-type experiences either involve a substantial involuntary increase in the access to one's unconscious mind or are indicative of an individual who has this access voluntarily. Following the arguments presented earlier, such access is essential and highly conducive to well-being.

I think this answer is correct and mostly complete. However, there is also something unsatisfactory about it: one might complain that we should be able to say something more specific about why mystical-type experiences are good for well-being. In particular, for the psychedelic mystical-type experiences, what part or aspect of the mind is being revealed that is so beneficial to well-being? If we wish, we can attempt an answer to this question, but this involves opening a Pandora's box of philosophical issues that is probably best left closed. Nevertheless, it is informative to see what happens if we take a peek inside.

To open the box is to ask: what about the mind is revealed during mystical-type experiences that is so conducive to well-being? We already have a hint as to what the answer might be, given the close parallel, if not identity, between mystical-type experiences and *satori*: one's true self is revealed in a mystical-type experience. Jung gives an excellent description of this idea in his discussion of *satori*:

> When one examines the Zen text attentively, one cannot escape the impression that, with all that is bizarre in it, *satori* is, in fact, a matter of *natural occurrence*, of something so very simple that one fails to see the wood for the trees, and in attempting to explain it, invariably says the very thing that drives others into the greatest confusion. Nukariya therefore is right when he says that any attempt to explain or analyze the contents of Zen with regard to enlightenment would be in vain. Nevertheless, this author does venture to say of enlightenment that it

embraces an insight into the nature of the self, and that it is an emancipation of the conscious from an illusory conception of self. The illusion regarding the nature of self is the common confusion of the ego with self. [...]

Jung 1949, p. 13

We see in this passage two important ideas that we've already come across: (i) the *ineffability* of the experience and (ii) an attempt to nevertheless articulate it (to open Pandora's box)—in this case, in terms of an insight into the nature of the self. We also get a third idea that we have not yet come across: a distinction between the *ego* and the self. Putting all this together, the fundamental idea that Jung is conveying in this passage is that *satori* is (or involves) the insight that the ego is not the self. Given the ineffability of *satori*, we should be wary of being committed to this idea, but we can tentatively venture that this point—or, at least, an attenuated version of it—may be true of mystical-type experiences.

What, exactly, is this insight that the ego is not the self? Obviously, this requires some explanation. Interestingly, Albert Einstein once gave a useful description of the insight we're trying to explain:

A human being is a spatially and temporally limited piece of the whole, what we call the 'Universe'. He experiences himself and his feelings as separate from the rest, an optical illusion of his consciousness. The quest for liberation from this bondage is the only object of true religion. Not nurturing the illusion but only overcoming it gives us the attainable measure of inner peace.

Einstein 1950

Here we get a bit more of what the idea is: we normally experience ourselves as in some sense being separate from everything else in the universe. However, this separated thing is an illusory self, and we make the mistake of thinking that it is one's self. As implied by the contrast that Einstein sets up, one's true self is something unbounded and universal—or, at the very least, something that is more expansive than the thing one typically identifies with. Although Einstein doesn't explain why, we also see the idea that overcoming the illusion is conducive to well-being ('the attainable measure of inner peace').

Jung (and probably Einstein as well) acquired this idea from Hindu and Buddhist philosophy:

Since the unconscious gives us the feeling that it is something alien, a non-ego, it is quite natural that it should be symbolized by an alien figure. Thus, on the one hand, it is the most insignificant of things, while on the other, so far as it potentially contains that 'round' wholeness which consciousness lacks, it is the most significant of all. This 'round' thing is the great treasure that lies hidden in the cave of the unconscious, and its personification is this personal being who represents the higher unity of conscious and unconscious. It is a figure comparable to Hiranyagarbha, Purusha, Atman, and the mystic Buddha. For this reason I have elected to call it the 'self', by which I understand a psychic totality and at the same time a centre, neither of which coincides with the ego but includes it, just as a larger circle encloses a smaller one.

Jung 1953, p. 247

The idea, then, is that the insight afforded by mystical-type experience is the dissolution of the ego illusion and a revelation of this larger psychic totality. In describing how the manifestation of this self relates to one's well-being, Coward 1979 writes:

It seems to have been Jung's view that as an isolated ego, a person would never succeed in reuniting the opposing forces [of good and evil]. Those forces within the personality would simply overpower one's ego, and chaos would ensue. What saves us from this fate, said Jung, is the fact that deep within each of us is the God-image which is the psychological foundation of our psyche. The God-image or archetype is inherent in the collective unconscious as the primal stratum or foundational matrix. The experiencing of the God archetype has a unifying effect upon the whole personality. Especially noticeable is the way in which the opposing tensions are brought together by the guiding influence of the God archetype over the individual ego. In Jung's view mysticism plays a large role in this whole process of uniting and balancing the opposing forces within experience. (In this context the term 'mysticism' is being used ... to mean the process of identifying with something more than the finite ego.)

Coward 1979, p. 325

In this passage, we start to get more of the picture. Not only do we see an elaboration of this distinction between the self and ego, but we also see why removing that illusion would contribute to one's well-being (because of its unifying effect on the mind).

We see the same idea endorsed by Maslow. In discussing this particular aspect of mystical-type experiences—the dissolution of the ego illusion, Maslow describes the insight in terms of *non-self*:

Loss of Ego: Self-Forgetfulness. Loss of Self-Consciousness. When you are totally absorbed in non-self, you tend to become less conscious of yourself, less self-aware. You are less apt to be observing yourself like a spectator or a critic. To use the language of psychodynamics, you become less dissociated than usual into a self-observing ego and an experiencing ego; i.e. you come much closer to being *all* experiencing ego. (You tend to lose the shyness and bashfulness of the adolescent, the painful awareness of being looked at, etc.) This in turn means more unifying, more oneness and integration of the person.

It also means less criticizing and editing, less evaluating, less selecting and rejecting, less judging and weighing, less splitting and analyzing of the experience.

This kind of self-forgetfulness is one of the paths to finding one's true identity, one's real self, one's authentic nature, one's deepest nature. It is almost always felt as pleasant and desirable. We needn't go so far as the Buddhists and Eastern thinkers do in talking about the 'accursed ego'; and yet there *is* something in what they say.

Maslow 1963, p. 63

The terminology here is slightly different—Maslow uses 'self-observing ego' and 'all-experiencing ego' to mark the distinction—but it is essentially the same idea being expressed: 'finding one's true identity, one's real self, one's authentic nature, one's deepest nature'. It is worth noting here that Maslow's description may seem paradoxical to some readers: after all, how can being self-forgetful help one find one's real self? This paradox can be resolved by understanding that the difference is the difference between experiencing the self with phenomenal opacity and with phenomenal transparency (Chapter 5). Represented opaquely, the self is experienced as an object that can be, for example, criticized by the mind. When experienced with transparency, the opaque self-representation is forgotten, and the self takes on an invisible quality to it that allows one's attentional resources to flow more freely and completely through that representation, thereby manifesting one's authentic self (Lyon and Farennikova 2022). In some cases, that shift from opacity to transparency then allows for a removal of the optical illusion of consciousness referred to by Einstein.[30] We also, again, get something of an explanation for why the removal of this illusion is good for well-being: it removes the unnecessary internal conflicts and divisions that hold us back from complete well-being.

So, we now have an answer as to what about the mind that mystical-type experiences reveal, and why this is beneficial to well-being. The basic idea is that such an experience involves a stripping away of the illusory identification of self with ego, so that one may glimpse the true, and deeper and more expansive, nature of one's self. Interestingly, many of the subjective reports from psychedelic therapy line up well with this answer. These reports vary from person to person and sometimes only involve an insight into the constructed nature of the usual sense of self (Letheby 2021). However, they also often involve a *positive* insight into the nature of the self—a sense of a true self lying behind the usual sense of self. For example, consider the following descriptions reported by Noorani et al. 2018, a pilot study on the effectiveness of using psilocybin to treat cigarette addiction.

---

[30] To be clear, an increase in transparency needn't entail a decrease in opacity. The shift can also be one from an experience that is *dominated* by opacity to one in which opacity and transparency are more balanced and in which the intellectual mind is in greater harmony with the larger system.

One patient describes a manifestation of a God-image and its identity with the patient's true self:

> I used to hide sitting on the air conditioning unit on the side of my house, when I used to smoke. And so the image was me sitting there, smoking, all hunched over, stupid, smoking. And the vine just rising up and this purply flower face thing looking down at me like, 'how ridiculous!' And then I'm not really that [person], I'm really this vine, that's really me, and the Goddess within me... how silly to think that [smoking]... was going to do anything or solve anything. So it was really just that rising up feeling, and that powerful feeling, and it just filled me with such beauty and strength and life.
>
> Noorani et al. 2018, p. 759

Another patient explicitly describes a true self being revealed:

> [It was] me revealing myself, like actually showing myself to the world. This is who I am, this is who I *really* am.
>
> Noorani et al. 2018, p. 765

Another patient's description highlights an increase in mindfulness—particularly the *memory* aspect of mindfulness—brought about by the experience that corresponded to the revelation of a lost aspect to the patient's self:

> I don't know if I really *learned*—it was more like letting back in stuff that I had blocked out?... I don't think I changed my values, just remembered more of them. Or just remembered to honour them more, or... *allow* them more.
>
> Noorani et al. 2018, p. 759

In summarizing these results, Noorani et al. report:

> Session experiences were described as revealing a deeper, better, or more essential self that either led to a decreased desire to smoke, or to smoking not making sense anymore. These psilocybin-occasioned insights into self-identity were reported by all of the five female interview participants, while only two of the seven male participants.
>
> Noorani et al. 2018, p. 759

One finds similar reports in other studies as well, for example:

> I feel more in touch with who I really am—my real self, myself that's connected to everyone and everything.
>
> Belser et al. 2017, p. 376

I just feel that definitely it [ayahuasca] got me more in touch with my spirit.... It brought it out more because it was there. But now it is there even more.

Argento et al. 2019, p. 784

Not God in some dogmatic way, a God-like archetype within your psyche, that is real and within you. I know this exists, I directly experienced it. I was suddenly taken in a rapture and I was floating in midair, with my eyes wide open and my mouth open, completely in a state of awe and ecstasy. It's a very powerful message to take away.

Watts et al. 2017, p. 535

I'm sort of discovering that God in yourself, so to speak.... So I think that's also opened up to me tremendously—a spiritual piece. And I've never been religious; I'm not religious particularly at all. And I feel like I've really connected with a spiritual side in myself as well... that adds another level of contentment and happiness.

Swift et al. 2017, p. 504

Similarly, in explaining the role that psychedelics play in the therapy for sexual trauma, Goldpaugh writes:

[...] Experiencing divinity through the self presents a direct challenge to the perception of the self as deficient or broken. [...] Once a survivor has had a direct felt sense of a divine presence, there is an advantageous opening where therapists may begin to question previous assumptions about being 'dirty', 'impure', or 'unlovable'.

Goldpaugh 2022, p. 5

Outside of the therapeutic research literature, we also find similar descriptions of one discovering or remembering one's self. For example:

[...] it is very common for drinkers [of ayahuasca] to report that under the intoxication they feel they are rediscovering a facet of their existence that is actually very basic, very much their own. It is as if life had estranged one from oneself and made one forget some very basic things pertaining to one's very essence. Time and again, drinkers say that the brew brings them 'back home'—to the true essence of their personality from which they have distanced themselves. Invariably, returning to this core is a delightfully comforting experience.

Shanon 2002, p. 62

Here we see, echoing Ellenberger's 1966 notion of a *pathogenic secret* (Chapter 3), the idea that regular life can lead one into a psychecryptic state in which one *forgets*, and becomes estranged and dissociated from, one's self. This coming 'back home' is a remembering, a revealing, of this lost self.

Thus, it seems that the source of well-being that a mystical-type experience provides lies in its ability to provide insight into the true nature of the self. In fact, this insight isn't just part of psychology, but a core element of many mystical traditions. For example, in Zen we find:

> The koan is not given as an object to understand. It is given to you to solve your own problem. Koan is given to manifest yourself as a perfect being. If you are completely free from everything, you don't need the koan.
>
> Sasaki 1974, p. 88

And:

> Buddhist philosophy tells us that man must return to his own real self, namely to non-ego. He must awaken to the fact that the self he normally considers to be his self or ego is a false self, full of ignorance and subject to suffering. He must get rid of this false self and see his real self. This real self is the Buddha-nature within every man.
>
> Kobori 1957, p. 48

And D. T. Suzuki gives a characterization of *satori* that is quite reminiscent of Shanon's description of ayahuasca bringing drinkers 'back home':

> Zen calls this 'returning to one's home'; for its followers will declare: 'You have now found yourself; from the very beginning nothing has been kept away from you. It was yourself that closed the eye to the fact'.
>
> D. T. Suzuki, 1927[31]

Similarly, the *Katha Upanishad* contains three verses that link the revelation of an inner self (ātman) to a release from suffering while also highlighting the ineffable character of this revelation and the fact that it can't be achieved by the intellect (alone):

> When he perceives this immense, all-pervading self,
> as bodiless within bodies,

---

[31] Suzuki 2014, p. 25. It should be noted that D. T. Suzuki didn't believe that psychedelics could induce these experiences. His main argument for this was that the Zen experience (*satori*) involves the manifestation of the 'true man' and that the experiences induced by psychedelics only consist of hallucinatory and illusory visions (Suzuki 1971). While this *can* be true of psychedelics (and is perhaps often true of them), a central thesis of this book is that this effect of theirs is not necessary, and when psychedelics induce experiences that are truly psychedelic, they begin to approximate the Zen experience.

as stable within unstable beings—
A wise man ceases to grieve.

This self cannot be grasped,
by teachings or by intelligence,
or even by great learning.
Only the man he chooses can grasp him,
whose body this self chooses as his own.

Not a man who has not quit his evil ways;
Nor a man who is not calm or composed;
Nor even a man who is without a tranquil mind;
Could ever secure it by his mere wit.

Katha Upanishad, Section 2, Verses 22–4[32]

This idea is also arguably the impetus behind the maxim *know thyself* that was inscribed at the temple of Apollo at Delphi.

With all that said, it is important to note that there is a popular view that runs contrary to the one I have just put forward. This view says that there are *no selves* to be revealed. For example, in the introduction to *Being No One*, Metzinger writes:

> [My] main thesis is that no such things as selves exist in the world: Nobody ever was or had a self. All that ever existed were conscious self-models that could not be recognized as models.
>
> Metzinger 2003, p. 1

According to this type of view, a mystical-type experience could only involve the revelation that *the self does not exist* (see also Letheby and Gerrans 2017 and Letheby 2021 for a view along these lines). Any other kind of "revelation" would be illusory in nature. There are a few reasons that can be marshalled in support of this view. First, for every subjective report about a revealed self, such as those quoted above from Noorani et al. 2018, one can find another report involving the "self" disappearing and the absence of any revealed self. Second, within various schools of Buddhist philosophy, this view is a popular interpretation of the Buddha's teaching of *anattā*, often translated as the doctrine of non-self and understood as the metaphysical claim that there is no self (of any kind). Third, Hume's influential argument that there is no self is also often appealed to in support of this view. Those in favour of this view may even say that an experience is not genuinely mystical (nor even of a mystical-type) if one is experiencing the presence of a self.

---

[32] Olivelle 1998, p. 387.

What are we to make of this? Unfortunately, any attempt to settle the debate will require another lengthy discussion and is likely to result in a stalemate. For example, an objection to Hume's argument is that it falsely assumes that if the self exists, then it would be easily observable (as a constant and simple impression) in the flow of experience. Some also point out that the standard interpretation of the Buddha's teaching of *anattā* can be seen as making a similar mistake (Wright 2017, pp. 119–29).[33] However, these Humeans and Buddhists can reply that their arguments are not meant to deductively entail that there is no self. Instead, the thought goes, these arguments should be seen as shifting the burden of proof to those who believe in the self. The Buddhists and Humeans may say: if you believe in a self, then tell us what it is, show us where it is, give us evidence for its existence. Appeals to subjective experiences of apparently authentic selves revealing themselves won't be sufficient for shifting the burden of proof back to the sceptic (and, similarly, pointing out that the self is ineffable[34] won't be of help). On the other hand, such subjective experiences will also be what prevents the sceptic from shifting the burden of proof to those who have had them. Those who experience revelations of a self may reply to the sceptics that it is *they* who haven't had a genuinely mystical experience. If we also add the premise that the ultimate experience of self is something ineffable, then we end up in a stalemate. So, it's not clear how this debate can be settled.

One reason for this stalemate may be that there is no objective fact to have a dispute over. For example, it may be that some people have true selves and others do not. Interestingly, Moore 2015 argues that the Socratic/Delphic sense of self-knowledge in the maxim *know thyself* involves the *construction* of the self. According to this view, responding appropriately to the maxim involves deliberately embarking on a process of self-constitution. It's possible that some people have made more progress than others in this respect.

Alternatively, perhaps some people have a better ability to have certain types of self-experiences than others do. For example, Whitfield 2021 has proposed that psychedelic-assisted psychotherapy should recognize a *spectrum* of selves, with three broad types of self corresponding to self as *content*, self as *process*, and self as *context*. Some of these may be more challenging for some people to experience, similar to how people vary in their ability to experience mental imagery, with some having aphantasia. Analogously some people may simply be blind in their mind's eye with respect to the self. Indeed, as we saw in Chapter 3, the Katha Upanishad says that only people of 'keen vision' can see the true self.

---

[33] It should be emphasized that this interpretation is subject to debate, and thus it is far from clear that the Buddha made this mistake. Similarly, it is not clear that Hume was talking about the same sense of self as we find in the above discussions. For Hume, the self was expected to be found, with relative ease, in regular conscious experience (impressions and ideas), whereas in many of the mystical traditions, the self is something that is *hidden* from (or in) regular conscious experience.

[34] For a defense of the idea that our awareness of the self is ineffable, see Jonas 2016, pp. 166–73.

One way to explain this possible variation is in terms of a variation in a disposition to identify with something other than one's usual sense of self (i.e. the ego). Perhaps one's usual sense of self is an arbitrary construction, and mystical-type experiences reveal this arbitrariness. This, in turn, creates an instability that ultimately collapses into one of two stable points: (i) a *unitive mystical experience*, in which one identifies with the oneness of the universe, and (ii) a *pure consciousness event*, in which any sense of identity becomes absent.[35] People may vary in their tendency to be drawn to these stable points. The disposition to resolve the arbitrariness one way or the other may also partly depend on one's background belief system. For example, as Nozick 1989 points out, Buddhist meditative practices are often *guided* by the doctrine of non-self (*anattā*), and thus their meditative experiences may, in a sense, be programmed by the doctrine (p. 142), which may affect how the instability is resolved. Nevertheless, regardless of how they come about, both kinds of experience, although radically different from each other, may nevertheless have a similar effect on well-being since they both involve a disintegration of the usual ego-based sense of self and its concomitant suffering.

However, there is a third kind of experience that is more complex than the first two. Accounts of this third kind of experience seem to vary in the literature. For example, Vervaeke and Ferraro 2016 propose that experiences of this third kind are a synergy of the experiences of the first two, while Forman 1999 argues that what is distinctive about these more complex experiences is that the intellect remains present in them. However, both agree that these experiences involve a revelation of *prajñā*. As usual, there are different renderings of *prajñā*, but a prominent one that is relevant to our discussion is that it is a form of wisdom that involves an ultimate knowledge of the self: a full understating of self-nature (Forman 1999). Obviously, that takes us back again to the idea of an underlying form of self that can be revealed in a mystical-type state. While I think we should be wary of analysing these states (see Chapter 10), I think it can be useful in this context to note that although *prajñā* cannot be realized via the intellect—and, indeed, transcends it—the intellect needn't cease to exist when *prajñā* is realized. Rather, as Forman argues, one is simply no longer caught inside the intellect—it continues to do its thing but with a kind of spaciousness and equanimity that one wasn't aware of

---

[35] For a discussion of these experiences and their distinction, see Forman 1999 and Vervaeke and Ferraro 2016. While these are often referred to as mystical experiences, I treat them here as mystical-type experiences and remain neutral as to whether they are genuinely mystical. Also, as an aside, it is worth noting that these two kinds of mystical-type experience may have two distinct neural correlates that are made available by the relaxing of the usual anti-correlation between the default mode network (DMN) and the dorsal attention network (DAN), which we came across in Chapter 5. In particular, the pure consciousness event may correspond to low activity in the DMN and DAN, and the unitive mystical experience may correspond to high activity in the two networks.

previously.[36] I would venture further that a similar point holds for the ego: one is no longer suffering from the illusion of the ego as the self, but the ego may still be present. Indeed, by remaining present, the ego can become more harmonious and better integrated with the larger form of being. Thus, while this third state is more complex than the first two, it is also more natural and wholesome and therefore has the potential to develop into an enduring flow of *eudaimonia*. Rather than simply being a temporary experience involving a revelation of some kind, it can become a permanent way of effortless being.

It is tempting to think that this third mystical state is more ultimate or real than the first two, with the first two being mere stepping stones or preparatory states (Vervaeke and Ferraro 2016). However, this third state could also just be another seemingly non-arbitrary way to resolve the instability (also driven by one's background belief system). Since there is a great deal of variation in humans in so many other ways, it is entirely possible that this is yet another way in which people can be different from one another. And so perhaps it makes little sense to try to settle this debate.[37]

Thanissaro Bhikkhu develops a similar line of thought in connection with the Buddhist doctrine of non-self:

> When Vacchagotta the wanderer asked [the Buddha] point-blank whether or not there is a self, the Buddha remained silent, which means that the question has no helpful answer. As he later explained to Ananda, to respond either yes or no to this question would be to side with opposite extremes of wrong view (Samyutta Nikaya 44.10). Some have argued that the Buddha didn't answer with 'no' because Vacchagotta wouldn't have understood the answer. But there's another passage where the Buddha advises all the monks to avoid getting involved in questions such as 'What am I?' 'Do I exist?' 'Do I not exist?' because they lead to answers like 'I have a self' and 'I have no self', both of which are a 'thicket of views, a writhing of views, a contortion of views' that get in the way of awakening (Majjhima Nikaya 2).
>
> Thanissaro 2014

As we will see in the next chapter, although ineffability is often understood as an inability to describe the experience, it may be more usefully understood as the

---

[36] As an aside, it may be that the kind of mystical experience that Forman 1999 focused on is a partial awareness of the union of Shiva and Shakti but with a strong tilt towards Shiva (thus missing a lot of energetic phenomena).

[37] There is much more to be said here than space permits. For a discussion of the history of the debate between Vedic and Buddhist philosophers embedded in the context of modern cognitive science and philosophy, see Thompson 2020, ch. 3. Also, see Albahari 2019 for a discussion of what cross-cultural facts about the self may be revealed through meditative practice.

insight that the experience *shouldn't* be described. In this case, trying to articulate what is or isn't revealed in a mystical-type experience may get in the way of others who wish to have such experiences and receive their benefits. In other words, there is a *normativity* to ineffability that often goes unappreciated. By respecting the ineffability of mystical experiences, we are better able to hold a (non-)conceptual space that allows for more inclusive conversations and diverse practices that can be tailored to the specific needs of different individuals (and groups). There is, thus, wisdom in leaving Pandora's box closed. We'll explore this line of thought in more detail in the next chapter.

9.7 Conclusion

We now have a better understanding of how psychedelic experience can promote well-being. The key idea is that to the extent that a psychedelic experience approximates mindfulness, it will result in the same benefits to well-being that a genuine increase in mindfulness typically yields. This mindfulness-based account naturally generalizes the simple answer we considered in the introduction of this chapter: that psychedelics have their therapeutic benefits because revealing hidden unconscious content can be beneficial to well-being. It also subsumes other proposals, such as those appealing to connectedness, flexibility, and changes in self-perception, since these are aspects or natural outcomes of increased mindfulness.

There are different methods for supplementing psychedelic experiences to help them approximate mindfulness. One would be for the individual in question to cultivate mindfulness via a sustained, disciplined mindfulness practice, such as meditation. Another way is for the individual to work closely with a therapist (or a guide), so that the therapist can play the role of a mindful mind while the individual undergoes the psychedelic experience. A salient hypothesis that falls out of this, which should be testable, is that the degree to which a psychedelic trip induces psychedelic experiences, combined with the extent to which such a trip is supplemented with mindfulness, should be predictive of the resulting beneficial outcomes to well-being. A similar hypothesis would hold for meditation-based interventions. Altogether, this gives us a clearer understanding of how the psychotherapeutic benefits of psychedelics and meditation can be explained in terms of their tendency to induce psychedelic, or mind-revealing, experiences.

It is important to note that we can accept this view without excluding the possibility that there are other ways by which psychedelics and meditation may be therapeutic. For example, it appears that some forms of depression are linked to inflammation and can be treated by drugs that target the immune system's inflammatory response mechanisms or their downstream consequences on the brain (Lee and Giuliani 2019). And there is growing evidence that psychedelics have anti-inflammatory effects and that so do various meditative practices.[38] It is therefore conceivable that these anti-inflammatory effects are responsible for some of the therapeutic benefits of psychedelics and meditation, and that these effects have little to do with the mind being revealed or made more mindful. In other words, it is not necessary for the explication of psychedelic experience to be involved in the explanation of *every* therapeutic effect of psychedelics and meditation. The fact that it can be used to explain some of the core effects is enough to help establish the fruitfulness of the explication.

Finally, we also considered the benefits to well-being that appear to be afforded by mystical-type experiences. As with other psychedelic experiences, there could be multiple ways in which these experiences are therapeutic. In this chapter, I identified and discussed one salient way: that mystical-type experiences enhance well-being because they reveal one's true self. There is good reason to be sympathetic to this view, but it is nevertheless a controversial one. Although it is an idea that should be appealing to many psychologists and psychotherapists, it will be a point of objection for others. The view will also be abhorrent to those Buddhists who understand *anattā* as the proposition that there is no self of any kind. Similarly, the view will be alien to those who have had psychedelic-induced mystical-type experiences that they take to reveal that they have no self (of any kind). As I pointed out, there is no easy way to resolve the debate between these two camps. It could well be that, just as humans are wildly different in so many other ways, perhaps some have hidden authentic selves and others do not. Because of this, I suggested that engaging in this debate might undermine the enterprise that is common to both camps, which is to ease suffering and enhance well-being as much as possible.

---

[38] For psychedelics, see Galvão-Coelho et al. 2020, Nau et al. 2013, Szabo 2015, Szabo and Frecska 2016, Flanagan and Nichols 2018, Szabo 2019, and Thompson and Szabo 2020, and for meditation, see Rosenkranz et al. 2013, Creswell et al. 2016, Bower and Irwin 2015, Buric et al. 2017, and Shields et al. 2020.

10
Mystical Experience

10.1 Introduction

Towards the end of the previous chapter, we touched upon the topic of mystical experience and sidestepped it by limiting our discussion to mystical-type experiences. In this chapter, we will tackle the subject of mystical experience head-on. The main reason for doing this is that psychedelics and meditation are often said to bring about mystical experiences, so it is natural for us to wonder whether such experiences are psychedelic. That is, are mystical experiences mind-revealing experiences? I will argue that we can't answer this question—at least, not in the way we might hope to—but also that there is much to be learned from understanding why this is so.

Before we get going, it will help to place this question within the larger context of this book. In the first four chapters, we were primarily concerned with what it means for an experience to be psychedelic and how we may articulate hypotheses concerning whether meditation and psychedelics reliably induce such experiences. In the following five chapters, we shifted away from purely philosophical issues to a more empirical focus. One way to think about these five chapters is that we were slowly moving from experiences that are *slightly* psychedelic to those that are *very* psychedelic. The sudden recollection of a lost memory (Chapter 6) is an experience that tends to be only slightly psychedelic—so much so that such an experience can easily happen without the assistance of meditation or psychedelics. The appearance of geometric hallucinations (Chapter 7) is a moderately psychedelic experience, so it tends to require some fairly substantial intervention on the mind, such as sensory deprivation, meditation, or the consumption of a psychedelic. The manifestation of creative insights (Chapter 8) and psychological insights (Chapter 9) in awareness also tends to be moderately psychedelic, but such insights can become very psychedelic, as the revelation of creative ideas transforms into the revelation of creative processes, and as the psychological insights transform into psychospiritual insights.

The culmination of this journey from the slightly psychedelic to the very psychedelic was the mystical-type experiences of the previous chapter, which appear to involve a highly novel revelation concerning one's self. We stayed neutral with respect to the question of whether these mystical-type experiences are genuinely mystical and relied on the fact that they can be understood in terms of psychometric scores, such as the Pahnke-Richards Mystical Experience

Questionnaire (Pahnke 1969, Richards 1975) and the Hood Mysticism Scale (Hood 1975, Hood et al. 2001, Spilka et al. 2005). This manoeuvre allowed us to philosophically engage with the experiences studied by scientists, but it also left the issue of genuinely mystical experiences largely unexplored. So, we will now consider such experiences and the question of whether they are psychedelic.[1]

However, in setting out to pursue this objective, we immediately run into a fundamental philosophical problem. To think about whether mystical experiences are psychedelic, we first need to know what mystical experiences *are*, and the problem is that there is no agreement as to how to define them. The use of the psychometric scores in the scientific literature may suggest the contrary, but they are based on the analysis of mystical experience from Stace 1960, which has received substantial criticism (Katz 1978). The scores themselves have also been criticized for smuggling in hidden assumptions about mysticism (Taves 2020, Sanders and Zijlmans 2021). However, an even more fundamental issue is that it is often said that a defining characteristic of mystical experiences is that they are *ineffable*. As William James put it:

> The handiest of the marks by which I classify a state of mind as mystical is negative. The subject of it immediately says that it defies expression, that no adequate report of its contents can be given in words. It follows from this that its quality must be directly experienced; it cannot be imparted or transferred to others.
>
> James 1902, p. 295

This creates a fundamental challenge for answering the question of whether mystical experiences are psychedelic. In order to answer the question, we need to know what mystical experiences are. However, if mystical experiences are ineffable, then we can't say what they are. Indeed, we don't even know if all the experiences that are being called 'mystical' are the same kind of experience.[2] This appears to make answering the most basic of questions about mystical experience impossible. For example, what does someone mean when they say they had a mystical experience during a psychedelic trip? How do they know what they are talking about? And how would we be able to tell if they are talking about the same thing as someone who says they had a mystical experience during a meditation retreat? If mystical experiences are ineffable, then it seems we have no way to answer these basic questions.

---

[1] Note that this is not the question of whether psychedelics induce genuinely mystical experiences (for discussion, see e.g. Zaehner 1957 and Smith 1964). Rather, the question here is whether genuinely mystical experiences are *mind-revealing* (or soul-manifesting), irrespective of what may trigger them.

[2] In the previous chapter, we came across three kinds of experience: unitive mystical experiences, pure consciousness events, and synergistic mystical experiences. There could be entirely other categories of experience that people report as being mystical and ineffable (e.g. kundalini experiences).

Another important consideration is that there is a sense in which ineffability is self-undermining, as St. Augustine observed (when contemplating the ineffability of God):

> Thus there arises a curious contradiction of words, because if the unspeakable is what cannot be spoken of, it is not unspeakable if it can be called unspeakable. And this opposition of words is rather to be avoided by silence than to be explained away by speech.
>
> Augustine 397 CE, *Christian Doctrine*, Book I, ch. 6[3]

Thus, it seems we can't even say that mystical experiences are ineffable, and so we should just resign ourselves to remaining silent about them.

However, I contend that Augustine presented a false dichotomy. Avoiding the issue with silence and explaining it away by speech are not our only options. A middle road is available: we can use words to better understand ineffability without explaining it away. One of the key ideas of this chapter is that by deepening our understanding of ineffability, we can come to understand mystical experiences (and whether they are psychedelic).

I propose that we can gain a deeper understanding of the ineffability of mystical experience by thinking about the ineffability of *pure uncertainty*. Mystical experience and pure uncertainty may seem like completely unrelated things, but it turns out they are deeply interrelated. By examining how our best theories of uncertainty—such as Bayesianism—fail to account for pure uncertainty, we will get a better handle on ineffability and, consequently, a deeper understanding of mystical experience. With that deeper understanding in place, we will then return to the question of whether mystical experiences are psychedelic.

The plan for the chapter is as follows. In Section 10.2, we'll examine some famous descriptions of mystical experiences. Although these descriptions run contrary to the ineffability of mystical experience, they will help those readers who may be unfamiliar with this topic to get a sense of what it might be about. In Section 10.3, we'll then examine some of the *theories* of mystical experience that have been put forward by philosophers. In that section, I will argue that such attempts to theorize about mystical experience are somewhat misguided because they do not sufficiently appreciate the significance of ineffability and that a more helpful way to advance our understanding is to allow for a *no-theory* theory of mystical experience. In Section 10.4, we will deepen our understanding of ineffability by exploring how it arises when we try to mathematically account for states of pure uncertainty. In Section 10.5, we'll then consider the question of whether mystical experiences are psychedelic. Although we won't be able to answer this question, strictly speaking, I'll argue that we can nevertheless attain some

---

[3] Green 2008, pp. 10–11.

important insights about it by framing the question in terms of how mystical experience may relate to *psychedelic space*. In Section 10.6, I will conclude with some final remarks about the relationship between analytic philosophy and mystical experience.

10.2 What Is Mystical Experience?

Out of context, the terms 'mystical' and 'mysticism' mean almost nothing (and are occasionally used as insults). The etymology of the terms can be traced back to the ancient Greek words *mystikos*, *mystēs*, and *myein*. These terms could take on meanings such as 'I conceal', 'one who has been initiated', but also 'to give first experience of something' (Bouyer 1980, Ogren 2016). That last meaning sounds like the sort of thing we're looking for: a particular expansion of awareness that consists in a revelatory experience. Nevertheless, the way these terms are used now, they can mean almost anything. So, in order to ask what mystical experiences are and whether they are psychedelic, we need to pin down what we're talking about.

Let's begin by considering some descriptions of experiences that have been said to be mystical. Although mystical experiences are often said to be ineffable, people still like to give descriptions of them. (More on this point later.) A natural starting point is with William James, who offered the first systematic study of mystical experience:

> Looking back on my own experiences, they all converge towards a kind of insight to which I cannot help ascribing some metaphysical significance. The keynote of it is invariably a reconciliation. It is as if the opposites of the world, whose contradictoriness and conflict make all our difficulties and troubles, were melted into unity. Not only do they, as contrasted species, belong to one and the same genus, but *one of the species*, the nobler and better one, *is itself the genus, and so soaks up and absorbs its opposite into itself*. This is a dark saying, I know, when thus expressed in terms of common logic, but I cannot wholly escape from its authority.
>
> James 1902, p. 388

Note that although James' description of his experience may sound somewhat confusing and incoherent, he is fully aware that such a description violates the usual rules of disciplined thought. Hence, his comment that his description 'is a dark saying' when 'expressed in terms of common logic'. That should give those who want to dismiss mystical experiences as nonsense at least some pause: James was no fool, and he was fully aware of his choice of words.

The next example highlights the contradictoriness associated with the experience perhaps even more explicitly:

Black does not cease to be black, nor white white. But black is white and white is black. The opposites coincide without ceasing to be what they are in themselves.

Otto 1932, p. 45

And we can find again a similar thought expressed by Meister Eckhart:

All that a man has here externally in multiplicity is intrinsically One. Here all blades of grass, wood, and stone, all things are One. This is the deepest depth.

Meister Eckhart[4]

These descriptions are somewhat restrained and written in the abstract. However, not all descriptions of mystical experiences are like this. For example, here is one that is much more personal and direct:

Suddenly I burst into a vast, new, indescribably wonderful universe. Although I am writing this over a year later, the thrill of the surprise and amazement, the awesomeness of the revelation, the engulfment in an overwhelming feeling-wave of gratitude and blessed wonderment, are as fresh, and the memory of the experience is as vivid, as if it had happened five minutes ago. And yet to concoct anything by way of description that would even hint at the magnitude, the sense of ultimate reality [...] seems such an impossible task. The knowledge which has infused and affected every aspect of my life came instantaneously and with such complete force of certainty that it was impossible, then or since, to doubt its validity.

Anonymous quoted in Harman 1963, pp. 10–11

And here is another example that is even more personal, with the individual comparing an MDMA experience he had with his addiction to sex and alcohol:

It really has an entirely different quality, like it's in some way outside all the time, outside of my life and my neuroses, literally a taste of the infinite bliss of being a conscious entity. In a very fundamental sense, it is the kind of experience that every conscious being really wants and needs. We get a sense of our true selves and how they are perfect, beautiful, whole, and complete. It fulfilled all of my childhood dreams, all of the unfulfilled longings, and all of the feelings of limitation and loss have been swept away by the sense of who I really am.

Anonymous quoted in Adamson and Metzner 1988, pp. 61–2

The above descriptions are all given by people who are largely in the tradition of Western thought. However, we can find similar descriptions in non-Western traditions. For example:

[4] As quoted in Otto 1932, p. 61.

[. . .] In Buddhist Emptiness there is no time, no space, no becoming, no-thing-ness; it is what makes all these things possible; it is a zero full of infinite possibilities, it is a void of inexhaustible contents.

Pure experience is the mind seeing itself as reflected in itself, it is an act of self-identification, a state of suchness. This is possible only when the mind is śūnyatā itself, that is, when the mind is devoid of all its possible contents except itself. [. . .]

Suzuki 1957, p. 28

The above descriptions are all fairly short, making them convenient to include given current limitations of space. However, one can also find much longer descriptions that offer a more nuanced picture of the experience. Indeed, there are entire works—such as the *Dao De Ching*—that can help one appreciate the nature of mystical experience.[5] Here, I will include one longer description by Arthur Koestler that is especially illuminating:

I was standing at the recessed window of cell No. 40 and with a piece of iron-spring that I had extracted from the wire mattress, was scratching mathematical formulae on the wall. Mathematics, in particular analytical geometry, had been the favorite hobby of my youth, neglected later on for many years. I was trying to remember how to derive the formula of the hyperbola, and was stumped; then I tried the ellipse and parabola, and to my delight succeeded. Next I went on to recall Euclid's proof that the number of primes is infinite. [. . .]

Since I had become acquainted with Euclid's proof at school, it had always filled me with a deep satisfaction that was aesthetic rather than intellectual. Now, as I recalled the method and scratched the symbols on the wall, I felt the same enchantment.

And then, for the first time, I suddenly understood the reason for this enchant-ment: the scribbled symbols on the wall represented one of the rare cases where a meaningful and comprehensive statement about the infinite is arrived at by precise and finite means. The infinite is a mystical mass shrouded in a haze; and yet it was possible to gain some knowledge of it without losing oneself in treacly ambiguities. The significance of this swept over me like a wave. The wave had originated in an articulate verbal insight; but this evaporated at once, leaving in its wake only a wordless essence, a fragrance of eternity, a quiver of the arrow in the blue. I must have stood there for some minutes, entranced, with a wordless awareness that 'this is perfect—perfect'; until I noticed some slight mental discomfort nagging at the back of my mind—some trivial circumstance that marred the perfection of the moment. Then I remembered the nature of that

---

[5] Although, in this context, the term 'experience' is a bit misleading. A better term would be 'insight' or 'way of being'. We will come back to this point at the end of the chapter.

irrelevant annoyance: I was, of course, in prison and might be shot. But this was immediately answered by a feeling whose verbal translation would be: 'So what? is that all? Have you got nothing more serious to worry about?'—an answer so spontaneous, fresh and amused as if the intruding annoyance had been the loss of a collar-stud. Then I was floating on my back in a river of peace, under bridges of silence. It came from nowhere and flowed nowhere. Then there was no river and no I. The I had ceased to exist.

[...] When I say 'the I had ceased to exist', I refer to a concrete experience that is verbally as incommunicable as the feeling aroused by a piano concerto, yet just as real—only much more real. In fact, its primary mark is the sensation that this state is more real than any other one has experienced before—that for the first time the veil has fallen and one is in touch with 'real reality' the hidden order of things, the X-ray texture of the world, normally obscured by layers of irrelevancy.

What distinguishes this type of experience from the emotional entrancements of music, landscapes or love is that the former has a definitely intellectual, or rather noumenal, content. It is meaningful, though not in verbal terms. Verbal transcriptions that come nearest to it are: the unity and interlocking of everything that exists, an interdependence like that of gravitational fields or communicating vessels. The 'I' ceases to exist because it has, by a kind of mental osmosis, established communication with, and been dissolved in, the universal pool. It is the process of dissolution and limitless expansion which is sensed as the 'oceanic feeling', as the draining of all tension, the absolute catharsis, the peace that passeth all understanding.

The coming-back to the lower order of reality I found to be gradual, like waking up from anaesthesia. There was the equation of the parabola scratched on the dirty wall, the iron bed and the iron table and the strip of blue Andalusian sky. But there was no unpleasant hangover as from other modes of intoxication. On the contrary: there remained a sustained and invigorating, serene and fear-dispelling after-effect that lasted for hours and days. It was as if a massive dose of vitamins had been injected into the veins. Or, to change the metaphor, I resumed my travels through my cell like an old car with its batteries freshly recharged.

Whether the experience had lasted for a few minutes or an hour, I never knew. In the beginning it occurred two or even three times a week, then the intervals became longer. It could never be voluntarily induced. After my liberation it recurred at even longer intervals, perhaps once or twice in a year. But by that time the groundwork for a change of personality was completed. I shall henceforth refer to these experiences as 'the hours by the window'.

Koestler 1954, pp. 404–7

There is a lot to contemplate in this beautiful description. We can see that Koestler's account is both profoundly personal, deeply moving, and yet also intellectually refined. And we see many of the themes we have come across already—those of unity, ineffability, certainty, ultimate reality, and ego dissolution (a dissolving of the 'I').

It is important for us to be clear that the point of including these descriptions is not that they will later serve as evidence for a theory of mystical experience. Nor is it because I think they are representative of all mystical experiences. The point of including them is simply to help orient those readers unfamiliar with mystical experiences so that they get *some* sense of what we're trying to understand—and also to help dispel some of the unhelpful associations that are often triggered by the term 'mystical'.

Now that we have a rough sense of what mystical experience may be, we can consider some of the theories of mystical experiences that have been put forward. Before we do, two brief terminological points are in order. Following Stace 1960, I'll say that someone is a *mystic* if they have had a mystical experience and take it seriously in some way. All of the authors quoted above are, therefore, mystics. It will also sometimes be convenient to speak loosely of *mysticism*. We can think of this roughly as an outlook that results from, and involves, taking mystical experience seriously. Nothing of substance will hang on these terminological choices. With that out of the way, let's now turn to the theories of mystical experience.

10.3 Theories of Mystical Experience

A popular theory of mystical experience is *perennialism*, which has its roots in the Renaissance and gets much of its popularity from Huxley 1945 and Stace 1960. There is a cluster of beliefs that perennialists tend to have, and these can vary somewhat, but a central belief of perennialism is that all mystical experiences are identical to each other or share a "common core". Another common perennialist belief is that all mystical experiences are experiences of *unity*, which can be thought of as the oneness of all reality and the interconnectedness of everything. These two beliefs typically form the foundation of perennialism, so they will be the focus here.[6]

It's worth exploring perennialism a bit further to get a sense of its appeal. The main appeal of the view is that unity appears to be a common element of most descriptions of mystical experiences *and* it also seems that unity can explain the other commonly reported aspects of mystical experience. Recall from the previous chapter that an experience is thought to be of a mystical-type to the extent that it involves: (i) unity, (ii) a noetic quality, (iii) a transcendence of time and space,

[6] A third perennialist belief is that mystical experience is the source of all religion and that all of the world's religions are somewhat crude, and potentially corrupt, attempts to articulate the content of mystical experience. I won't discuss this third belief here since its sociological character places it beyond the scope of this book.

(iv) ineffability, (v) paradox, (vi) sacredness, and (vii) positive feelings of bliss, joy, wonder, and awe. Each of these factors can be explained to some degree by unity.

Regarding (ii), unity is, roughly speaking, a metaphysical statement about reality that runs contrary to our usual understanding of the world, and so an apparent experience of unity would have a noetic quality to it.

Regarding (iii), as Bertrand Russell once pointed out, a denial of division entails a denial of time:

> A third mark of almost all mystical metaphysics is the denial of the reality of Time. This is an outcome of the denial of division; if all is one, the distinction of past and future must be illusory.
>
> Russell 1910b, p. 10

The same is also true of space, and so we can see why an experience of unity would be an experience that transcends time and space.

Regarding (iv), Plotinus made a similar observation concerning the description of mystical experience:

> [...] No doubt we should not speak of seeing; but we cannot help talking in dualities, seen and seer, instead of, boldly, the achievement of unity. In this seeing, we neither hold an object nor trace distinction; there is no two. [...] only in separation is there duality [...] This is why the vision baffles telling; we cannot detach the Supreme to state it; if we have seen something thus detached we have failed of the Supreme which is to be known only as one with ourselves.
>
> Plotinus, *Ennead VI*, 9:10[7]

The thought is that all factive language, even the simplest sentence, involves duality, and so there is no way to express unity. For example, if you ascribe a predicate F to an object a, then you reject its negation *not Fa*. For a similar reason, we can see why unity would entail that the experience involves (v) paradox: this occurs when the mind tries to think logically, which necessarily involves duality, about something that has no duality.

Regarding (vi), unity can explain the sacredness of mystical experience in terms of the dissolving of the usual boundary between the self—or what is erroneously assumed to be the self (the ego)—and the rest of the universe. For example, Happold writes:

> Bound up with the sense of oneness and the sense of timelessness there is another characteristic of mystical experience, the conviction that the familiar phenomenal ego is not the real I.

---

[7] MacKenna 1952, pp. 359–60.

This conviction finds expression in one form in the Atman doctrine of Hinduism. The self, the *ego* of which we are normally conscious, it is asserted, is not the true self. It is conscious only by fits and starts; it is bound up with bodily organizations and mental happenings which are subject to change and decay; it is, therefore, only an ephemeral, phenomenal self.

In man there is another self, the true Self, which is not affected by ordinary happenings and which gives him a sense of identity through numerous bodily and mental transformations. It does not change in the slow changes of the organism, in the flux of sensations, in the dissipation of ideas, or in the fading of memories. This true Self Hinduism calls the *Atman*. The Atman is immortal, constant, and unchanging, and is not bound by space-time. It is not only an individual self, it also has a universal quality. It is 'that by which the universe is pervaded, which nothing pervades, which causes all things to shine, but which all things cannot make to shine'. In its nature, moreover, this True or Greater Self is divine. 'The knowledge that Brahman and Atman are one and the same' wrote Sankara, 'is true knowledge'.

Happold 1963, p. 48

As Happold also goes on to note, the sacredness of mystical experience can be accounted for by other traditions as well. For example, Meister Eckhart writes:

> There is in the soul something which is above the soul, Divine, simple, a pure nothing; rather nameless than named, unknown than known. . . . It is absolute and free from all names and all forms, just as God is free and absolute in Himself. It is higher than knowledge, higher than love, higher than grace. For in these there is still distinction. In this power God doth blossom and flourish with all his Godhead and the spirit flourisheth in God.

Meister Eckhart[8]

We see here, again, that the idea of unity (the lack of distinction) plays a key role in defining the thing that Eckhart says is 'above the soul'.

Finally, unity can also explain (vii) the positive feelings of bliss, joy, wonder, and awe, because it entails that mystical experience involves, as James described, the melting into a unity of 'the opposites of the world, whose contradictoriness and conflict make all our difficulties and troubles'. We also saw this idea in the previous chapter, from Jung and Maslow—that is, that much suffering and impediments to increased well-being stem from internal conflicts and divisions. In Buddhism, the process of unifying the mind can involve open wonder (beginner's mind) and can lead to levels of absorption known as *jhanas*, with the early *jhanas* involving experiences of bliss and joy (according to some *jhana* systems).

---

[8] Quoted by Happold 1963, p. 49.

Although these explanations are quick and rely on particular conceptions of mystical experience, they are enough for us to appreciate the appeal of unity to perennialists and why many believe that unity is the core feature of mystical experience. It should be noted, though, that the significance of unity can easily be overemphasized—or, at least, not all mystics are in agreement about its importance. For example, Shinryū Suzuki pointed out that:

> Sometimes people put stress on oneness, but this is not our understanding. We do not emphasize any point in particular, even oneness. Oneness is valuable, but variety is also wonderful. Ignoring variety, people emphasize the one absolute existence, but this is a one-sided understanding. [...]
>
> This kind of experience is something beyond our thinking. In the thinking realm there is a difference between oneness and variety; but in actual experience, variety and unity are the same. Because you create some idea of unity or variety, you are caught by the idea. And you have to continue the endless thinking, although actually there is no need to think.
>
> Suzuki 1970, pp. 119–20

Thus, there is a sense in which thinking of these experiences in terms of unity—or, indeed, any feature that may be considered characteristic of them—can involve a distortion of them and a fundamental misunderstanding of their nature. This is an important point that we will come back to in a moment.

The other dominant theory of mystical experience is *contextualism*. In contrast to perennialism, contextualism denies that there is a common core to all mystical experiences and argues that the content of any given mystical experience is specific to the individual in question and highly dependent on their cultural context. This view, which is also sometimes called *constructivism*, is largely due to Katz 1978, who criticized Stace's arguments for perennialism and unity. One of Katz's main criticisms is that the descriptions of mystical experience are not as unified as perennialists make them out to be. For example, Katz points out that Stace's cross-cultural analysis does not assign sufficient weight to important mystical traditions such as Kabbalah, whose descriptions of mystical experience are at odds with those that Stace selected for his analysis. Moreover, Katz argues that Stace is not justified in treating as equivalent many of the core concepts that he finds in his selected descriptions, such as the Self in Advaita Vedanta, Emptiness in Zen, and God in medieval Christian mysticism. Altogether, Katz argues that a proper analysis of the descriptions of mystical experiences that have been given across cultures and throughout the ages shows that they lack a common core, and moreover, that the nature of a given mystical experience depends on the context in which it occurs.

At this point, it would be natural for us to consider how a perennialist may reply to the contextualist. However, I think it is more fruitful to point out something odd about this debate. The oddness is that the debate about the nature of mystical experience boils down to a debate about how we ought to interpret the various *descriptions* of mystical experience, almost all of which include some statement about the *ineffability* of the experience. Curiously, both Stace and Katz diminish the significance of ineffability. Although Stace is adamant that mystics are not mistaken about their mystical experiences, he nevertheless goes on to argue that they *are* mistaken about the ineffability of their experiences (Stace 1960, p. 305).[9] And Katz explicitly states that the project is to analyse *descriptions* of mystical experience:

> [... T]he only evidence we have, if we are not mystics ourselves, and even mystics really do not have a privileged position here, is the account given by mystics of their experience. These are the data of study and analysis.
>
> Katz 1983, p. 5

Presumably, the reason for adopting this attitude towards ineffability is that there is nothing else that can be done—descriptions of mystical experiences are the only things that scholars of mysticism have to work with. By taking the descriptions of mystical experiences as the data, we are able to put ourselves in the position of analysts who are simply trying to systematize and explain the objective data. It makes the project of understanding mystical experience objective, scientific, and naturalistically acceptable. So, from a strategic perspective, this methodological assumption makes perfect sense.

However, how are we to reconcile this methodological assumption with the ineffability that many of the descriptions themselves contain? We've seen some examples already, but there are many more. For example, consider D. T. Suzuki on the ineffability of the transcendental world (*lokottara*):

> When language is forced to be used for things of this world, lokottara, it becomes warped and assumes all kinds of crookedness: oxymora, paradoxes, contradictions, absurdities, oddities, ambiguities, and irrationalities. Language itself is not to be blamed for it. It is we ourselves who, ignorant of its proper functions, try to apply it to that for which it was never intended.
>
> Suzuki 1957, p. 51

And Grof's description of LSD-induced mystical experience:

> This experience is boundless, unfathomable, and ineffable; it is existence itself. Verbal communication and the symbolic structure of our everyday language

---

[9] Stace's argument for this claim is somewhat convoluted, so I won't include a proper discussion of it here. Very briefly: Stace grants that mystical experiences are ineffable and argues that *remembered* mystical experiences are not, and that alleged descriptions of mystical experiences are in fact descriptions of remembered mystical experiences (pp. 297–306). However, even if we grant all of these premises, it follows that Stace can only give a theory of remembered mystical experiences and not of mystical experiences themselves.

seem to be a ridiculously inadequate means to capture and convey its nature and quality.

Grof 1975, p. 203

And Koestler, following up on his statement that 'the I had ceased to exist', wrote:

It is extremely embarrassing to write down a phrase like that when one has read *The Meaning of Meaning* and nibbled at logical positivism and aims at verbal precision and dislikes nebulous gushings. Yet, 'mystical' experiences, as we dubiously call them, are not nebulous, vague or maudlin—they only become so when we debase them by verbalisation.

Koestler 1954, pp. 405–6

Note that these descriptions do not contain statements about one being at a loss for words. Instead, the descriptions express a stronger notion of ineffability: to verbalize the experience is to *debase* it, and language is not suited for capturing the experience. Therefore, according to these descriptions, we can't understand what the experience is by analysing descriptions of it. To put it another way, if we are to take the descriptions seriously, as both Stace and Katz say we should, then it follows that we shouldn't take them seriously. The idea of trying to understand mystical experiences by analysing descriptions of them is, therefore, a fundamental mistake.

To be fair, Katz is keenly aware of this point about ineffability and what it entails:

[I]f words mean anything my position seems to be the only reasonable one to adopt. Many students of mysticism might see this remark as their 'escape hatch' for avoiding my conclusion. After all, they might argue, all mystics are wary about using language to describe their experience, and many are absolutely opposed to its employment, arguing a form of 'I don't mean what I say and I don't say what I mean'. Also, we are sure to be reminded of the well-known mystical penchant for paradox and ineffability as relevant at this point. However, this 'escape' is no escape at all. It fails to provide the desired way out because it fails to realize that, if the mystic does not mean what he says and his words have no literal meaning whatsoever, then not only is it impossible to establish my pluralistic view, but it is also logically impossible to establish any view [e.g. perennialism] whatsoever. If none of the mystics' utterances carry any literal meaning then they cannot serve as the data for any position, not mine, and certainly not the view that all mystical experiences are the same, or reducible to a small class of phenomenological categories.

Katz 1978, p. 40

Katz is entirely correct here, except for one thing: the implicit assumption that one ought to have a view (a theory) of mystical experience in the first place. The problem is that this is exactly what the statements of ineffability are warning us against. For example, in Zen, this point is often made rather explicitly:

> Zen has nothing to do with letters, words, or sutras. It only requests you to grasp the point directly and therein to find your peaceful abode. When the mind is disturbed, the understanding is stirred, things are recognized, notions are entertained, ghostly spirits are conjured, and prejudices grow rampant. Zen will then forever be lost in the maze.
>
> Suzuki 1964, p. 46

And:

> Followers of the Way, if you want insight into dharma as it is, just don't be taken in by the deluded views of others. Whatever you encounter, either within or without, slay it at once. On meeting a buddha slay the buddha, on meeting a patriarch slay the patriarch, on meeting an arhat slay the arhat, on meeting your parents slay your parents, on meeting your kinsman slay your kinsman, and you attain emancipation. By not cleaving to things, you freely pass through.
>
> Linji Yixuan[10]

It seems fairly clear, then, that we are not going to understand mystical experience by ignoring its ineffability and proceeding to analyse the descriptions that mystics warn us against analysing. Indeed, since the statements of ineffability undermine the possibility of establishing any theory whatsoever, they lead us inexorably to what we may call a *no-theory* theory (or a no-view view) of mystical experience.

There are seven common objections to this argument for a no-theory theory of mystical experience. The first objection is that our goal is to develop an understanding of mystical experiences, and so a no-theory theory of mystical experience can't help us with that goal—only a positive theory, such as perennialism or contextualism, can. There are two replies to this objection. First, there is a proof by demonstration: in the next section, we will see how we can develop an understanding of mystical experience without committing to a theory of it. Second, it is a mistake to think that all understanding must come by way of a theory. As Maslow put it:

> Our conscious intellect is too exclusively analytic, rational, numerical, atomistic, conceptual and so it misses a great deal of reality, especially within ourselves.
>
> Maslow 1963, p. 69

---

[10] Sasaki 2009, p. 22.

This is a common theme in many mystical writings: there is a realm of understanding that exists beyond the scope of language. So we're not justified in assuming that all understanding must come by way of a theory.

The second objection is that ineffability is self-undermining, and so we can—and should—ignore statements of ineffability in the descriptions of mystical experience. This manoeuvre then frees us to analyse and theorize to our heart's content about the descriptions' remnants. The reason for thinking that ineffability is self-undermining is the same idea we saw from St. Augustine in Section 10.1: to say that mystical experience is ineffable is to say something about mystical experience, which would contradict its ineffability. Although it is correct that ineffability is self-undermining in this way, it doesn't follow that we're licensed to ignore it and focus on the remnants of the descriptions. To do so would be an almost *deliberate* failure to understand what the mystics are saying. To limit ourselves to analysing the descriptions of mystical experiences would be a mistake similar to choosing not to look through a Magic Eye picture and concluding that it doesn't contain a hidden image. In Buddhist philosophy, this is the mistake of only looking at a finger pointing to the moon: if you just look at the finger (the teaching), you'll fail to see the moon (the wisdom) to which it is pointing.[11]

The third objection is that if we don't take the descriptions of mystical experiences as data to be analysed, then we can't approach this topic as naturalists. Replying properly to this objection requires a lengthy discussion of naturalism since it is notoriously difficult to define. However, two brief remarks can be made here. The first stems from the fact that naturalism can be thought of in terms of *epistemic humility*: we shouldn't believe in entities or properties that go beyond our best scientific theories or the available empirical evidence. When we don't have evidence with respect to some theory (or hypothesis), then we should refrain from forming a belief in that theory. From this perspective, a no-theory theory of mystical experience is the only naturalistically acceptable position. Since we lack any data upon which we can base a theory of mystical experience, we ought not to be committed to any theory of it. The second remark is again that the proof is in the pudding: in the next section, when we unpack the idea of ineffability to get a better understanding of mystical experience, there won't be anything non-naturalistic—no gods, spirits, grand metaphysical claims, etc. In short, although mysticism is often thought of as running contrary to naturalistic principles, this is based (at least in part) on a failure to understand the ineffability of mystical experience.

Relatedly, the fourth objection makes the point that an ineffable experience must manifest as something ineffable at the level of the brain and that this would run counter to naturalism. This objection is mistaken for at least two reasons. First, the physical correlate of an ineffable experience could be something as mundane as

---

[11] See Murphy 1996 for a similar take on the epistemological status of the mystical language of Meister Eckhart.

a disruption to brain regions or networks responsible for speech production, such as Broca's area (Winkelman 2017), allowing the brain to enter patterns of activity that lie outside those associated with discursive thought. Second, ineffability at the level of the brain wouldn't necessarily contradict naturalism. For example, consider the view that scientific descriptions (hypotheses, models, theories) are, among other things, compressions of observed data points that satisfy key theoretical virtues, such as simplicity, statistical fit, precision, unification, explanatory power, etc.[12] According to this view, an indescribable data set is one that is too complex to be compressed into a form that is explanatorily valuable to us. That is, as we collect more data, we find it increasingly difficult to provide simple descriptions that are precise and explanatorily useful. In such cases, the solution is to abstract away from the data (sacrificing precision and perhaps statistical fit) for a gain in simplicity and explanatory power. For example, we see this in statistical mechanics: the microphysical data are far too complex for us to describe in any useful way, so we abstract away from them and give summary descriptions in terms of higher-level concepts such as probability and entropy. Interestingly, that is exactly what we have seen so far in psychedelic science, with one of the leading ideas being that psychedelics increase the brain's entropy, often measured in terms of signal complexity (Carhart-Harris 2018). Therefore, one could potentially argue that, far from running counter to naturalism, the no-theory theory of mystical experience fits rather neatly with current empirical findings.[13]

The fifth objection argues that, although it may be correct that we can't use descriptions of mystical experience as data, it doesn't follow that there are no data at all. For example, one might try to say that there are data from neuroimaging studies of mystical experiences. However, without a definition of mystical experience, how can we know which neuroimaging studies target mystical experiences, as opposed to some other kind of experience? We can't. Alternatively, one might try to say that there are *first-person* data: someone who has had a mystical experience can use that experience as a data point for their theory. The problem with this proposal is that it gives up on the idea of the data being *objective*. Theories are shared enterprises: part of the point of having them is that there can be a community of researchers developing and evaluating them together. We, therefore, give up on that enterprise by allowing the data to be subjective. This, in itself, is not a problem. The problem is that it is all too easy for people with different theories of subjective data to make the mistake of thinking that they are having a real disagreement about the correct theory of objective data.

The sixth objection points out that some descriptions of mystical experiences do not involve statements of ineffability, and so we can't conclude that *all* mystical

---

[12] For recent discussions of theoretical virtues, see Keas 2018 and Schindler 2022.

[13] To be clear, this argument is just a proof of concept. The point here is only that ineffability doesn't *necessarily* run counter to naturalism.

experiences are ineffable. This objection is similar in spirit to Katz's criticism of Stace's argument (that unity is the core of all mystical experiences). In this vein, one could also argue that the supposed ineffability of mystical experience is itself contextual and thus relative to a culture or a certain kind of religious thought, etc. Let us suppose this is true. Then it follows that we have two classes of descriptions: those that involve ineffability and those that do not. Further, let us suppose that both are deserving of the name 'mystical' (whatever that amounts to—see the end of this chapter). Thus, perhaps there are two kinds of mystical experiences. Nevertheless, we're still left with the task of grappling with those mystical experiences that are ineffable.

Finally, the seventh objection is that mystics themselves don't seem to take ineffability all that seriously. As the satirical poet Po Chü-i wrote:

> 'He who talks doesn't know
> he who knows doesn't talk':
> that is what Lao-tzu told us,
> in a book of five thousand words
> If he was the one who knew,
> how could he have been such a blabbermouth?
>
> Po Chü-i[14]

And so we may wonder: why take the mystics' statements of ineffability seriously, if they themselves do not? And if we don't have to, then perhaps we *can* usefully analyse descriptions of mystical experience.[15] One reply to this objection is that we don't know how representative the blabbermouths are: we don't know how many mystics have remained silent about their experiences. Perhaps the blabbermouths are a minority, and perhaps they don't fully understand what they are trying to describe. That is, since Lao-tzu chose to write about the Dao, perhaps it follows he didn't fully understand it.

In some cases, there may be something to this reply. For example, perhaps for some cases of psychedelic-induced mystical experiences—without any supporting context or framework for disciplined thought—it is reasonable to say that the experience wasn't fully understood. However, a better reply is that ineffability doesn't preclude *any* use of words when helping people understand mystical experiences. For example, it is entirely compatible with ineffability that words can be used to help *guide* someone towards a mystical experience. From this perspective, many of the writings of mystics are better seen as a kind of literary charades: they point to

---

[14] Quoted in Mitchell 1988, p. 89.
[15] Following similar reasoning, Yaden et al. 2015 provide a quantitive linguistic analysis of 777 descriptions of mystical experiences.

that which cannot be spoken of directly. For example, much of the *Dao De Ching* reads like this, and the playful language of *Zhuangzi* is arguably intended to allow language to become phenomenally transparent so that the reader can be directed towards the Dao without it being described explicitly (Vrubliauskaite 2014).

Alternatively, the writings may try to point people *away* from what mystical experience *is not*—following the *via negativa* (apophatic) strategy that many mystics have pursued. Similarly, the koans of Zen are often used as "thought roadblocks" that are designed to force the student into a new way of thinking (or a new way of not thinking). Plato's allegory of the cave in *Republic* can also be read this way: the point of education is not to *transfer* truths to people, but to teach them how to see truths for themselves (not unlike Zen's notion of *special transmission*). It is also worth noting in this regard that the Eleusinian mystery rites were guarded with the utmost secrecy (sharing their details was a capital punishment). While there is some debate as to what was kept secret (the details of the rituals, some doctrinal truth, etc.), one possibility is that the secrecy was simply a way of protecting the ineffable experience of the final revelation from the linguistic distortion that would inevitability arise in common discourse. Etymologically, then, it could be that a 'mystical experience' is an experience that shouldn't be spoken about by those without expert training (due to its high value and ineffability). At any rate, essentially the same principle is in place: words can be used to guide people towards mystical experience, even if they can't be used to describe the experience directly.

Now that we have a better sense of how we can approach the issue of mystical experience, let's now explore ineffability more carefully. This, in turn, will help us develop a better understanding of mystical experiences.

10.4 Ineffability

As we've seen already, the ineffability of mystical experience involves more than people simply being at a loss to describe the experience. Rather, it seems there is something inappropriate about language as a means for conveying the nature of the experience. As Koestler 1954 put it: we *debase* mystical experiences when we try to verbalize them. And, paraphrasing Suzuki: when we force descriptions upon mystical experience, we necessarily distort the experience, and this error is not due to language itself, but rather due to our ignorant misapplication of it. Thus, there is a *normative* aspect to ineffability.

There is actually a second, closely related, source of normativity: while the *speaker* necessarily distorts the experience with language, the *listener* also has their role to play in its distortion. Douglas Shrader captured this well in recounting his attempts to describe his mystical experience:

Any description that I could provide of the experience, once I surrendered, will be inadequate at best. Worse, my words are as likely to obscure and mislead as they are to inform and illuminate. [...]

Whenever I spoke of the experience, I tried to be intellectually cautious and spiritually responsible. Whatever I offered with one hand, I took back with the other. I found myself incessantly repeating the following refrain: 'It was like this, but not really. It was sort of like that, but not in the way that you might initially think'. Unfortunately, as I quickly learned, people heard what they wanted to hear and disregarded the rest. What I offered as fumbling, grossly inadequate descriptions became concretized in their minds as authoritative expressions of firsthand experience. Gradually I shied away from providing any description at all, drew nourishment from the experience that was—inexplicably and paradoxically—still with me, and began to explore the paths of contemplation and inward reflection.

Shrader 2008, p. 5

We also see the same idea attributed to the Buddha in the *Sallekha Sutta*:

Others will adhere to their own views, hold on to them tenaciously, and relinquish them with difficulty; we shall not adhere to our own views or hold on to them tenaciously, but shall relinquish them easily: effacement should be practiced thus.

Nanamoli and Bodhi 1995, p. 127

In short, people will hear what they want to hear. Of course, people hear what they want to hear all the time, but the point is that this disposition is particularly pernicious when it comes to mystical experience.

Let's call these two aspects of ineffability the *problem of language* (speaker distortion) and the *problem of communication* (listener distortion) for mystical experience. The two problems are related but distinct. The first problem is that there is no way to represent mystical experience using language without distorting it in some way. The second problem is that, for a given linguistic representation, people will lock on to some part of it as authoritative and disregard the rest.[16] By observing these two problems and thinking about them more carefully, we can better understand ineffability and, in turn, better understand mystical experience.

One way to think about these two aspects of ineffability more carefully is to see if they arise in another context. Interestingly, it appears that this is the case. A fundamental problem in the theory of uncertainty concerns how we can mathematically represent *maximal uncertainty*. In Bayesianism, this is known

---

[16] These are two manifestations of an underlying problem: that language traps the mind in a discursive form of thought and thereby prevents the mind from attaining the non-discursive insight of mystical experience.

as *the problem of priors*. We can think of this as analogous to the problem of linguistically representing mystical experience. It turns out that when we try to represent maximal uncertainty using mathematical language, two sub-problems emerge that are analogous to the problems of language and communication for mystical experience. We'll see how this works in a moment, but before we do, it will also help to see that there are some interesting and independent reasons to think that maximal uncertainty might have some useful similarities to mystical experience. To put it another way, there are some reasons to think that we can use maximal uncertainty as a kind of *model* for mystical experience.

The previous sentence may trigger an alarm bell for some readers: if we use maximal uncertainty as a model for mystical experience, then doesn't that contradict the point from the previous section that we should have a no-theory theory of mystical experience? This is a perfectly reasonable concern to have at this point, and we'll come back to it later on, but the short answer is that it does not. The trick in avoiding the contradiction involves how we use the model. If we intend for it to be descriptively accurate of mystical experience, then we do have a contradiction. However, if we only use the model to guide our thinking in a particular direction, then there is no contradiction. As I said, we'll come back to this point later on. Let's first see the motivation for the model and how the problem of representing maximal uncertainty can shed some new light on the ineffability of mystical experience.

One motivation for thinking that maximal uncertainty can be used as a model for mystical experience stems from the entropic brain hypothesis: psychedelics are thought to increase the entropy of one's brain and, correspondingly, one's state of uncertainty (Carhart-Harris et al. 2014).[17] If mystical experiences are maximally psychedelic experiences (or approximations of them), then they may correspond to states of maximal entropy and thus states of maximal uncertainty. A similar motivation stems from the REBUS model of psychedelics: psychedelics are thought to relax the strength of priors in the predictive hierarchy of Bayesian priors (Carhart-Harris and Friston 2019). So, if mystical experiences are maximally psychedelic experiences, then they may involve a maximal relaxation of these priors, which may correspond to a predictive state that is maximally uncertain. Of course, there is a big assumption behind these two motivations: that mystical experiences are maximally psychedelic (or come close to being maximally psychedelic). However, within the confines of these particular frameworks for thinking about psychedelic experiences, this doesn't seem to be an unreasonable assumption to make.

These two motivations stem from psychedelic science, but we can also find motivation for the model from the mystical traditions: mystics often indicate that

---

[17] Roughly speaking, entropy in this context is a measure of uncertainty: more uncertainty, more entropy.

maximal uncertainty is part of the enlightened state or functions as a gateway to it. For example, in the *Dao De Ching*:

> Not knowing is true knowledge.
> Presuming to know is a disease.
> First realize that you are sick;
> then you can move toward health.
> The Master is her own physician.
> She has healed herself of all knowing.
> Thus she is truly whole.
>
> Chapter 71, *Dao De Ching*[18]

And also in Zen with Boshan's notion of *Great Doubt*:

> In Zen practice, the essential point is to rouse doubt. What is this doubt? When you are born, for example, where do you come from? You cannot help but remain in doubt about this. When you die, where do you go? Again, you cannot help but remain in doubt. Since you cannot pierce this barrier of life and death, suddenly doubt will coalesce right before your eyes. Try to put it down, you cannot; try to push it away, you cannot. Eventually you will break through this doubt block and realise what a worthless notion life and death is—ha! As the old worthies said: 'Great doubt, great awakening; small doubt, small awakening; no doubt, no awakening'.
>
> Shore 2016, p. 10

We see the same idea in *Don't-Know Mind*:

> This don't know is your true master. Always keep the mind that doesn't know and soon you will attain enlightenment.
>
> Kyong Ho Sunim[19]

And in the second chapter of the *Kena Upanishad*:

> To whomsoever it is not known, to him it is known: to whomsoever it is known, he does not know. It is not understood by those who understand it; it is understood by those who do not understand it.[20]

---

[18] Mitchell 1988. It is useful to compare Mitchell's (somewhat controversial) rendering of Chapter 71 with this translation by Ames and Hall 2002: 'Knowing that one does not know is knowing at its best; But not knowing that one knows is suffering from a disease. Thus, the reason the sages are free of disease; Is because they recognize the disease as a disease. This is why they are not afflicted'. This translation (and their commentary) highlights an important point that isn't clear in Mitchell's rendering, which is that the not-knowing clears the way for an alternative (and more valuable) form of knowing.
[19] Quoted in Sahn 2012, p. 647.   [20] Radhakrishnan 1968, p. 585.

We also find this idea in Western mysticism. It appears perhaps most famously in *The Cloud of Unknowing*, but also, for example, in the sermons of Meister Eckhart:

> So in truth, no creaturely skill, nor your own wisdom nor all your knowledge can enable you to know God divinely. For you to know God in God's way, your knowing must become a pure unknowing, and a forgetting of yourself and all creatures.
>
> Meister Eckhart, Sermon 4[21]

In summary, there is reason—from both science and the mystical traditions—to think that we may learn something useful by treating maximal uncertainty as a model of mystical experience.

So, let's now take a moment to think about the problem of representing maximal uncertainty. To help avoid the discussion becoming too abstract, we'll work within a particular theory of uncertainty: Bayesian probability theory. This choice is convenient since it is probably the most popular theory and it allows us to examine the problems that interest us. Despite its popularity, the Bayesian theory of uncertainty has a well-known problem at its foundations: it isn't obvious how a state of maximal uncertainty can be represented with a probability distribution. There's a famous paradox, known as Bertrand's paradox, that highlights this problem. We'll consider a simplified version of the paradox that is adapted from van Fraassen 1989. The paradox itself doesn't quite involve maximal uncertainty, but it nevertheless nicely exemplifies the problems we run into as we approach maximal uncertainty.

Here's an example of the paradox. Imagine a factory that produces boxes that are perfect cubes with side lengths between 1 and 3 meters. Based on this information, what probability should you assign to the next box the factory produces having a side length between 1 and 2 meters? It seems that the only reasonable probability is 50%, since you have no reason to think that 1-to-2 meters is more or less likely than 2-to-3 meters. That's the answer most people give. Now imagine another factory that produces boxes that are perfect cubes with face areas between 1 and 9 square meters. Based on this information, what probability should you assign to the next box the factory produces having a face area between 1 and 4 square meters? It seems in this case, it is reasonable to assign a probability less than 50%, since the range of 1 to 4 is smaller than the range of 4 to 9. More specifically, it seems one should assign a probability of $(4 - 1)/(9 - 1) \times 100\% = 37.5\%$.

For both factories, the answers of 50% and 37.5% are the intuitive answers that most people give. They are also the answers dictated by the *principle of indifference*, which says that if you have no reason to think one possibility is more likely than

[21] Walshe 2009, p. 56.

another, then you should assign them equal probability.[22] The paradox arises when we notice that there is no difference in the imagined factories: a factory that produces boxes with side lengths between 1 and 3 meters is a factory that produces boxes with face areas between 1 and 9 square meters (and vice versa). And, more specifically, the event of the next box having a side length between 1 and 2 meters is the same as the event of it having a face area between 1 and 4 square meters. This means we assigned two different probabilities—50% and 37.5%—to the same event.

This paradox highlights the problem that interests us: in general, there is no way to represent maximal uncertainty with a probability distribution. In both ways of imaging the box factory, you have no information about what the next box will be like. Besides the constraints given, you have no information about its side length or face area. Within those constraints, you are maximally uncertain about the next box. When you imagine the box factory in terms of side lengths, you have the intuition that 50% probability reflects your state of maximal uncertainty. This seemed reasonable because assigning a probability of 50% appears to avoid taking a stand that goes beyond what you know about the side lengths. However, what you didn't realize—if you're like most people and didn't know the trap was coming—was that by trying to not take a stand with respect to the *side lengths*, you inadvertently took a stand with respect to the *face areas*. This means that there is no way to express your maximal uncertainty using a probability function. If you think you've done it for side lengths, then you've failed to do it for face areas—and vice versa.

There is a large literature on this problem of representing maximal uncertainty in the Bayesian framework. Some principles have been advanced that are meant to overcome the shortcomings of the principle of indifference (Jaynes 1973); however, they never completely solve the problem (van Fraassen 1989). The general upshot is that there is no way to represent maximal uncertainty within the Bayesian framework (Joyce 2010). However, this is not a problem that is specific to Bayesianism. It can be proven that *any* theory of uncertainty that satisfies minimal plausible conditions will suffer from a version of this problem (Titelbaum 2011). In the literature, the problem has become known as the *problem of language dependence*. The problem is that we have a strong intuition that there should be a way of expressing our uncertainty in a way that is independent of how we describe the space of possibilities, but there isn't. There is, therefore, an ineffability of maximal uncertainty. In the box factory example, this arises when we describe the box factory in terms of side areas and face areas.

Thus, we can now see how the ineffability of maximal uncertainty is similar to the ineffability of mystical experiences. To borrow D.T. Suzuki's words from before: when probability theory is forced to be used for states of maximal uncertainty, it

---

[22] The principle of indifference can be understood as a special case of the more general principle of maximizing entropy (Jaynes 1973).

becomes warped and assumes all kinds of crookedness. And this is not because of a defect with the Bayesian framework—it is due to our ignorant misapplication of the framework. The crucial fact that is so easy for us to miss is that when we use *any* substantive theory to represent our uncertainty, we necessarily take a stance that goes beyond what we actually know (Titelbaum 2011). And a big part of the problem is that we do this unwittingly: we don't realize that we're adding something substantial to the situation, even in simple examples such as those of the box factory, let alone the complex scenarios we encounter in daily life. To put the point in other words, we have two problems: (i) there is no way for us to formally represent maximal uncertainty without distorting it, and (ii) we're strongly disposed to do so without realizing it.

The first problem is a direct analogue of our problem of language for mystical experience. The second problem becomes a direct analogue of the problem for communication when we see that the strong disposition causes communication problems. Suppose there is a box factory like the one in our example, and I want to tell you about it. Being fully aware of the problem of language dependence, I do the right thing and just say that there is a box factory that produces side lengths between 1 and 3 meters—that is, I refrain from saying anything about a probability distribution. However, I should know better: because you're a Bayesian (let's suppose), you will assign some probability distribution or other and thereby add more to the situation than I intended to communicate. Moreover, by choosing to speak in terms of side lengths, I've unwittingly primed you to assign a particular probability distribution.[23] Unless I take appropriate precautions—for example, to warn you about the problem of language dependence—you're likely (if you're like most people) to over-interpret my description of the state of uncertainty. And so we see how the two aspects of ineffability (the problems of language and communication) arise for states of maximum uncertainty.

There are other advantages to modelling mystical experience as a state of maximal uncertainty. For example, we can see how the debate between perennialists and contextualists about mystical experience reflects the debate between objective and subjective Bayesians about maximal uncertainty. Objective Bayesians believe that for any state of uncertainty, there is *one* probability function that correctly represents it and that maximal uncertainty is represented by a *uniform* distribution. This principle is also known as the Uniqueness Thesis (see Kopec and Titelbaum 2016). In contrast, subjective Bayesians believe that a given state of uncertainty can be equally well represented by different probability functions for different agents, with the matter being partly settled by subjective choice.

We can also see how the problems we've been discussing arise in a new form when we think about the learning experience that is required to transform one's

---

[23] Indeed, there is evidence that this 'partition priming' happens in real-life situations (Fox and Clemen 2005).

current state of uncertainty into a state of maximal uncertainty. For example, I'm uncertain of many things, but I also know some things, and there are also some things that I think I know but really don't. To enter a state of maximal uncertainty, I would have to have an experience that causes me to unlearn everything I know and everything I think I know. Let's call the totality of what I have to unlearn P. The same is true for you, except that what you have to unlearn is different from what I have to unlearn—so let's call that Q. Now suppose I have experienced a state of maximal uncertainty, and you haven't, but you'd like to. It would be foolish of me to tell you that all you have to do is unlearn P (or worse: to learn that P is false). Suppose I did tell you this, and you believed me. I would thereby have misled you: you'd spend a lot of time trying to unlearn P when what you need to do is unlearn Q.

We see, then, that an important driving force behind ineffability is *humility*. It is a recognition that in attempting to describe mystical experiences, one will inevitably mislead others. And it's important to recognize that there's no way out of this situation. For example, let's suppose that I'm a little less foolish: I recognize that whereas I had to unlearn P, you need to unlearn Q, and I also recognize that there is a substantial overlap between P and Q—let's call this overlap R. I could then say that you need to unlearn R, plus some other knowledge specific to you. The problem with this is that I don't know where R begins or ends. Perhaps I can identify some fragments—for example, we both know the sky is blue. However, there are other substantial fragments that I can't be sure are in R. For instance, I don't know the nature of your self-conception. There will always be such fragments because I don't have perfect access to your mind. Indeed, I don't even have perfect access to my own mind, so I also don't know what P is. I'm bound to make some error in trying to guess what R is. Alternatively, I could try saying that you need to unlearn everything you know and think you know. However, you already know that—what else would the transformation to a state of maximal uncertainty involve? It seems, then, that the best I can do if I want to say something substantial is to name some of the things I unlearned—perhaps those that were most surprising—and take great pains to warn you that you may have to unlearn something rather different.

In thinking through the problems of communicating these transformative experiences, we see analogues of the perennialist and contextualist views of mystical experience. The "perennialist" gets something right: the state of maximal uncertainty is the same for everyone, even though it may be *represented* in different ways (for example, using probability functions). The "contextualist" also gets something right: the experience that leads to maximal uncertainty is specific to the individual. By applying the analogues of these views to maximal uncertainty, we can see how the two views both get something right. However, we can also see what they get wrong about maximal uncertainty. The "perennialist" makes the mistake of thinking they can give a unique and undistorted representation of maximal uncertainty, and the "contextualist" conflates properties of the individually specific *process* and representational plurality with those of the universal *outcome* (which, remember, may not be achievable).

The model can also help us appreciate how one may become better at sharing one's experiences involving maximal uncertainty. By learning how different people tend to react to different attempts at description, one can begin to anticipate what will be misleading about a given description for a given person. Some have argued that this is one of the morals of the story of the Buddha's silence in response to Vacchagotta (Chapter 9). The thought is that either answer (of 'yes' or 'no') to Vacchagotta's question of whether the self exists would mislead Vacchagotta—and so the Buddha chose to remain silent in response to his question. However, the Buddha had no problem with explaining this to Ananda—presumably, because Ananda's mind had been sufficiently prepared to receive the explanation. The other main interpretation, which we briefly saw in the previous chapter, is that any attempt to discursively engage with the mystical can all too easily land one in a 'thicket of views, a writhing of views, a contortion of views'. In my opinion, both interpretations are correct (or can be useful) and compatible with each other. For example, imagine someone who has experienced a state of maximal uncertainty and can perfectly read the minds of others. Because of this mind-reading ability, this person can describe to any given individual exactly what they need to unlearn in order to transform into a state of maximal uncertainty. Although the problem of language dependence would still be a problem for this person, the problem of communication would not. Of course, none of us are close to being perfect mind-readers, but we can take small steps in that direction by becoming more empathetic and learning more about how each other's minds work. With this point in mind, I think we can say that in this lesson about maximal uncertainty, there is—ineffably—a lesson about mystical experience.

There is one final point worth making about this model of mystical experience as a state of maximal uncertainty before we move on. This point concerns the relationship between maximal uncertainty and concepts. In the example I gave earlier of the box factory, we didn't quite have a state of maximal uncertainty. It was only a state of maximal uncertainty with respect to a specific issue (of the size of the next box). We still knew a lot of stuff: that there would be a next box, that there is a factory, that it produces boxes that satisfy certain constraints, and so on. We also knew of different ways to think about the boxes: we can think about them in terms of their side lengths, face areas, volumes, etc. And we knew about the relationships between these different ways of thinking about the boxes—for example, that face area is side length squared. So, we were quite far from considering a genuine case of maximal uncertainty. If we were to somehow strip out all of this knowledge from the example, we wouldn't even be able to conceptualize the space of possibilities, let alone divide them up into events or assign probabilities. Thus, we see another similarity between maximal uncertainty and mystical experience and begin to see how some of the strange descriptions of mystical experience can make sense, for example:

> Black does not cease to be black, nor white white. But black is white and white is black. The opposites coincide without ceasing to be what they are in themselves.
>
> Otto 1932, p. 45

In our example: even though we wouldn't be able to divide the world up into boxes of various side lengths in a state of maximal uncertainty, there would still *be* boxes with side lengths. If we were to temporarily enter such a state of genuine maximal uncertainty and then return to a normal state, in which we can conceptualize the box factory example, our attempts to describe what it was like to experience maximal uncertainty would sound a lot like Otto's description of opposites coinciding without ceasing to be what they are in themselves.[24]

Our model of mystical experience as maximal uncertainty has now served its purpose. We have begun to see more clearly what ineffability amounts to and why descriptions of mystical experience tend to have their seemingly nonsensical and paradoxical nature. Now that we are done with the model, it is time for us to let it go. This is *absolutely crucial*, because if we fail to let it go, we would be discarding the very lessons that the model has helped us learn.[25] The *Alagaddupama Sutta* attributes this manoeuvre of letting go (of a useful way of thinking) to the Buddha:

> Bhikkhus, I shall show you how the Dhamma [teaching] is similar to a raft, being for the purpose of crossing over, not for the purpose of grasping. [...]
>
> Bhikkhus, when you know the Dhamma to be similar to a raft, you should abandon even the teachings, how much more so things contrary to the teachings.[26]

We also see the same idea in Verse 18 of the *Amritabindu Upanishad*:

> Having studied books, the wise man, solely devoted to knowledge and wisdom, should give up the books entirely, like the man who, seeking for rice, gives up the husk.[27]

---

[24] Rayo 2011 has also noticed the problem of representing the extreme uncertainty that arises from ineffability and argues for a "localist" way of modelling ineffability with probability functions that is congenial to the approach proposed here. This stripping away of all knowledge, including conceptual knowledge, is also part of the Buddhist realization of emptiness (*śūnyatā*).

[25] In the same way as in Buddhism, one must not only realize emptiness, but also the emptiness of emptiness.

[26] Nanamoli and Bodhi 1995, p. 135.   [27] Sastri 1921, p. 74.

And it is arguably the same idea with which Wittgenstein concluded the *Tractatus Logico-Philosophicus*:

> My propositions are elucidatory in this way: he who understands me finally recognizes them as senseless, when he has climbed out through them, on them, over them. (He must so to speak throw away the ladder, after he has climbed up on it.)
> He must surmount these propositions; then he sees the world rightly.
> Whereof one cannot speak, thereof one must remain silent.
>
> Wittgenstein 1921, 6.54[28]

Wittgenstein made his point using propositions (and logic and images) because these were the primary forms of representation in his time. We now have probability theory (and information theory built upon it). Since these are now the dominant forms of representation in many fields of inquiry (including psychedelics research), I've used a model built with these particular tools to make the same point. However, contained in that point is the point that we must let go of the model, even though it is has been elucidatory of mystical experience.

Because we've spent a great deal of time considering the model, we should take a moment to see why it would be a mistake to cling to it. In this regard, it is important to point out that mystical experiences are often construed as anything *but* involving maximal uncertainty. For instance, *satori* is often described as a comprehension, an understanding, and an insight into one's true nature (and ultimate reality). This hardly sounds like a state of maximal uncertainty. Similarly, consider James' general description of mystical states:

> They are states of insight into depths of truth unplumbed by the discursive intellect. They are illuminations, full of significance and importance, all inarticulate though they may remain; and as a rule they carry with them a curious sense of authority for after-time.
>
> James 1902, p. 416

Again, such a construal of mystical experience seems quite distant from the experience being a state of maximal uncertainty. This is one important reason why we need to let go of the model.

One word of caution: in letting go of the model, we avoid making one mistake, but we should also make sure we avoid making the opposite mistake. We need to let the model go, but we don't need to reject it. In this regard, it helps to observe

---

[28] Ogden 1999, p. 108. It should be noted that the interpretation of the *Tractatus* is subject to much debate. For useful discussions about Wittgenstein's alleged mysticism behind the *Tractatus*, see McGuinness 1966, Morris and Dodd 2007, Lugg 2014, and Engelmann 2018.

that these different construals of mystical experience—being a state of maximal uncertainty and involving deep, authoritative insight—are not necessarily at odds with each other. For example, it may be that a state of maximal uncertainty *allows* for deep insight. In other words, it may be that in order to have deep insight, you have to let yourself not know. This is the Zen idea of *shoshin*, or beginner's mind:

> The practice of Zen mind is beginner's mind. The innocence of the first inquiry—what am I?–is needed throughout Zen practice. The mind of the beginner is empty, free of the habits of the expert, ready to accept, to doubt, and open to all possibilities. It is the kind of mind which can see things as they are, which step by step and in a flash can realize the original nature of everything.
>
> Suzuki 1970, p. xiv

And we saw earlier with Boshan's notion of Great Doubt that 'if you doubt fully you will awaken fully' and from Verse 18 of the *Amritabindu Upanishad* that letting go of lower knowledge (based on words) is necessary for the attainment of higher knowledge (that is beyond words). We also saw this same idea in Meister Eckhart's sermon quoted above: 'for you to know God in God's way, your knowing must become a pure unknowing'. We also see the same idea described by Bertrand Russell:

> All who are capable of absorption in an inward passion must have experienced at times the strange feeling of unreality in common objects, the loss of contact with daily things, in which the solidity of the outer world is lost, and the soul seems, in utter loneliness, to bring forth, out of its own depths, the mad dance of fantastic phantoms which have hitherto appeared as independently real and living. This is the negative side of the mystic's initiation: the doubt concerning common knowledge, preparing the way for the reception of what seems a higher wisdom. Many men to whom this negative experience is familiar do not pass beyond it, but for the mystic it is merely the gateway to an ampler world.
>
> The mystic insight begins with the sense of a mystery unveiled, of a hidden wisdom now suddenly become certain beyond the possibility of a doubt. The sense of certainty and revelation comes earlier than any definite belief. The definite beliefs at which mystics arrive are the result of reflection upon the inarticulate experience gained in the moment of insight. [...]
>
> Russell 1910b, pp. 35–6

So, while the model of mystical experience as maximal uncertainty can help us appreciate the ineffability of mystical experience and thus mystical experience itself, we need to be careful to let the model go, and we also need to be careful not to reject it.

There are three concluding remarks about ineffability that will be helpful before we move on to the question of whether mystical experiences are psychedelic (in the next section).

The first is that the humility behind the ineffability of mystical experience is a natural continuation of the fundamental idea of person-centred psychotherapy. This fundamental idea is that individuals have the capacity to self-heal, and so, in many cases (but not all), the job of the therapist is primarily to facilitate this process—for example, by creating a safe and supportive environment for the individual and making sure that their basic needs are satisfied. There is, thus, a kind of humility at the core of person-centred psychotherapy: it is a recognition that the individual is often in a better position than the therapist to sort themselves out. This is the same humility that lies behind the ineffability of mystical experience. The spectrum of well-being continues beyond the treatment of pathological conditions, towards flourishing, individuation, self-transcendence, etc. Just as the individual has the innate capacity to self-heal, the individual also has the innate capacity to self-transcend. And just as the therapist should avoid interfering with the process of self-healing as much as possible, the mystic should avoid interfering with the process of self-transcendence as much as possible.[29] The recognition that it is all too easy to mislead the individual applies no matter where the individual is on the spectrum of well-being.

The second remark is that by recognizing the humility that lies behind ineffability, we can see how the practice of meditation has the sorts of effects that would lead one towards a mystical experience. For example, a common effect during the initial stages of a meditative practice is that one begins to see how the mind reacts to various situations with a speed that is so fast that it renders the reactions, and the driving forces behind them, invisible. We all have these reactions, but we tend to notice them only in extreme situations, such as when they have become particularly self-destructive or when there is an outside intervention—for example, when a close friend points one of them out to you. The practice of meditation helps slow down these patterns and create some space between them. This then allows one to take different steps and change one's patterns of thought. This process thereby helps weaken our strong disposition for thinking in particular ways. For example, it helps reveal what it is that we want to hear and why we want to hear it. Weakening this disposition makes it easier to hear the message behind the words of the mystic (to look through the Magic Eye painting).

Similarly, we can see how the consumption of psychedelics will tend to lead to the same outcome. The consumption of psychedelics appears to have similar effects to meditation in this respect—that is, they tend to disrupt one's usual patterns of

---

[29] This is why I remained neutral as to what self-transcendence consists of and what mystical-type experiences reveal about the self. To make a claim about such things would be to make the mistake that I'm arguing we should avoid making.

thought and make new ones available. The main difference, of course, is that the effects of psychedelics tend to be more dramatic, rapid, noisy, and less controllable than those of meditation.[30]

To be clear, this isn't to say that meditation and psychedelics reliably induce mystical experiences. The point is that some of the effects of these interventions are the sorts of effects that may make it easier for one to understand mystical experiences. We are highly prone to misinterpret attempts to describe or point to mystical experiences with no awareness that we are doing so.[31] By better understanding how deep our inability to listen goes, we can thereby increase our chance of understanding mystical experiences.

The third (and final) concluding remark is that just as we needed to let go of the model of mystical experience as a state of maximal uncertainty, we also need to let go of the idea that mystical experiences are ineffable. In other words, all of this talk about ineffability is itself misleading. Recall from the previous section that ineffability is self-undermining, and the point is to *see through* the words being used to describe mystical experiences. The self-undermining aspect of ineffability manifests here in several ways. For example, ineffability implies for many people the kind of "mystical nonsense" that naturalists are right to reject. More importantly, it implies that it is *impossible* to say *anything* about mystical experiences. However, as we saw with the ineffability of maximal uncertainty, this is not entirely correct—the ability to describe the experience rests, in part, on an understanding of the person to whom one is describing the experience. Thus, the upshot is that although we can't say what mystical experiences are, we can *sort of* say what they are—we just need to be mindful of the lessons learned by thinking carefully about ineffability. To put this overall point in another way, the self-undermining feature of ineffability can be construed as *the ineffability of ineffability* and so it can be seen to parallel the emptiness of emptiness.

With this mindset in place, we're now in a position to consider whether mystical experiences are psychedelic—that is, whether they are mind-revealing.

10.5 Are Mystical Experiences Psychedelic?

In his last publication, just before his passing in 1910, William James hypothesized that mystical experiences are psychedelic:

---

[30] It is important to remember, from Chapter 4, that such statements should be understood to have implicit qualifications. The precise effects of a psychedelic are highly dependent on a host of factors. For example, the experience of a highly mindful individual on a low dose of psilocybin while meditating at a meditation retreat will likely be radically different from the experience of an individual who is lacking mindfulness and has taken a strong dose of DMT at a music festival.

[31] The issue here is similar to the phenomenon of false memories that we saw in Chapter 6. For example, in the DRM paradigm, people not only falsely believe the lure word was presented, but they also report remembering *seeing* it. It's difficult to realize you're wrong when you think you can call to mind a memory of the perceptual experience that justifies your belief.

My hypothesis is that a movement of the threshold downwards will similarly bring a mass of subconscious memories, conceptions, emotional feelings, and perceptions of relation, etc., into view all at once; and that if this enlargement of the nimbus that surrounds the sensational present is vast enough, while no one of the items it contains attracts our attention singly, we shall have the conditions fulfilled for a kind of consciousness in all essential respects like that termed mystical.

James 1910, pp. 86–7

I think we can use this hypothesis to shed some light on our central question of whether mystical experiences are psychedelic. The point of this section is not to argue or assume that James' hypothesis is true, but rather to use it as another tool to help us consider whether mystical experiences are psychedelic.

It may be tempting to conclude, based on the ineffability of mystical experience, that we simply can't answer our central question. Although there is a sense in which this is true, we've also seen that there is a sense in which it isn't, since ineffability also precludes the statement that one can't say anything about mystical experience. For lack of a better way of putting it, we can get something of an answer by dancing around the question. One way to dance around the question is to think about where mystical experiences may be located in psychedelic space. In the previous chapter, we considered various reasons for thinking that mystical-type experiences are experiences that are *very* psychedelic—that is, they score very high on the dimensions of scope, novelty, clarity, and duration.[32] Perhaps, then, we can think of genuine mystical experiences as being maximally psychedelic. In other words, can we think of mystical experiences as perfect revelations of the entire mind?

In terms of James' hypothesis, we might think this question amounts to the following: is mystical experience a maximal enlargement of the nimbus that surrounds the sensational present? However, this is not quite the same question. Note that in James' hypothesis, there is an additional constraint: that no one of the items in the 'enlarged nimbus' *attracts our attention*. The reason for this is that if an item attracted attention, then the scope of awareness would collapse back to its non-mystical mode, and the experience would no longer be mystical:

[The experience's] form will be intuitive or perceptual, not conceptual, for the remembered or conceived objects in the enlarged field are supposed not to attract the attention singly, but only to give the sense of a tremendous *muchness* suddenly

---

[32] Recall that a mystical-type experience is just one that scores sufficiently high on the usual psychometric measures of mystical experience. A given mystical-type experience may or may not be a mystical experience.

revealed. If they attracted attention separately, we should have the ordinary steep-waved consciousness, and the mystical character would depart.

James 1910, p. 87

So we can see how there is an important difference between a mystical experience (as hypothesized by James) and other psychedelic experiences we have been considering, including mystical-type experiences. For example, during a psychedelic trip, one may attain a psycho-spiritual insight that attracts the bulk of one's attention. Indeed, this insight may capture so much attention that one may become completely absorbed in it. Such an experience would not be mystical, according to James' hypothesis. Importantly, this would be true even if the content of the experience may be described as having mystical elements—such as a belief that everything is one, etc. Therefore, attention plays an important role in James' hypothesis regarding mystical experience: attention must be uniformly, and therefore maximally, diffused across the items of the unconscious. If any item separately attracted attention to any degree, then the distribution would be non-uniform.

This fits well with our hypothesis from Chapter 5 that psychedelics and meditation reveal the mind via their effects on attention. Very briefly, the idea there was that both interventions alter the usual patterns of the mind's allocation of attentional resources. The practice of meditation does this in a gradual and controlled manner, and psychedelics do this in a more explosive and disruptive way. A *complete* removal of the mind's usual patterns of assigning attentional resources would constitute a necessary condition for an experience to be mystical (according to James' hypothesis). Thus, we can see how meditation and psychedelics could potentially give rise to a mystical experience (so construed).

On the one hand, it sounds like such an experience should count as being psychedelic, since a mass of unconscious material would be brought into awareness, and this effect involving attention is a natural extension of what we have considered earlier. On the other hand, if attention is maximally diffused across this mass of unconscious material, which is presumably large in size, we may wonder whether the material actually appears in awareness. Perhaps it does, but only to a minimal degree, and so maybe a mystical experience is one that is maximal in scope but minimal in clarity. That would mean that mystical experiences are psychedelic, but would it also entail that they are not maximally psychedelic? Not necessarily, since there may be in-principle tradeoffs between the dimensions. Given that the human brain is a finite system that is contained by physical laws, it is plausible that there are strict limitations on how much the dimensions may be increased simultaneously. And so, there may be a limit to how much scope and clarity an experience can have simultaneously. If so, then the structure of psychedelic space would be such that there are several maximal points (corresponding to several maximally psychedelic experiences) rather than a single one. However, it could also be objected that in such a state of maximally diffused attention, nothing receives enough attention to properly appear in awareness (and only gives a sense of the tremendous muchness revealed). If so, then awareness would be devoid of any content, and so the experience would not be psychedelic to any degree.

In considering these two options, we see that there is a conceptual tension. On the one hand, attention is distributed over everything, but on the other hand, everything receives hardly any attention. It's almost as though the entire unconscious is revealed while conscious experience remains completely empty. A natural thought to have at this point is that our regular concepts of awareness, attention, representation, and consciousness are simply not equipped to handle such an unusual situation. There's another paradox in probability theory, known as de Finetti's lottery, which provides us with a close analogue of this situation. The paradox goes as follows. Suppose you've been entered into a lottery that has a countably infinite number of tickets, with the tickets consecutively numbered 1, 2, 3, and so on. And suppose you've been told that the lottery is *fair*—that is, no ticket is more likely than any other to be drawn as the winning ticket. It seems, then, that you should assign equal probability to each ticket being the winning ticket. However, it turns out that there is no way of doing this. You could try assigning each ticket some positive probability, ϵ. However, that means the probability that *some* ticket wins is ϵ summed infinitely many times, which results in a probability greater than 1, thus violating the axioms of probability. Alternatively, you could try assigning each ticket a probability of 0. However, that means the probability that any ticket wins is 0 summed infinitely many times, which results in a probability of 0, and which therefore also violates the axioms of probability—since the probability that *a* ticket wins is 1. And so we have a paradox: there's no way to assign probability uniformly across each of the infinite possibilities. There's a large literature on this paradox and how to resolve it (e.g. Bartha 2004, Elliot 2020, Norton 2020), but the basic upshot is that our usual concepts of probability don't apply neatly to this kind of unusual scenario.

The thought, then, is that perhaps something similar is happening with mystical experience: that is, that there is no way to uniformly distribute what we normally think of as attention. One specific way to make this precise is to say that it is constitutive of attention that it is *selective*, and so if attention is distributed uniformly (across all of the mind), then it isn't selective of anything, and so it isn't attention anymore. This idea lines up quite neatly with the non-duality that mystical-type experiences are often said to involve (which is sometimes described in terms of ego-dissolution, unity, emptiness, pure awareness, etc.). Selective attention implies an attentional object—some object that receives more attention than something else—which in turn implies a distinction between subject and object. The breaking down of attention, or the transformation of it, is thus necessary, and perhaps sufficient, for an experience to be mystical. (However, as always: we should be wary of saying something about mystical experience.)

So, where does this leave us with our question of whether mystical experiences are psychedelic? In attempting to answer this question, it may be helpful to say that mystical experiences are so psychedelic that they transcend the category of psychedelic experience. This answer fits well with the ineffability of mystical experiences. Mystical experiences are psychedelic, but they are also not. In this regard, it helps to remind ourselves of some of the descriptions of mystical experience we saw earlier:

> Black does not cease to be black, nor white white. But black is white and white is black. The opposites coincide without ceasing to be what they are in themselves.
>
> Otto 1932, p. 45

And:

> The keynote of it is invariably a reconciliation. It is as if the opposites of the world, whose contradictoriness and conflict make all our difficulties and troubles, were melted into unity. Not only do they, as contrasted species, belong to one and the same genus, but one of the species, the nobler and better one, is itself the genus, and so soaks up and absorbs its opposite into itself.
>
> James 1902, p. 388

And:

> Whenever I spoke of the experience, I tried to be intellectually cautious and spiritually responsible. Whatever I offered with one hand, I took back with the other. I found myself incessantly repeating the following refrain: 'It was like this, but not really. It was sort of like that, but not in the way that you might initially think'. [...]
>
> Shrader 2008, p. 5

The first two descriptions are sometimes used to support perennialism, with its commitment to unity being the core of mystical experience (for example, Stace 1960), since the transcendence of categories is taken to follow from unity. However, unity is itself a category: a commitment that unity is the core of mystical experience entails a commitment to a duality, since it rejects any duality of mystical experience. There is a sense, then, in which ineffability (when properly understood) is more true to the unity of mystical experience than a commitment to unity itself is. This is frustrating if we insist on a definitive answer to our question of whether mystical experiences are psychedelic. However, if we can somehow let ourselves not know the answer to the question, we can thereby get an answer to it. In short, mystical experience may be sort of psychedelic, and even sort of *maximally* psychedelic, but perhaps not in the way we might initially think.

10.6 Conclusion

The central question of this chapter has been whether mystical experiences are psychedelic experiences—that is, whether they are mind-revealing experiences. To answer this question, we had to take seriously the problem of defining what a mystical experience is. And to do that, we found that we had to grapple with the ineffability of mystical experience. I argued that because of this ineffability, we should not try to analyse descriptions of purported mystical experiences. This would be a fundamental methodological mistake—one that has been made by perennialists and contextualists (Stace 1960, Katz 1978). The only way to avoid this mistake is to embrace a *no-theory* theory of mystical experience. That is, the best way we can understand mystical experience is to forego having a theory of it. This is not a new idea—mystics have been advising as such for millennia—however, it seems to have been forgotten, or at least under-appreciated in contemporary academic discussions.

I've also argued that one way we can better understand mystical experience is to develop a better appreciation of its ineffability. It is easy to misunderstand ineffability as simply being the inability to describe the experience and as a kind of failing of the individual in question: if they were more intelligent or more articulate, they would figure out a way to describe the experience. To help dispel that misunderstanding, we explored how ineffability arises in connection with states of maximal uncertainty, and we saw how this has nothing to do with intelligence or articulacy. Ineffability arises from such experiences in two ways: (i) the content of the transformative experience is highly specific to the individual undergoing it, and (ii) there is no language-independent way of taking a substantial epistemic attitude towards such an experience. As a result of (i), we can see how ineffability is a form of *humility*—and not some sort of linguistic failing. Part of the ineffability of maximal uncertainty is a recognition, a noetic insight, that the transformation required is specific to you and that it will be specific in a different way for someone else, and so you are not in a position to tell them what the experience is. And as a result of (ii), we can see how language itself can lack resources that we may have expected it to have. We saw how this manifests specifically in the Bayesian framework, but the point holds for any framework of uncertainty. The point, then, is that we can get a better understanding of the ineffability of mystical experience by comparing it to the ineffability of maximal uncertainty. This comparison helps us see how the ineffability of mystical experience is much more substantial than simply being at a loss for words.

Although it is helpful to use maximal uncertainty as a model for mystical experience in this way, we need to recognize that in doing so, we run afoul of ineffability. That is, we're bound to say something about mystical experiences that is highly misleading. For this reason, it is essential to note that mystical experiences are often characterized as involving a high degree of *certainty*. For instance, they are often said to seem "realer than real" and involve some form of profound insight into the ultimate nature of self and reality. That hardly sounds like a state of maximal uncertainty. And so, although the model can help us develop an appreciation for ineffability, we should be aware that holding on to it is just as mistaken as holding on to a particular theory or description of mystical experience.

With this understanding of mystical experience thus established, we were then able to turn to the question of whether mystical experiences are psychedelic. Not surprisingly, the answer to this question is indefinite. By pursuing James' hypothesis about mystical experiences (Section 10.5), I hoped to show that the answer is that mystical experiences are psychedelic, and also that they are not. That may seem a bit anti-climactic, but that is only because we began this adventure motivated by the question of whether mystical experiences are psychedelic. However, if we look at the result from the perspective of trying to understand these experiences—the psychedelic and the mystical—then the outcome is more substantial. We see how revealing all of the mind—or as much of it as possible—may involve, or lead to, the revelation of something else.[33]

From a strictly analytic perspective, this chapter has been mostly pointless. Whereas previous chapters offered conceptual explications, hypotheses, arguments, and conclusions, this chapter doesn't offer any of that. This is because if I've done my job correctly, I've managed to say nothing of the sort about mystical experiences—except the general point that we ought to take their ineffability seriously. However, the fundamental idea here is that mystical experience is something that we can understand without being committed to such things. It's a kind of understanding that is beyond the realm of analytic philosophy (and science) but also one that is not in conflict with it. Indeed, one goal of this chapter has been to show how analytic philosophy can bring value to discussions about mystical experience. Nevertheless, it is important to recognize that mystical experience is a kind of singularity for analytic philosophy. The usual rules of the game, at least as they are traditionally conceived, break down at the point of mystical experience. It can therefore be tempting to dismiss mystical experiences as nonsense, but there is no good reason for doing this. There's no reason why analytic philosophers cannot engage with mystical experiences while also preserving everything that is good about their tradition.

---

[33] For James, this was the 'tremendous *muchness*', but we may allow for other possibilities, such as pure awareness, or self-nature, etc., as well as allowing for the case that these are not distinct possibilities.

To this point, at the end of his *Modes of Thought* lectures, Alfred North Whitehead wrote:

> If you like to phrase it so, philosophy is mystical. For mysticism is direct insight into depths as yet unspoken. But the purpose of philosophy is to rationalize mysticism: not by explaining it away, but by the introduction of novel verbal characterizations, rationally coördinated.
>
> Whitehead 1938, p. 174

This is what I've tried to do in this chapter, except I would say that Whitehead didn't *quite* get mysticism right. Mysticism is not just insight into depths *as yet* unspoken, it is also insight into depths that *cannot* or *should not* be spoken. As Pseudo-Dionysius the Areopagite put it:

> For the higher we soar in contemplation the more limited become our expressions of that which is purely intelligible; even as now, when plunging into the Darkness that is above the intellect, we pass not merely into brevity of speech, but even into absolute silence of thoughts and of words. Thus, in the former discourse, our contemplations descended from the highest to the lowest, embracing an ever-widening number of conceptions, which increased at each stage of the descent; but in the present discourse we mount upwards from below to that which is the highest, and, according to the degree of transcendence, so our speech is restrained until, the entire ascent being accomplished, we become wholly voiceless, inasmuch as we are absorbed in it that is totally ineffable.
>
> Pseudo-Dionysius the Areopagite 5–6c. CE, *The Mystical Theology*, ch. 3[34]

Nevertheless, philosophy is still mystical in the sense that Whitehead describes, since we can introduce new verbal characterizations that are rationally coordinated around the mystical. We see a similar idea expressed by Bertrand Russell:

> [T]he greatest men who have been philosophers have felt the need both of science and of mysticism: the attempt to harmonise the two was what made their life, and what always must, for all its arduous uncertainty, make philosophy, to some minds, a greater thing than either science or religion.
>
> Russell 1910b, p. 19

Such a harmonization is one of the central goals of this book: by using the philosophical explication of psychedelic experience in terms of psychedelic space, we can unite a wide range of disparate empirically observable phenomena (involving

---

[34] Quoted in Nieli 1987.

meditation and psychedelics) with mystical experience in a way that respects the scruples of both science and mysticism.

One way of summarizing the main point of this chapter is that mystical experiences are deeply, intrinsically, paradoxically, transformatively, and noetically ineffable. They are deeply ineffable because their ineffability is deeper than that of regular experience. They are intrinsically ineffable since their ineffability is their defining feature. They are paradoxically ineffable because ineffability is itself a description. They are transformatively ineffable because truly understanding their ineffability requires a transformation of one's mind. And, finally, they are noetically ineffable, because there is a form of knowledge that comes along with that transformation—the wisdom that arises from allowing one's self to not know.

To conclude this chapter, there is one final point that we should consider. It is actually the most important point, and it gives us another way of understanding mystical experiences. The point is that *naming* mystical experiences has many of the same problems that descriptions and theories of the experiences suffer from. For example, consider the name we have been using: 'mystical experience'. This name has at least two substantial problems with it. First, it implies that what we're talking about is a kind of *experience*, but we could just as well think of it as a sort of *knowledge*, or a form of *understanding*, or a kind of *apprehension*, or a way of *being* (there is also a sense in which it is the *world* that is mystical). For some reason, the concept of experience has become the default one to use, and we should be wary of that. For example, the concept of experience involves a duality between the experiencer and the experienced. Second, the term 'mystical' raises associations that make it difficult for many people to think clearly about this topic. Indeed, it is probably fair to say that the typical associations around the term 'mystical' are worse in this respect than those surrounding the term 'psychedelic'. So, the name 'mystical experience' is probably doing more harm than good. However, it is not as though some other name will do better. The point is that any name will be just as problematic.

In this regard, it helps to be mindful that mystics have also warned us about the use of names—in addition to descriptions. For example, we can see this point in the first chapter of the *Dao De Ching*:

> Words that describe Tao, do not capture the real Tao;
> Names that represent Tao, do not express the eternal Tao.
> The nameless is the source of heaven and earth;
> The named is the source of all particular things.
> Through desirelessness, the unnamed is experienced as oneness;
> Through desire, the named is experienced as manifested things.
> The nameless and the named are alike because they originate from the
>   same source;
> They are diverse because they are described differently;

Their ineffable source is a deep cosmic mystery;
One who comprehends this profound connection between the nameless
and the named attains total wisdom.[35]

To be clear, the warning here is not that we shouldn't use names. Rather, we should be mindful of what is happening when we use a name.

How can this point about names give us another way of understanding mystical experience? One way to see how is to consider what happens if we try to give it a name that may seem innocuous and completely free of any preconceptions. So, for example, let's call it 'X'. Although this name still has problems—for example, it implies there is one thing or one kind of thing that we can call 'X' (recall the discussion in Section 10.2)—it shines a different light on the questions we've been considering in this chapter. For example, using this new name, the central question of this chapter is whether X is psychedelic. That seems like a strange question to ask, and appreciating its strangeness can help us understand X: any question about it is based on something of a *non sequitur*—how did we find ourselves asking something about X? Nevertheless, let's put this aside and push on: to answer our central question of whether X is psychedelic, we need to know what X is. But how can we do that? Perhaps we have in mind some idea of X to which we can point. For example, we might try to say that X tends to happen when people take psychedelics and/or meditate for long periods of time. But how do we know this is true of X? And how would we reply to someone who disagreed? Indeed, how do we even get the idea that there is something we might try to call 'X' and potentially disagree with other people about? If you have questions similar to any of these, ask yourself: why are you asking them? Perhaps the answer is because you want to have X. But then what is it that you want? How do you know it is real? And how do you know you want it? Thus, although the name 'X' is still problematic, it has tremendous value: it highlights the deep uncertainty that must be grappled with.

To be clear, the point is not to raise scepticism about X—although these are the sorts of questions that a good sceptic about X will ask. The point is that these questions help reveal a path towards X: a path that is made out of the kind of doubt that is wonder. They reveal the cloud of uncertainty that the individual must pass through, and which only the individual can pass through, in order to understand X.

---

[35] Malhotra 2006, p. 4.

11
Psychedelic Philosophy

Wisdom springs from meditation; without meditation wisdom wanes. Having known these two paths of progress and decline, let a man so conduct himself that his wisdom may increase.

Dhammapada, Maggavagga 282[1]

11.1 Introduction

So far, the main goal of this book has been to use the tools of philosophy to help us understand the phenomenon of psychedelic experience. In this penultimate chapter, we're going to flip things around: we will see how psychedelic experiences can help us do philosophy. Indeed, I'll make the case that there is a distinctive way of doing philosophy, which I call *psychedelic philosophy*, that involves the regular engagement with psychedelic experiences.

I use the term 'philosophy' here broadly and in its original sense as the love of wisdom. I also use the term 'wisdom' rather inclusively, with the broad constraint that wisdom concerns how to live well (similar to Kekes 1983 and Nozick 1989). This may involve anything from being able to make good decisions in daily life, to having knowledge of important topics, such as metaphysics, mathematics, and science, to knowing how to take care of one's soul (if such a thing exists).[2] As such, the implications of this chapter are rather far-reaching and not limited to academic philosophy.

The main idea of this chapter is that there are valuable methods of doing philosophy—of pursuing wisdom—that involve a regular engagement with psychedelic experiences. I call these methods *psychedelic methods*. In the coming sections, I will argue that these methods can help us do better philosophy—and, thus, become wiser and live better lives. Despite their philosophical value,

---

[1] Buddharakkhita 1996.

[2] Some readers may be concerned that this understanding of philosophy renders many contemporary academic philosophers as not "real" philosophers, and instead implies that they are something else—technical specialists, perhaps. However, I don't think that thought is correct, for there is such a great variety of ways to live well and perhaps an even greater variety of points from which we all start. Nothing in the definition rules out, for example, that having a specialist expertise in modal logic counts as having wisdom.

psychedelic methods seem to be largely missing from contemporary Western philosophy. Perhaps some philosophers already use them, but do so in secret because of the controversial reputation from which psychedelics and meditation (and related practices) have suffered (especially since the late 1960s). Some philosophers have confessed as much in personal communication, but they seem to be the exception rather than the norm. Therefore, one of the goals of this chapter is to shine some light on these methods and help remove some of their stigma.

Before we get going, it is important to sort out some potential confusions. As throughout this book, I use the term 'psychedelic experience' to refer to a *mind-revealing experience*. Such an experience can be brought about via the consumption of certain substances, but it can also be brought about via other means, such as the practice of meditation. Indeed, consuming a so-called psychedelic substance may not always be the best way to have a psychedelic experience. It will depend on a host of other factors, such as the nature of the substance, the psychological condition of the individual in question, their intentions, their environment, their relationships and responsibilities, the legal jurisdiction under which they resign, and so on. Therefore, it is important to be clear at the outset that psychedelic philosophy is not about consuming certain substances for the sake of doing philosophy. The primary focus instead is on how engaging with psychedelic *experiences* can help us do philosophy.

A related issue that will be helpful to clear up right away is that this chapter is not about the hypothesis that the origins of philosophy stem from the use of psychedelic substances in ancient times. It has been argued that various philosophical traditions were borne out of the ritualistic use of psychedelics. For example, Vedic philosophy may have been grounded in the consumption of *soma*, possibly a psychedelic mushroom tea or an ayahuasca-like brew (Clark 2017, Muraresku 2020). Closer to home, Western philosophy appears to have its roots in the consumption of *kykeon*, likely either a drink made out of *ergot* or another ayahuasca analogue (Hillman 2008, Clark 2017, Muraresku 2020). The thesis that philosophers, such as Socrates, Plato, and Aristotle, participated in the Eleusinian Mysteries also seems compelling (especially given the references to the mystery rites in Plato's dialogues). Relatedly, there is some evidence that the priestess Pythia, the oracle of Delphi, entered psychedelic trances by inhaling ethylene (Boer et al. 2001, Spiller et al. 2002). Although these historical claims may be probable, my case for the merits of psychedelic philosophy does not rest upon them. With that said, I will occasionally refer to these historical points, but only to acknowledge that psychedelic philosophy is almost certainly not a new idea—it has likely been around in some form or other for thousands of years.

The plan for this chapter is as follows. In Section 11.2, I will discuss in more detail what wisdom is and why it is important to pursue. This will provide some useful connections to other important notions we have already come across—such as mindfulness and well-being. In Section 11.3, I will make the case for psychedelic philosophy. This will involve drawing a distinction between its methods for pursuing wisdom and those of analytic philosophy and natural philosophy (i.e. science). In Section 11.4, I will propose that the best way of doing philosophy is one that integrates the methods of all three approaches (as well as others, such as those from the discipline of phenomenology). In Section 11.5, I will briefly consider whether psychedelic philosophy has distinctive objects as its own philosophical pursuits. In Section 11.6, I will discuss the empirical evidence that the methods of psychedelic philosophy can help us become wiser, drawing upon the operationalizations of wisdom established in Section 11.2. I'll then conclude in Section 11.7.

11.2 Philosophy as the Pursuit of Wisdom

The term 'philosophy' derives from the words *philo* and *sophia*, and is often translated as the love, or pursuit, of wisdom. Generally speaking, wisdom concerns knowing how to live a good life. This is often thought to include such things as avoiding poor health, living an ethical life, making good decisions, having a love for learning, and progressing towards the higher end of the spectrum of well-being (through self-actualization, individuation, transcendence, care for the soul, etc.).

Over the years, philosophers have attempted to define more precisely what being wise involves. Here, we'll look at three major historical definitions, as they will be most relevant for our discussion later on.[3]

The first definition is often known as *theoretical* wisdom, which is another common translation for *sophia*.[4] This form of wisdom consists in knowing truths that are universal, timeless, abstract, or in some sense higher than other truths. There is some debate about which sorts of truths fall into this classification, but common examples include the truths of mathematics, logic, science, ethics, metaphysics, political theory, poetry, music, etc. However, theoretical wisdom is also sometimes thought to only concern truths that are *a priori* in nature—roughly speaking, those that can be known independently of experience. This classification would rule out knowledge of scientific truths, for example, as theoretical wisdom. However, we needn't get caught up in such debates here. One way of resolving this issue is to follow Plato and understand *sophia* as involving beautiful knowledge that brings one closer to contemplation of Beauty itself. This, then, can permit a degree of subjectivity regarding *sophia*. For some people, poetry is the best place to start their ascent; for others, it will be mathematics, the laws of physics, the

---

[3] For reasons of space, I'll limit the discussion to these three definitions. For more recent work on this topic in philosophy, see Ryan 2020 for an overview, and within psychology in the form of the Berlin Wisdom Paradigm, see Baltes 2004 and Banicki 2009 for an overview.

[4] Some care is needed in making such translations. Part of the reason for this is that there is rarely any clear separation between our concepts and our theories of our concepts, and the meaning of *sophia* evolved over time, from Pythagoras, through Heraclitus and Plato's dialogues, to Aristotle's *Metaphysics* and *Nicomachean Ethics*, and beyond (see Moore 2019 for a discussion of the historical evolution of the meaning of these terms).

workings of the biological world, etc. For our purposes, it suffices to note that there is a form of wisdom known as *sophia* or theoretical wisdom, and that this involves having knowledge of important truths—many of which may be known *a priori*.

The second historical conception of wisdom is the one that Plato depicts Socrates articulating in *Apologia*. This form of wisdom consists in being aware of the limits of one's knowledge—not thinking one knows something when one does not. To put it another way, wisdom involves being aware of one's actual uncertainty. As is well known, Plato's dialogues often involve a familiar outcome: because of Socrates' relentless questioning (his method of *elenchos*), his interlocutors come to realize that they lack knowledge about some important matter (for example, what it means to be courageous).[5] This realization constitutes an experience of *aporia*— a state of profound doubt and an awareness of one's true uncertainty. By having such an experience, one becomes a little wiser in this sense. Moreover, if one is a philosopher, then one will emerge from this experience with an even stronger passion (*eros*) for *sophia*. There's a sense, then, in which *aporia* is a purifying experience that is not unlike the kind of experience one may have with psychedelics. The process of transformation can be deeply unpleasant, but the result is a freedom from one's previous delusions that allows one to better pursue wisdom.

Although this conception of wisdom is often attributed to Socrates, we can see it—or close analogues of it—in other schools of thought. We see it in Zen with beginner's mind (*shoshin*) and Boshan's notion of Great Doubt, which we encountered in the previous chapter: 'if you doubt fully, you will waken fully'. Indeed, there is a moment in the *Apologia* where Socrates likens his philosophical activity (of inducing *aporia* with *elenchos*) to that of waking up his fellow Athenians and helping them take better care of their souls. The idea is, arguably, also present in the *Analects of Confucius* (Book II), the *Dao De Ching* (Chapter 71), the Upanishads, and numerous texts of Christian mysticism. It is plausible that many mystics and philosophers throughout history have independently (or somewhat independently) perceived this form of wisdom. Certainly, a common theme across many traditions is that we suffer from not only our ignorance but our ignorance of our ignorance. The latter prevents us from even trying to address our ignorance and keeps us trapped in a prison that we can't see. Thus, there is wisdom in understanding that this is our condition and therefore allowing one's self to be uncertain—to sit in an extended state of profound doubt and wonder. For convenience, I will refer to this as the wisdom of *aporia*, or *aporetic wisdom*.

In more modern times, this form of wisdom—or, rather, the lack of it—has come to be understood in terms of *overconfidence* (Dunning 2011). There are different ways to measure overconfidence, but a common one is in terms of the *calibration* of one's subjective probabilities (or levels of confidence). The basic idea is that if you

---

[5] Or, on another way to read the dialogues, the interlocutor doesn't necessarily come to this realization, but *the reader* does.

are aware of your true state of uncertainty, then your probabilities will tend to be well calibrated: they won't be too high, which would count as overconfidence, and they won't be too low either, which would count as underconfidence. Although there are these two ways to fail at being calibrated, it is widely recognized that people tend to err on the side of overconfidence. For example:

> Overconfidence is found in most tasks; that is, people tend to overestimate how much they know.
>
> Lichtenstein et al. 1982, p. iv

And we see this observation echoed throughout history:

> One of the painful things about our time is that those who feel certainty are stupid, and those with any imagination and understanding are filled with doubt and indecision.
>
> Russell 1951, pp. 4–5

And:

> [. . .] the over-weening conceit which the greater part of men have of their own abilities, is an ancient evil remarked by the philosophers and moralists of all ages.
>
> Smith 1776, p. 109

It seems that our inability to be wise in this respect is robust and timeless. Indeed, the psychologist Daniel Kahneman has even said that overconfidence is the most damaging of all biases and the one he would most like to eliminate if he had a magic wand (Shariatmadari 2015). To make matters worse, there is some evidence that overconfidence can spread through populations like a contagious disease (Cheng et al. 2020). It is an understatement, then, to say that we would all benefit from some new methods (or the revival of some ancient ones) for tackling this pervasive, deeply ingrained, and destructive psychological condition.

The third and final conception of wisdom is the notion of *phronēsis*, which is often translated as 'practical wisdom'. This form of wisdom is often associated with Aristotle's discussion of the concept in his *Nicomachean Ethics* (NE) but the idea was clearly present before his time, and Plato's dialogues contain important discussions of the concept (Stern 1997). Nevertheless, it is probably fair to say that Aristotle was the first to attempt to articulate a precise analysis of *phronēsis* and to draw a clear distinction between it and *sophia*. The concept of *phronēsis* is difficult to define explicitly, and Aristotle's analysis is subject to much debate. It is also not entirely clear if Aristotle had only one concept of *phronēsis* or if he was perhaps working with two (Curnow 2011). Nevertheless, *phronēsis* is commonly thought to involve the following features:

- Making good decisions and performing good actions (NE 1140a25–30).[6]
- Knowing what is good for one's self, for others, for collectives, and for any self in the abstract (NE 1140b, 1141b–1142a).
- Being able to perceive the details of any situation that are relevant for good decision-making (NE 1141b4–16).
- Having learned lessons from a diverse set of life experiences (NE 1142a12–16, 1143b).
- Being able to deliberate well about what to do in a given situation (NE 1140a25).

It is also often thought that *phronēsis*, in an important sense, can't be taught, but it can nonetheless be learned and developed over time.

Although it is difficult to say exactly what *phronēsis* amounts to in practical terms, it seems to have some clear similarities with mindfulness. Indeed, McEvilley 2002 has argued that a better translation of *phronēsis* is *mindfulness*, understood as the Buddhist concept of *sati* (see Chapters 6 and 9). Weiss 2017 also argues for understanding *phronēsis* in terms of mindfulness. If correct, this would partly explain why it is difficult to define *phronēsis* since, as we have seen, it is also difficult to say precisely what mindfulness is (see Chapters 6 and 9). Nevertheless, even if the two concepts are not the same, it is clear that there are some strong similarities between them. We can see this by examining the features of *phronēsis* listed above: many of them are also features of mindfulness. For example, being able to apprehend the relevant details of a given situation is part of what it means to have lucid awareness of the present moment. The same goes for knowing what outcomes are good for one's self. As another example, being able to deliberate well involves having a good working memory, which is part of the memory aspect of *sati* (Dreyfus 2011). So it seems there is a good case to be made that *phronēsis* and *sati* are very similar, if not identical.

However, although there are these points of similarity, there is at least one important difference: *phronēsis* involves being experienced in life, whereas that doesn't seem to be required of mindfulness. As Aristotle points out, young people will tend to lack *phronēsis* because they lack life experience (NE 1142a12–16). In contrast, it doesn't seem that lacking life experience would prevent a young person from being mindful. This difference, however, is immaterial: we can say that *phronēsis* ≈ mindfulness + life experience, to capture the core idea that there is a deep similarity between *phronēsis* and mindfulness. There is also reason to suspect that there may be an interesting interaction between mindfulness and life experience. Several researchers have thought that increases in mindfulness should result in increases in the core personality trait of openness (to experience), which should, in turn, result in one becoming more experienced (in the sense relevant for *phronēsis*) as one progresses through life (see Barner and Barner 2011

---

[6] All references to the NE are based on Crisp 2000.

for a review). However, the empirical evidence for this hypothesis is currently unclear.[7] Nevertheless, we can recognize that there is a strong similarity between the *phronēsis* and mindfulness of an individual and that this similarity will become stronger as one moves through life (all else being equal). This close relationship between *phronēsis* and mindfulness will be important later on, when we consider how psychedelic experience can be used to enhance the former.[8]

Although the above discussion is only a brief overview of these three important conceptions of wisdom, we have enough detail for our purposes. It is worth noting, though, that all three conceptions of wisdom are not entirely distinct. For example, Aristotle commented that Socrates was correct in saying that all moral excellences implied practical wisdom (NE 1144b), and that *phronēsis* involves, or requires guidance from, *sophia* (NE 1141b4–16).[9] And, writing before Socrates and Aristotle, Heraclitus interwove aspects of these different forms of wisdom:

> Many fail to grasp what they have seen,
> and cannot judge what they have learned,
> although they tell themselves they know.
>
> Heraclitus ca. 475 BCE[10]

Whether *aporia* and *phronēsis* are the same (or coextensive) is an interesting question that I won't pursue here. Nonetheless, it's worth noting that together they highlight a deep tension that must be overcome in order to live well. As Bertrand Russell put it:

> [. . .] it is not enough to recognize that all our knowledge is, in a greater or less degree, uncertain and vague; it is necessary, at the same time, to learn to act upon the best hypothesis without dogmatically believing it.
>
> Russell 1950, p. 43

---

[7] There is evidence that mindfulness positively correlates with openness (Brown and Ryan 2003, Baer et al. 2004, Thompson and Waltz 2007, Giluk 2009, Haliwa et al. 2020). However, the strongest association between mindfulness and the core personality traits appears to be a negative correlation with neuroticism, followed by positive correlations for conscientiousness, agreeableness, openness, and extraversion (Haliwa et al. 2020), with conscientiousness potentially being the strongest positive association (Giluk 2009). There is also evidence that experience with meditative practices is positively correlated with openness to experience (Hurk et al. 2011, Pokorski and Suchorzynska 2018), but we can't tell from this correlation whether people with high openness tend to be attracted to meditation or whether meditation increases openness (or both). One small study on patients with multiple sclerosis found that 8 weeks of mindfulness-based stress reduction (MBSR) had no significant effect on openness (or on neuroticism, extraversion, and agreeableness) but a positive effect on conscientiousness (Crescentini et al. 2018), in line with the results of Giluk 2009. Using a between-subjects design, Chan and Wang 2019 found that 10 minutes of mindful meditation resulted in increased openness in comparison to mind-wandering and inert control groups.

[8] Another possibility worth mentioning is that *phronēsis* develops as one pursues the Noble Eightfold Path (see Chapter 9). If so, its relationship to mindfulness is even more difficult to state explicitly, but it would still be the case that mindfulness is necessary, and highly conducive, for *phronēsis*.

[9] See also Curnow 2011 for a discussion of this issue.   [10] Haxton 2001.

This highlights nicely how the aporetic and practical conceptions of wisdom are entangled and how they are both essential for wisdom in general. Similarly, a case could be made that there is an important relationship between *aporia* and *sophia*, especially if the latter, in its ultimate form, has similarities to other, ineffable forms of wisdom, such as *prajñā* (Coe 1983). Indeed, *aporia* can be seen as necessary for the ineffable wisdom that may be revealed in a mystical experience (Chapter 10)— for example, the letting go of *apara vidya* (lower, conceptual knowledge) for the sake of attaining *para vidya* (upper, non-conceptual knowledge).[11] Since this has already been covered in the previous two chapters, I'll focus here on the more tangible forms of wisdom, especially those easily recognizable to analytic philosophers and scientists.

To summarize: we have three important conceptions of wisdom that are likely interrelated but nevertheless worth keeping distinct: (i) *sophia* (theoretical wisdom), (ii) *aporia* (aporetic wisdom), and (iii) *phronēsis* (practical wisdom). Now that we have a better sense of what it can mean to be wise, let's consider how engaging with psychedelic experiences can help us grow in wisdom.

11.3 Psychedelic Methods

We have already come across some hints for how psychedelic experiences may help us cultivate wisdom in the three respects we have considered. First, our *theoretical* wisdom can be enhanced via insight. As I argued in Chapter 8, psychedelic experiences can promote insights by revealing hidden ideas and creative processes that we can deploy to generate more insights.[12] Second, our *aporetic* wisdom is enhanced when we are made aware of our lack of knowledge, which is a revelation of our true state of uncertainty. So, if psychedelic experiences reveal our hidden

---

[11] Indeed, there is a key moment in Plato's *Symposium* in which Diotima of Mantinea indicates that Socrates may be sufficiently prepared (in his *aporia*) to progress from the lower Mysteries to the higher ones.

[12] It is worth noting that there is a richer sense in which psychedelic experience can help us cultivate *sophia* in Plato's dialogues that is connected to his theory of *anamnēsis*. For example, in *Phaedrus*, we find:

> That process is the recollection of the things our soul saw when it was traveling with god, when it disregarded the things we now call real and lifted up its head to what is truly real instead.
>
> For just this reason it is fair that only a philosopher's mind grows wings, since its memory always keeps it as close as possible to those realities by being close to which the gods are divine. A man who uses reminders of these things correctly is always at the highest, most perfect level of initiation, and he is the only one who is perfect as perfect can be. He stands outside human concerns and draws close to the divine; ordinary people think he is disturbed and rebuke him for this, unaware that he is possessed by god.
>
> Socrates in *Phaedrus*, 249c–249d (Reeve 2012)

For Plato, there are (at least) two ways to remember and process this knowledge: through dialogue and through contemplation of ever more perfect forms of beauty.

lack of knowledge, they will tend to dissolve our ignorance and improve our wisdom in this respect. Third, our *practical* wisdom will tend to improve as we become more mindful, due to the positive relationship between *sati* and *phronēsis* discussed in Section 11.2. Since psychedelic experiences can be good temporary approximations to increases in mindfulness (Chapter 9), they facilitate similar benefits to well-being in the long run. Such benefits are exactly what we would expect to result from improvements to our practical wisdom.

So, we already have a rough feel for how psychedelic experiences may help us become wiser. In this section, I'll make a more detailed case for thinking that there is a distinctively psychedelic way of doing philosophy, which has its own advantages and disadvantages and which should be integrated with the other ways of doing philosophy. To help build this argument, let's first consider what distinguishes one way of doing philosophy from another.

One way to distinguish the different ways of doing philosophy is to see if there is anything distinctive about their *methods* and *objects*. For example, analytic philosophy tends to focus on concepts as its objects and uses methods of analysis to unpack and clarify them. In contrast, *natural philosophy*—that is, science[13]—tends to focus on the truths of the empirically observable world as its objects and the use of statistical methods to acquire knowledge of these truths. As another contrast, the distinction between analytic and continental philosophy is sometimes characterized in terms of the two traditions placing a different emphasis on the methods of analysis and synthesis, as well as difference in the objects they tend to focus on, with continental philosophy tending to focus more on phenomenological, social, and political issues (Prado 2003).[14] To be sure, these characterizations are extremely rough, and the distinctions between the approaches to philosophy are far from clear-cut. For example, Quine 1960 famously argued that analytic philosophy is continuous with the sciences. Nevertheless, despite the fuzziness, there are useful distinctions to be made between the different ways of doing philosophy, and recognizing them will help us appreciate how psychedelic philosophy is yet another approach to philosophy, with its own methods (and maybe also objects).

Based on this way of thinking, to define psychedelic philosophy (or to explain what sets it apart), we must consider its methods and objects. However, in order to make the case that psychedelic philosophy is a valuable way of doing philosophy, I'm going to focus primarily on its *methods* and show how they can be used to pursue the objects of analytic philosophy and science. This is a dialectical choice. Although psychedelic philosophy may have its own distinctive objects, which I will discuss briefly in Section 11.5, the value in pursuing these objects may not be

---

[13] One may argue that science is an offspring of natural philosophy, perhaps made distinct by its reliance on the peer-review method. That may be a useful distinction to make, but the general point of this chapter will still apply (i.e. that psychedelic methods can be used to advance science).

[14] A useful analogy that helps capture the distinction likens analytic philosophy to physics and continental philosophy to the arts (Levy 2003).

recognized by those immersed in the traditions of analytic philosophy and science. So, in order to demonstrate the value of psychedelic philosophy to this audience, I'll focus on how the merits of its methods can be evaluated in terms of achieving familiar objectives: theoretical, aporetic, and practical wisdom.

The key distinction between analytic philosophy and science, on the one hand, and psychedelic philosophy, on the other, is that the former rely heavily on analytic methods for thinking and the latter relies on what I will call *psychedelic methods*. This distinction between analytic and psychedelic methods is similar to the distinction between analytic-based and insight-based strategies for creative problem-solving we saw in Chapter 8. That helps us get a feel for where we're going, but it will pay to lay out the distinction more carefully.

The characteristic feature of analytic methods—which could also be called *discursive* methods—is that they involve the serial, rule-based manipulation of linguistic or symbolic representations of the objects of study (building valid arguments, making precise inferences, etc.). The quintessential analytic method is that of logical deduction, which was first systematically developed by Aristotle and recorded in his work *Prior Analytics*. Another class of analytic methods is that of probability theory, statistics, and decision theory—these are all systems of rules that help us manage uncertainty. Yet another class involves methods of conceptual analysis, explication, and engineering—these are all methods for helping us improve our concepts, which are the basic building blocks for analytic thinking.[15] What these methods have in common is that they all involve the rigorous, sequential application of language-based rules of thought and a strong emphasis on precision, clarity, and consistency.[16]

In some cases, the rules of an analytic method are strict, such as those of logical deduction, and in other cases, the rules are more flexible, such as those of conceptual explication. Another class of analytic methods for which the rules are less strict is *philosophical heuristics* (Hájek 2014, 2016, 2018). These can be thought of as "rules of thumb" for analytic thinking, and we came across an example of them in Chapter 8 when we considered the possibility that some creative processes are not hidden from awareness. That example involved systematically exploring different combinations of old ideas to find new good ideas, a process that can be of great use to philosophy. Hájek has developed an extensive catalogue of such heuristics. As another example, whenever you use a definite description of the form 'the X' ('the cause', 'the true', 'the biggest', etc.), you should check for two ways in which your thinking may have failed: (i) there could be *no* X, or (ii) there could be *multiple* Xs. It's easy to miss these possibilities, and it's easy for them to cause

---

[15] Recall, from Chapter 2, that my definition of psychedelic experience in terms of psychedelic space is an example of conceptual explication.

[16] It is important to note that for each class of method, there can be substantial disagreements about what the correct rules are. For example, there are different systems of logic that may be competing or complementary (Beall and Restall 2006) and alternative axiomatizations of probability with different advantages and disadvantages (Lyon 2016).

problems in our reasoning. So, it is a good heuristic to check for them whenever our thinking about a topic involves a definite description.[17] Such heuristics are, thus, another class of analytic methods that can help us do philosophy.

There's another example of a philosophical heuristic that is useful for us to consider because it provides us with a convenient way to pivot from analytic methods of philosophy to psychedelic ones. Bertrand Russell describes this heuristic and explains how it can help us think about ethical issues in a way that protects us from our emotional biases:

> There is another intellectual virtue, which is that of generality or impartiality. I recommend the following exercise: When, in a sentence expressing political opinion, there are words that arouse powerful but different emotions in different readers, try replacing them by symbols, A, B, C, and so on and forgetting the particular significance of the symbols. Suppose A is England, B is Germany and C is Russia. So long as you remember what the letters mean, most of the things you will believe will depend upon whether you are English, German or Russian, which is logically irrelevant. When, in elementary algebra, you do problems about A, B and C going up a mountain, you have no emotional interest in the gentlemen concerned, and you do your best to work out the solution with impersonal correctness. But if you thought that A was yourself, B your hated rival and C the schoolmaster who set the problem, your calculations would go askew, and you would be sure to find that A was first and C was last. In thinking about political problems this kind of emotional bias is bound to be present, and only care and practice can enable you to think as objectively as you do in the algebraic problem.
>
> Russell 1950, pp. 47–8

This heuristic of abstracting away from the emotionally charged aspects of an issue appears many times throughout the history of philosophy—perhaps most famously with Rawls' (1971) *veil of ignorance*.[18] The reason why this provides us with a convenient way to pivot from analytic methods to psychedelic methods is that Russell goes on to describe another way by which we may think with ethical generality:

> Thinking in abstract terms is of course not the only way to achieve ethical generality; it can be achieved as well, or perhaps even better, if you can feel generalized emotions. But to most people this is difficult. If you are hungry, you will make great exertions, if necessary, to get food; if your children are hungry, you may feel an even greater urgency. If a friend is starving, you will probably

---

[17] We saw an example of this at work in Chapter 7: while many authors refer to 'the' bifurcation parameter of the Ermentrout and Cowan 1979 model, the model actually has *many* bifurcation parameters.

[18] To be clear, neither the heuristic nor the veil of ignorance entails Rawls' meta-ethical conclusions.

exert yourself to relieve his distress. But if you hear that some millions of Indians or Chinese are in danger of death from malnutrition, the problem is so vast and so distant that unless you have some official responsibility you probably soon forget all about it. Nevertheless, if you have the emotional capacity to feel distant evils acutely, you can achieve ethical generality through feeling. If you have not this rather rare gift, the habit of viewing practical problems abstractly as well as concretely is the best available substitute.

Russell 1950, p. 48

This example highlights two key points that can help us see how psychedelic methods have particular advantages over analytic ones. So let's unpack each point.

The first point is that—as observed by Russell—the difficulty with achieving ethical generality is that we tend to easily *forget* the suffering of those who are distant from us. Upon learning about their suffering, we may be able to empathize in a way we do for those who are closer to us (children, friends, colleagues, compatriots, etc.). However, because of the great distance between them and us, we soon lose this state of extended empathy. The distance needn't be geographical— it could be cultural, political, economic, or even temporal. Whatever the nature of the distance, it has the effect of increasing (or maintaining) the level of one's phenomenal opacity with respect to those in need (Chapter 5). We can think of this loss of empathy simply as forgetting, as Russell does, but we can also think of it as a shrinking or collapsing of awareness—that is, as a psychecryptic experience. This way of framing the phenomenon can help us appreciate how a psychedelic experience may facilitate the emotional capacity for feeling distant evils acutely. Reversing the psychecryptic experience and, in particular, increasing one's phenomenal transparency, facilitates the flow of attentional resources through one's representations to a deeper, more connected awareness of the issue at hand (Chapter 5).[19]

The second point is that even though we tend to be stuck in the psychecryptic state (of not empathizing with those who are distant and suffering), not all is lost: we can still use the analytic method of treating the problem abstractly to arrive at the ethically general conclusion. This gives us a feel for an important aspect of the difference between psychedelic and analytic methods. The best scenario would be one in which we could just feel the generalized emotions. Failing that, we can fall back to an analytic method to get to the same outcome.[20] The situation is similar to searching for something in a dark closet. It would be best if you could just *see* what you're looking for. However, if the light is broken, then that won't be possible.

---

[19] In both cases, increasing opacity or transparency, the result is that all people are treated with equanimity.

[20] To be clear, the claim here is not that we should feel generalized emotions all the time. Rather, the claim is that we would be better off if we *could* feel them when doing so would serve us well.

Nevertheless, you can still find what you're looking for by systematically reaching around for the objects and evaluating whether what you're touching feels right. In other words, analytic methods can help us find our way through the dark, but it would be much easier if we could just turn on the light.

An important point that is missing from Russell's passage is that there are methods that can help us feel generalized emotions. Russell simply notes that the ability is rare and difficult for most people to achieve. He doesn't provide any guidance for how we may cultivate the ability. In contrast, he does describe a method for controlling for our emotional biases—namely, the heuristic of approaching the problem abstractly. This glaring absence is, I think, representative of much of contemporary philosophy: there is often little discussion of methods that may help us turn on the light (or see in the dark). But there are such methods. In this particular case, perhaps the most obvious methods involve the practice of compassion and loving-kindness meditation. As Vervaeke and Ferraro 2016 have pointed out, these meditative practices are oriented towards increasing phenomenal transparency (Chapter 5) and, in particular, *connectedness* and *unity* with other beings, which can help our emotions generalize. (In contrast, Russell's method of abstraction is oriented towards increasing phenomenal opacity.) Furthermore, we also have accumulating evidence that psychedelics regularly induce increases of phenomenal transparency, particularly in the form of experiences of increased connectedness and unity.[21] Although these experiences are temporary, occurring during psychedelic trips, they appear to continue to have some degree of reverberation beyond the trip, and may produce long-lasting changes to one's awareness.

Clearly, then, there are methods that can help us feel generalized emotions. And, as Russell indicates, there is a sense in which this is a *better* way to achieve ethical generality. One could perhaps make the case that the reason why it is better is because feeling the generalized emotions is itself more ethical than reasoning about the problem abstractly. However, a more minimal claim is sufficient for our purposes. Being able to feel generalized emotions is better because it is easier to think with ethical generality than it is to reason abstractly about an ethical issue. That is, there's a sense in which the psychedelic method is more *efficient* than the analytic one.

Let's consider another example that illustrates this point about efficiency: Descartes' search for a foundation of all knowledge. In order to find this foundation, Descartes employed his *method of doubt*: he argued that any belief that can be reasonably doubted can't be part of the foundation. To identify which beliefs can be doubted, he carefully worked his way through various lengthy chains of reasoning. Famously, this led him to *cogito ergo sum* (I think, therefore I am).

---

[21] For example, see Belser et al. 2017, Nour et al. 2017, Malone et al. 2018, Carhart-Harris et al. 2018, Noorani et al. 2018, Argento et al. 2019, Forstmann et al. 2020, Gregorio et al. 2021, and Breeksema et al. 2020 for a review.

However, his laborious method of arriving at this conclusion gave rise to a point of criticism, with Gassendi complaining that it would have been easier for Descartes to simply regard all his previous knowledge as uncertain, in one fell swoop. In response to this criticism, Descartes replied:

> You say that you approve of my project for freeing my mind from preconceived opinions; and indeed no one can pretend that such a project should not be approved of. But you would have preferred me to have carried it out by making a 'simple and brief statement'—that is, only in a perfunctory fashion. Is it really so easy to free ourselves from all the errors which we have soaked up since our infancy? Can we really be *too* careful in carrying out a project which everyone agrees should be performed?
>
> Descartes 1641[22]

The key point here is that the task of freeing our minds from preconceived opinions can appear deceptively simple, whereas in reality, it is extremely difficult and so requires careful and detailed argument or reasoning.

However, there is another way to arrive at the same result that is much more efficient. A common experience people have during psychedelic trips is to become aware of how little they actually know. For example, people become aware of how radically misleading their sensory experience can be. They also often have insights into the uncertain nature of the rest of their beliefs and assumptions. In other words, there appears to be an increase in their aporetic wisdom: their ignorance is dissolved, and they become more aware of the true state of their uncertainty. Also, as we have seen in previous chapters, there appears to be a general increase in the uncertainty (entropy) of their conscious state (Carhart-Harris et al. 2014, Carhart-Harris and Friston 2019). Closely related to this point is the observation that, in addition to increasing phenomenal transparency (as we saw in the previous example), psychedelics also regularly increase phenomenal *opacity*. These increases in opacity are accompanied by feelings of optionality and even unreality—for example, one may experience that one's usual sense of self may not be real or necessary (Letheby 2021). Once one has had such an experience, it becomes much easier to see that there is very little, if anything, that we can truly claim to know with certainty. Consequently, there is much less of a need to convince oneself of this by argument (which is not to say that the method of doubt has no value).

Indeed, this psychedelic method is better than Descartes' method of doubt in another way. As mentioned, Descartes arrived at the conclusion that the only thing he knew with certainty was *cogito*, 'I think', and the entailment, *sum*,

[22] Cottingham 1985, p. 241. For Gassendi's objection, see p. 180.

'I exist'. However, as many who have had an experience of psychedelic-induced ego dissolution can attest, it is entirely possible to be uncertain about the existence of an 'I'. Insights along these lines are not uncommon in high-dose psychedelic trips, and it is received wisdom for many Buddhists that the practice of meditation can bring about similar insights.[23] Therefore, it would seem that even by taking as much care as he did with his arguments, Descartes was still unable to completely free his mind from his preconceived opinions. A better conclusion for Descartes to arrive at would have been something along the lines of 'there is thinking' rather than attributing the thinking to an 'I' (an important point made by Gassendi 1641, Nietzsche 1886, Russell 1945, and Lichtenberg 1971). To be clear, the point here is not that the statement 'I think' is false. The point is only that it is something that can be *doubted*—and debated, as many philosophers have.[24]

We've now seen two examples for how psychedelic methods may help us achieve objectives that fall under the remit of analytic philosophy—thinking with ethical generality and becoming aware of how even our most basic beliefs are subject to at least some degree of doubt. These are major examples from the history of philosophy, and I think there are many others we could explore. These include William James' experience with nitrous oxide and his insights about Hegel's absolute idealism (James 1882); Hume's arguments about personal identity and Buddhist doctrine of *anattā*, or non-self (Wright 2017, pp. 82–102); the role of *eros* in philosophy as explored in Plato's *Symposium* and the aesthetics of experiences induced by psychedelic drugs; the New Riddle of Induction (Goodman 1955) and the Buddhist notion of *śūnyatā* (emptiness); or the the hard problem of consciousness (Chalmers 1996), non-dual awareness, and Spinoza's substance monism (Sjöstedt-Hughes 2022). Each example is worth exploring; however, we will have to put them aside since they can come with their own sets of controversies, which we lack the space to discuss here. Moreover, they can easily divert us from the main issue. So, I think it is more fruitful to turn our attention to how psychedelic methods can also help us with the "daily grind" of doing philosophy (and science, engineering, business, etc.).

As an example, let's consider open-monitoring meditation. Recall that this is the practice of allowing thoughts and sensations to arise and then allowing them to pass without reacting to them. One of the benefits of this practice of meditation is that it slows down one's mental processes and creates space between one's thoughts and sensations, allowing us to break free from our habitual patterns of thinking. Here's a nice description:

[23] There is a subtlety here that we should be mindful of, which is that it is possible to recognize the proposition 'I think' as something one can know, but where the concept of 'I' is quite different from usual one we use in everyday life—it would be the more expansive/inclusive notion of Self that one finds in traditions such as Advaita Vedanta, some threads of Buddhist philosophy, and Jungian psychology.

[24] For example, see Metzinger 2003, Strawson 2009, Peacocke 2012, Prinz 2012, Siderits et al. 2011, Nida-Rümelin 2017, and Zahavi and Kriegel 2016.

The senses perceive the object, which then the mental consciousness instantly conceptualizes in a manner conditioned by all of our past experience, and superimposes this conceptualized version back onto the originally neutral data of our senses—all of this occurring so fast that we don't even notice the process, and are only left in the end with the mind's conceptual version of things that we take to be reality.

Namgyal 2011[25]

And compare with the following description:

Such spontaneous or automatic inferences, which the subject cannot help make, take him via presuppositions he is unaware of relying upon to conclusions he finds intuitively compelling regardless of what warrant he has for them.

Fischer 2011, p. 4

The first passage is taken from the introduction to Thrangu's translation of *The Ninth Karmapa's Ocean of Definitive Meaning*, an important text in Vajrayana Buddhism, and the second is taken from Fischer's *Philosophical Delusion and its Therapy: Outline of a Philosophical Revolution*, a book squarely in the tradition of analytic philosophy. However, despite the fact that these two works are from completely different traditions, they have much in common. Fischer's central thesis is that, unbeknownst to us, much of our philosophical thinking is erroneously shaped by our preconceptions, beliefs, desires, etc., and that it is difficult for us to become aware of these hidden forces and how they influence our reasoning. Open-monitoring meditation can help us become aware of these hidden processes and develop the ability to break free from them. And this is true regardless of the philosophical issue we might be working on. (For example, someone's atheistic or religious beliefs may shape their philosophical thinking about some seemingly unrelated matter—economics, say.)

Here's another example of how an established practice of open-monitoring meditation can help that will be familiar to most philosophers. Much of philosophical progress involves introducing novel distinctions that have previously gone unrecognized. The reason why new distinctions can be valuable is that without them, we are prone to conflate ideas or concepts that should be kept distinct in our thinking. Conflation often happens because we think too quickly and don't put enough (or any) space between our thoughts. The process of discovering a new distinction that needs to be made, or recognizing the value of an existing one, often involves reasoning analytically to resolve a tension in our thinking. In such cases, we feel that something has gone wrong and so we look for ways to break our concepts up to give us more flexibility for resolving the tension. This method is perfectly adequate. However, the practice of open-monitoring

[25] Namgyal 2011, p. 1.

meditation provides us with an alternative: by creating more space between our thoughts, it helps us to see the distinctions that need to be made *before* the tension arises. And, as with the previous examples of psychedelic methods, there are some respects in which this is a better method. There is a sense in which it is more efficient, since it reduces some of the need for analytic thinking, thus freeing up conscious resources for other tasks. It is also proactive, rather than reactive, since it helps one see the relevant distinctions and avoid the conflations before a problem arises in the first place.

There are other ways that open-monitoring meditation can help with philosophy. For example, as we saw in Chapter 8, this form of meditation appears to promote insight-based solutions to creative problems, and a lot of philosophical activity is a form of creative problem-solving. Especially when it comes to constructing philosophical arguments or objections, it can help to have more novel and far-reaching insights (novelty and scope), insights that are more precise in detail (clarity), and to be able to hold such insights in awareness for sufficient periods of time (duration). Similarly, to jump back to psychedelics, a psychedelic trip may facilitate creative insights or improve the ability to shift to different perspectives on a given issue, or to come up with highly novel thought experiments. As such, there are many ways in which psychedelic methods can help us with the process of philosophy. These methods are not limited to helping us have profound insights about major issues, such as the nature of our knowledge. They can also help us with smaller-scale philosophical objectives, such as observing subtle distinctions.

Now that we've seen some examples of psychedelic methods, we can turn to how we may give a general characterization of them. One key criterion is that, whereas the analytic methods are inferential, the psychedelic ones are experiential.[26] A second key criterion is that, while the analytic methods operate at the level of our conscious intellect, the psychedelic methods help us tap into our unconscious cognitive and sensorimotor resources. To use an analogy, consider the distinction between a CPU, which is optimized for serial computation, and a GPU, which is optimized for parallel computation. Our analytic methods run on our "CPUs", and the psychedelic methods help us access our "GPUs".[27] Another analogy comes from statistics and data science: one shouldn't rely exclusively on statistical analyses; instead, one should also *look* at the data—and in as many ways as possible. By looking at the data, we take advantage of our visual and cognitive modes of comprehension that are left unutilized by our methods of statistical analysis.

---

[26] As I noted in Chapter 3, we should be careful about the distinction between inference and experience, since experience itself can be thought of as a kind of inference. Nevertheless, if experience is a form of inference, there is still a useful distinction to be made between our experiential inferences and our non-experiential inferences.

[27] Note that the distinction here is not quite the usual system 1 vs. system 2 (dual process) distinction (Gilbert 1999, Kahneman and Frederick 2002). One way to think about it is that we rely on system 2 to use our analytic methods, and one thing our psychedelic methods can do is help us create novel integrations between system 1 and system 2. This idea is similar to the argument that lucid dreaming can be used as a method for creative problem-solving (Stumbrys and Daniels 2010, Smith 2014).

The distinction between analytic and psychedelic methods is similar: analytic methods are vital for good philosophy, but we shouldn't rely exclusively on them; we should also make use of our psychedelic methods to *look*. A third key criterion of psychedelic methods is, of course, that they should be mind-revealing. This is an important point. It's not enough for some method to merely not be analytic for it to count as psychedelic. The method must reveal the mind in some way—by revealing hidden knowledge, hidden uncertainty, a hidden desire, a hidden thought process, a hidden perspective, and so on. Finally, as a fourth key criterion, the method should have a tendency to enhance wisdom in some way, which is the ultimate goal of philosophy.

The thought, then, is that philosophy could be substantially improved if we integrated psychedelic methods with our analytic ones.[28] Just as good creative problem-solving requires both analytic- and insight-based strategies, good philosophy requires both analytic and psychedelic methods. This is also a point that has been made about our general well-being—recall Maslow's claim from the previous chapter:

> Our conscious intellect is too exclusively analytic, rational, numerical, atomistic, conceptual and so it misses a great deal of reality, especially within ourselves.
>
> Maslow 1963, p. 69

Maslow's remarks about creative problem-solving and human well-being carry over to philosophy. In a way, this shouldn't be a novel point, since the bulk of contemporary philosophical activity is a form of creative problem-solving, and the ultimate goal of philosophy is to cultivate wisdom, which is about living well. However, psychedelic methods are rarely, if ever, taught by philosophy departments. To be sure, some classes on topics such as Buddhist philosophy may teach meditative practices, and some may touch upon the general idea of not relying exclusively on our analytic methods. However, at least to my knowledge, psychedelic methods are not taught as a package in any systematic way (even by another name), and certainly not in the way that our analytic methods are taught.[29]

So far, I've focused on methods that involve meditation and psychedelics, but it is worth noting that there are other psychedelic methods that involve other kinds of interventions on the brain/mind. These may include or involve sensory deprivation, dreaming, various yogic practices, alcohol, exercise, sauna, scents,

---

[28] Another way of framing this idea is that the use of psychedelic methods can help counterbalance the so-called *linguistic turn* that philosophy took in the early twentieth century (Rorty 1967). Roughly speaking, the linguistic turn was a shift from trying to understand the nature of reality to studying how our concepts work.

[29] It's worth noting in this regard that philosophical heuristics (one class of analytic methods) are also not widely taught. A plausible explanation for this is that the heuristics have only recently been explicitly identified as something that *can* be taught (Hájek 2014, 2016, 2018). However, it's also worth noting that philosophical methods in general are rarely taught in any explicit and systematic way—although there are some notable exceptions (Daly 2010, Sytsma and Livengood 2015, Steinhart 2017).

dance, sex, fasting, etc. One feature common to all of the methods discussed so far that may stand out to some readers is that they have a substantial physiological aspect to them. However, this is not an essential feature of what makes for a psychedelic method. To make this clear, let's briefly consider two examples that are unlike the others in this respect: (i) engagement with myth and (ii) engagement with aesthetic experience.

From an analytic perspective, engaging with myth would seem to be another opposite of philosophical inquiry. However, it is well known that Plato made extensive use of myth (*mythos*) and mythological characters throughout his dialogues. There are different theories for why Plato relied so heavily on myth, and there is probably no single, unified explanation (Collobert et al. 2012). However, it seems plausible that at least in many cases, Plato used myth as a way of uncovering hidden truths. This view about the function of myth was discussed by Jung:

> Myths are original revelations of the preconscious psyche, involuntary statements about unconscious psychic happenings, and anything but allegories of physical processes.
>
> Jung 1959, p. 261

To be clear, we needn't be committed to the view that all stories that are commonly called 'myth' fit this function, or even if they do, that they then must have philosophical value. However, it seems plausible that the careful construction of a myth, or the careful recording of an experienced myth, can be deployed usefully to serve philosophical purposes. Myths can be used to tap into the power of unconscious processes for philosophical investigation (similar to the power of visualizing data instead of relying only on statistical analyses of it) or for sharing philosophical insights that may be resisted if communicated via analytic means. Whereas analytic methods (or *logos*, which is historically contrasted from *mythos*) take advantage of the serial processes of the conscious, *mythos* takes advantage of the massively parallel and associative threads of the unconscious.

This can be seen with Hemingway's "iceberg" technique of writing: the mind is relied on to fill in the missing pieces, thus creating rich landscapes and backstories far better than the author's own words can. One example that is effective at demonstrating the power of this technique is the following short story—often considered the *shortest* story (and erroneously attributed to Hemingway):

For sale: baby shoes, never worn.

This single sentence provokes the mind, causing it to rush in with a story and its concomitant emotions. The result is remarkably effective. Similarly, the power of *myth* stems from this disposition of the mind to uncover, explore, and share ideas that are already deep in the mind. For many philosophical questions, this can be much more effective than any analytic method. Compare, for example, the power of Homer's story of *Ulysses and the Sirens* and Aristotle's discussion of *akrasia* in *Nicomachean Ethics*. Both are about the same phenomenon—weakness of the will, which is a form of psychecryptic experience—but the former strikes a deeper chord in the mind.

To be clear, this doesn't mean that *mythos* should be used to the exclusion of *logos*. The best wisdom would result from studying both Homer and Aristotle—as well as the latest science on human behaviour and decision-making. The methods, therefore, are not rivals. They are complementary. However, they do need to be integrated. From this perspective, Plato's dialogues, laden with both myth and reason, appear to be a particularly sophisticated integration of the methods of *mythos* and *logos*.[30]

The second psychedelic method that isn't physiological also contrasts with *logos*: it involves the engagement with aesthetic experience. There are different theories of aesthetic experience, and it is not clear if aesthetic experiences form a unified kind. However, a common thought is that they involve *aesthetic attention*. For example, a minimal definition of aesthetic experience is that it involves attending to an object's features for their own sake, independently of the utility they may have (Levinson 2016, pp. 28–42).[31] Similarly, some aesthetic experiences may involve focusing attention on an object while simultaneously distributing attention across its features (Nanay 2016a, pp. 12–35). As such, many (if not all) aesthetic experiences involve a disruption of the usual patterns of attentional resource allocation.

This puts aesthetic experiences and the experiences typically induced by meditation and psychedelics in the same ballpark (Chapter 5). Although this doesn't entail that all aesthetic experiences are psychedelic experiences, it does suggest that many are, and so there may be substantial overlap between the two kinds of experience.[32] By disrupting our usual patterns of attentional resource allocation, aesthetic experiences involve the creation of a surplus of attentional resources. Indeed, Aqil and Roseman 2023 propose that the therapeutic benefits

[30] Another important point I lack the space to discuss concerns the connections between myths that create a mythological world, as Bremmer 1986 observed: 'myth evokes further myths . . . it is almost true that every Greek myth is ultimately connected in a chain of association with every other Greek myth' (p. 6). The thought, then, is that a familiarity with the mythological world, combined with a balanced application of psychedelic and analytic methods, would have a profound effect on one's wisdom in the regular world.

[31] This is closely related to Kant's notion of aesthetic disinterestedness. Indeed, Kant's view on the relationship between morality and aesthetics closely parallels the view offered here. On Kant's view, aesthetic experiences help us understand moral ideas by presenting them in a sensible form and motivate us appropriately to fulfil our moral duties. Similarly, psychedelic experiences help us understand abstract philosophical ideas by presenting them in a sensory (and somatic) form and motivate us appropriately to implement them in our lives. The basic insight is also arguably what is behind various tantric and shamanic practices.

[32] For Plato (particularly in *Symposium* and *Phaedrus*), increasingly abstract aesthetic experiences involving beauty are what enables one to ascend to the highest form of wisdom—contemplation of, and creation in, the Beautiful.

of psychedelics may be driven by their aesthetic effects. The basic thought is that an intense and absorbing aesthetic experience will draw attention away from self-oriented cognition and thereby deactivate and disintegrate the DMN (and its usual relations to other networks). This attentional surplus can then be allocated to our representations of the world, thus helping us see it in a different way, as Nanay points out:

> Why do we pay large sums of money to put ourselves in a position to have an aesthetic experience (which, as we have seen, doesn't always then materialize)? If we accept my claim about the centrality of aesthetic attention in understanding aesthetic experience, the answer will be straightforward: because aesthetic experiences allow us to see and then attend to the world differently: in a way that we don't, and couldn't, see it otherwise.
>
> Nanay 2016a, p. 35

Although these experiences reveal something new about the world, some of them may also be psychedelic experiences if they involve the revelation of unconscious representations of the world that would otherwise be hidden from our awareness.

However, there is another class of aesthetic experiences that will count as psychedelic that may be even more important—at least for the purpose of doing philosophy. While the attentional surplus of an aesthetic experience can end up allocated to our representations of the world, it can also flow to other parts or aspects of the mind. Therefore, such an experience can also help us to see *our minds* in a way that is difficult (if not impossible) for us to do otherwise.[33] Moreover, and this is the crucial point for our purposes, aesthetic experiences can be *designed* so that they are psychedelic in particular ways. Whereas interventions involving meditation and psychedelics typically result in an attentional surplus that is largely undirected, some aesthetic experiences can be designed to guide attentional surplus to particular ideas, themes, associations, and so on (which is arguably what is happening in tantric and shamanic practices). As an example, consider what happens when you aesthetically attend to Bosch's *The Garden of Earthly Delights*, or consider how the aesthetic properties of churches and other religious buildings disrupt attention and direct it towards particular religious ideas. Similarly, aesthetically attending to objects, such as Buddha statues, Zen rock gardens, mandalas, etc., can help bring to awareness parts and aspects of the mind that

---

[33] An interesting side note here is that meditation and psychedelics should help us have aesthetic experiences, which, as Nanay points out, are not always easy to have. Moreover, they should also enhance our normally occurring aesthetic experiences. In this regard, it is worth noting that this is how Aldous Huxley described one of his experiences while on mescaline (Huxley 1954, pp. 21–2).

are otherwise difficult to experience.[34] This makes the engagement with aesthetic experience another distinctive psychedelic method for doing philosophy.[35]

To summarize, we see how there are psychedelic methods of philosophy that don't involve anything especially physiological. Reading a mythical tale or looking at a work of art is no more physiological than sitting down to read an academic paper. We can also see how these methods may be combined in various ways. For example, one may spend some time contemplating particular myths, then spend some time meditating, and then engage with particular aesthetic objects that relate to the contemplated myths, perhaps while under the influence of a psychedelic substance.[36] From the perspective of the literature on psychedelics, such a process would be understood in terms of carefully designing the set and setting for a psychedelic session. However, this perspective would render the process of designing the set and setting as secondary to the psychedelic session. I suggest that, instead of thinking of the set and setting as affecting a psychedelic session, it may be more useful to understand the psychedelic session as *revealing* the importance of set and setting in regular life. Therefore, a better perspective might be to view the process of designing the set and setting as involving its own psychedelic methods, and consider it as important and valuable as a psychedelic session itself.[37]

11.4 Relationships with Other Philosophical Methods

Now that we have a feel for what psychedelic methods of philosophy look like, we should consider how they relate to other philosophical methods.

Probably the most important point to make in this regard is that psychedelic methods should be integrated with analytic methods. A major reason for this is that the results that arise from psychedelic methods—insights, for instance—have no guarantee of being true. They can fail to be true for at least two reasons: (i) the experiences that give rise to them lack *clarity*, and (ii) the experiences may involve the revelation of content that is *false* (a hidden false belief, for example).[38] Moreover, the products of psychedelic experiences (for example, insights) often come along with an unshakable conviction—people often report a 'veil' being

---

[34] On this note, recall also the psychedelic effects of *deity meditation* (which involves the memorization and subsequent visualization of a visual scene involving a deity) from Chapter 5.

[35] This point can also help us understand the role that beauty plays for the philosopher in Plato's dialogues, especially in *Symposium* and *Phaedrus* (Chapter 3).

[36] Such a process may resemble the processes of mystical initiations, such as the lower and higher initiations of the Eleusinian Mysteries and those of ancient Egypt.

[37] Although Metzner and Leary 1967 focus on such psychedelic methods for the purpose of programming a psychedelic experience, much of their discussion highlights how these methods are psychedelic in their own right—see, for example, their discussion of focusing visual attention on a *mandala* (p. 9).

[38] Indeed, false insights can be deliberately induced in controlled settings (Laukkonen et al. 2020).

lifted and true Reality being revealed. So, we should make sure to be wary of the epistemological status of any results that come out of psychedelic experiences. That doesn't mean that we should disregard them; it just means that we should treat them like any other source of information. That is, we should check if they align with our larger belief system (prior to the experience). We should also see if they can be given independent justification, and presented in a logical form that would convince other people. Moreover, if the outcomes of the experiences have empirical content, we should check them against established scientific evidence and theory. In other words, we need to make sure that psychedelic methods are kept in check by analytic methods.

The point about 'being kept in check' doesn't fully reflect the relationship between the two methods. It gives the impression that psychedelic methods are only methods of *discovery* and analytic methods are only methods for *justification*. However, this way of partitioning the methods would be incorrect: analytic methods can be used for discovery, and psychedelic ones can be used for justification.

We have already seen examples of the former: the use of creativity heuristics to aid the discovery of new philosophical ideas and Socrates' method of *elenchos* for discovering one's actual state of ignorance. Analytic philosophers also spend a lot of time carefully constructing thought experiments that can expose latent philosophical intuitions. We can also find examples of the latter—of psychedelic methods supporting justification. For example, by practising mindfulness, one can better implement Russell's strategy of abstracting away from emotionally charged specifics—for instance, by noticing when one has failed to make one's reasoning sufficiently abstract. Relatedly, by being more aware of how one's emotions and hidden biases influence one's thought processes, one can be more discerning about the quality of one's reasoning on any given occasion. Psychedelic methods can also spur insights that can be used to support conclusions, such as Poincare's intuitive mathematical breakthroughs (Chapter 8). Finally, if we're willing to expand our usual notion of justification so that it itself is more psychedelic, then we can see how psychedelic methods can be used to justify conclusions and decisions by revealing their alignment with our deepest values and most authentic sources of motivation.

Instead of splitting them up in terms of justification and discovery, we can think of the analytic and psychedelic methods as techniques for tackling philosophy from different angles. As Hájek is careful to point out about philosophical heuristics:

The heuristics are no substitute for depth. I am not promising wisdom, or profound insight. But I hasten to add that what I offer is not antithetical to them, either, and indeed I think it helps rather than hinders progress to such wisdom or insight.

Hájek 2014, p. 6

By the same token, the psychedelic methods are no substitute for *justification*. However, they are not antithetical to it either, and they can help us improve the justification of our beliefs—for example, by helping us be more empathic with those who have opposing views. In other words, the best kind of philosophy involves a mastery of both kinds of method and their integration. The Persian mystic-philosopher Suhrawardi made a similar point when describing what he referred to as *intuitive philosophy*:

> The best student is the student of both intuitive [mystical] philosophy and discursive [analytic] philosophy. Next is the student of intuitive philosophy, and then the student of discursive philosophy.
>
> Suhrawardi 1186, p. 3[39]

Intuitive philosophy, also known as the philosophy of illumination, can be understood as a specific form of psychedelic philosophy that focuses on experiences that are mystical in nature. So, this idea that philosophy can be improved by incorporating psychedelic methods and integrating them with our analytic (or discursive) methods is not a new one. However, it is fair to say that the psychedelic renaissance we are currently witnessing shines new light on this old idea. Obviously, much more can, and should, be said about the relationship between psychedelic and analytic methods, but this suffices for our present purposes.[40] The key point is that the different kinds of method are complementary, mutually supportive, and should be integrated into a unified approach to philosophy.

Another important relationship is the one between psychedelic philosophy and the philosophical discipline of *phenomenology*—as developed by Husserl, Heidegger, Sartre, Merleau-Ponty, and others in the continental tradition, as well as those in the Buddhist and Hindu traditions. Very briefly, phenomenology is the study of the structure of conscious experience, whereas psychedelic philosophy is about bringing hidden parts or aspects of the mind into conscious experience in the service of pursuing wisdom. The two modes of inquiry are different, but they are interrelated and mutually supportive. For example, psychedelic experiences can provide novel and important data for phenomenological investigation, thereby functioning as a method of discovery. Some parts of Sartre's *Nausea*, for instance, were motivated by his experiences with mescaline. Going in the other direction, by better understanding the structures of conscious experience with the help of phenomenological theory, it is possible to have psychedelic experiences that are

---

[39] Walbridge and Ziai 1999.

[40] One further point worth flagging is that the distinction between the kinds of method admits boundary cases. For example, Socrates' method of *elenchos* is arguably both analytic and psychedelic. Also, the methods deployed in *Dharma combat* in Zen are often discursive in nature (though perhaps without being analytic) and yet also often have psychedelic effects. Similarly, various writing techniques, such as journaling and free writing, can have psychedelic effects.

more effective in the pursuit of wisdom. For example, Buddhist conceptual systems of *jhānas* (understood, roughly speaking, as different states of absorption) are phenomenological theories that serve this purpose. Similarly, the *chakra* and *nadi* systems of tantric yoga are phenomenological theories that facilitate the awareness, and management, of *prāna* (subtle energy). Another example, which is from analytic philosophy but nevertheless phenomenological, is that of the distinction between phenomenal opacity and transparency (Chapter 5). Knowledge of these two concepts and how they apply to the mind can be used to navigate through one's psychedelic and meditative experiences with greater precision and sophistication.

Finally, we should consider the relationship between psychedelic methods and those of Buddhism. One difficulty in considering this relationship is that there is no one thing that is Buddhist philosophy, and there is a great deal of variation between Buddhist schools of thought. Some Buddhists are against the consumption of mind-altering substances (with perhaps the exception of tea), while some are not. This could then be a potential source of contrast (between psychedelic and Buddhist philosophy) but, given the variation in Buddhism, it is not guaranteed. A similar point holds for many other methods—for example, some forms of Buddhism incorporate yogic practices, while others do not. However, perhaps it could be said that in comparison to any particular school of Buddhist thought, psychedelic philosophy would be more ecumenical in its methods. A second potential difference that may hold with some generality is that psychedelic philosophy is not tied to particular traditions, texts, teachers, or teachings, and it is open to incorporating entirely novel methods (for example, some new methods we haven't discussed could involve biofeedback and machine learning). Thus, it could be considered more forward-looking in a way that some Buddhist schools of thought are not. With that said, as I pointed out in Chapter 2, some schools of Buddhist thought (as well as other mystical traditions, particularly those of Hinduism) are quite explicit that they are not tied to any particular teaching or practice. So, teasing out the distinction is by no means straightforward. Nevertheless, there is substantial overlap between the view advocated here and the argument that Western philosophy (analytic and continental) would benefit greatly from a healthy injection of Zen practice (Coe 1983).

Now that we have a sense for how psychedelic methods relate to those of other approaches to philosophy, let's consider briefly the *objects* of psychedelic philosophy.

11.5 Objects of Psychedelic Philosophy

So far, our discussion has been focused on psychedelic methods that can be used to pursue the same philosophical objects as those of analytic philosophy and science (both understood as ways of doing philosophy). The reason for this is mostly dialectical: in order to demonstrate the value of psychedelic methods to analytic philosophers and scientists, it makes sense to focus on showing how the methods can be used to achieve aims that have recognizable value for those traditions. So we've considered how psychedelic methods can help us: have insights about issues within analytic philosophy and science, safeguard ourselves against fallacious reasoning, better appreciate what we are uncertain of, and make good decisions. In the next section, we'll consider what evidence there is to support these claims, but before we get to that, we should briefly consider whether psychedelic philosophy has its own distinctive objects.

With respect to its objects, psychedelic philosophy occupies territory that overlaps with analytic philosophy on the one hand, and Buddhism and other mystical traditions on the other hand. As we have seen in the Bertrand Russell example, it can address the same questions using different means. However, there are important differences. From the perspective of analytic philosophy and science, psychedelic philosophy is different because it can include as its objects personal transformations that allow for entirely new forms of wisdom and well-being (Kaufman 2020). Such transformations include enlightenment or awakening, but also the kinds of psychological and psycho-spiritual insights we encountered in previous chapters.

From the perspective of Buddhism and other mystical traditions, psychedelic philosophy is different because it includes as its objects anything that is conducive to the various kinds of wisdom that we considered (*sophia, aporia*, and *phronēsis*). As such, the objects of psychedelic philosophy can include a great variety of things, such as insights about mathematics, solutions to engineering problems, insights about unknown unknowns about geopolitical events, how to run a better business, and so on. All these things can be conducive to the pursuit of wisdom.

Another way to put the same point is that what makes psychedelic philosophy distinctive is primarily its methods involving psychedelic experience and its ecumenical approach to philosophy in general, being open-minded as to what objects can be pursued.

11.6 Evidence

If the arguments in Sections 11.2 and 11.3 are correct, then it should be possible to observe empirically that the use of psychedelic methods can help us cultivate wisdom. As usual, the connection between philosophical ideas and the empirical world is often indirect, but it seems that in this case, we have some plausible and fairly clear connections. As Kekes 1983 puts it, 'wisdom ought also to show in the behaviour of the man who has it' (p. 281). In particular, we should see evidence that the practice of meditation and the consumption of psychedelics tend to do things such as: help us have insights that constitute, or reflect, increases in theoretical wisdom; help us become aware of our ignorance, thus enhancing our aporetic wisdom; and help us become more mindful and/or more experienced, thus enhancing our practical wisdom. Since we have already considered the evidence that psychedelics and meditation may promote creative insights (Chapter 8), which can enhance theoretical wisdom, I'll focus here on whether they can also enhance aporetic and practical wisdom.

We have two kinds of intervention (those involving psychedelics and meditation), which can pair up with two kinds of effect (improvements in *aporia* and *phronēsis*), so there are four possible connections to consider. Let's start with the connection between psychedelics and aporetic wisdom.

The anecdotal evidence that psychedelics make people more aware of what they don't know is compelling. Here is one example from a recent psilocybin study:

> I mean, it's really hard to describe. You just know, but you feel it in a very intense way because part of it is in the process of knowing, you realize that you didn't know before.
>
> Belser et al. 2017, p. 371

Such reports appear to be quite common for psychedelic trips and psychedelic-assisted psychotherapy. While such anecdotal reports abound, the objective evidence is largely lacking. To my knowledge, there has so far only been one study that systematically investigated the effects of a psychedelic on overconfidence. Lyons and Carhart-Harris 2018 found that psilocybin sessions resulted in depressed subjects making more accurate forecasts about their life events. Before the psilocybin sessions, the subjects had an overly pessimistic outlook: they were too confident that bad things would happen. After the sessions, the subjects became better calibrated in their forecasts. At this stage, we don't yet know whether or how this would generalize to healthy subjects. It could be that the psilocybin sessions resulted in a removal of bias or, alternatively, a general increase in optimism. If the latter, then psychedelics may increase overconfidence in healthy subjects— for example, those who are already too confident that *good* things will happen. However, given the anecdotal evidence just mentioned, it is entirely possible that overconfidence is reduced instead.

Another potential line of evidence that psychedelics reduce our overconfidence and increase *aporia* stems from the evidence that they ease our fear of death (e.g. Griffiths et al. 2016, Yaden et al. 2017). Indeed, Moreton et al. 2020 have proposed that this may be a key psychotherapeutic mechanism of psychedelics. The connection between this effect and aporetic wisdom may seem stretched at first, but consider Socrates' comment on the subject during his trial:

> To fear death, gentlemen, is no other than to think oneself wise when one is not, to think one knows what one does not know. No one knows whether death may

not be the greatest of all blessings for a man, yet men fear it as if they knew that it is the greatest of evils. And surely it is the most blameworthy ignorance to believe that one knows what one does not know. It is perhaps on this point and in this respect, gentlemen, that I differ from the majority of men, and if I were to claim that I am wiser than anyone in anything, it would be in this, that, as I have no adequate knowledge of things in the underworld, so I do not think I have.

Socrates, *Apologia*, 29a–b[41]

This could be part of what is going on when a psychedelic session eases one's fear of death—namely, the realization that there is little justification for one's prior conceptions, explicit or implicit, about death. To be sure, the change in attitude could stem from having an experience of unity, connectedness, and self-transcendence, and so the effect could be explained by an arrival of new beliefs about death rather than the removal of the old, overconfident ones. However, even if this is the case, it could still be argued that it is not the new beliefs doing the therapeutic work, but rather the sense of deep uncertainty—and grand wonder—that these experiences help uncover. For example, consider Roland Griffiths' summary of this effect of psilocybin:

There is something about the core of this experience that opens people up to the great mystery of what it is that we don't know. It is not that everybody comes out of it and says, 'Oh, now I believe in life after death'. That needn't be the case at all. But the psilocybin experience enables a sense of deeper meaning, and an understanding that in the largest frame everything is fine and that there is nothing to be fearful of. There is a buoyancy that comes of that which is quite remarkable. To see people who are so beaten down by this illness, and they start actually providing reassurance to the people who love them most, telling them 'it is all okay and there is no need to worry'—when a dying person can provide that type of clarity for their caretakers, even we researchers are left with a sense of wonder.

Griffiths, interviewed by Schiffman 2016

This sounds quite similar to how Socrates describes his wisdom. Moreover, Griffiths' description of how the transformed people provide reassurance to their caretakers bears a striking resemblance to Plato's depiction in *Phaedo* of Socrates providing reassurance to his friends during his final hours.[42] One important

---

[41] Cooper and Hutchinson 1997.

[42] One study involving a comparison of Buddhists and other religious and nonreligious groups found evidence in tension with this basic idea. Nichols et al. 2018 found that Monastic Tibetan Buddhists had a higher fear of death than other groups (Christians, Hindus, non-religious, etc.) despite having a stronger reported commitment to the doctrine of non-self. One potential explanation for this result that Nichols et al. consider is that the participants were not long-term meditators, and so while they may have eliminated a *philosophical* grasping of the self, it's possible they hadn't yet eliminated an

difference, though, is that for the patients, this is a sudden transformation brought about by the psilocybin sessions, whereas for Socrates, this was an enduring state he had cultivated through his practice of philosophy: 'those who practice philosophy in the right way are in training for dying and they fear death least of all men' (*Phaedo*, 67e).[43]

Another line of evidence stems from the neuroimaging studies that indicate that the brain increases in entropy (Carhart-Harris et al. 2014, Carhart-Harris 2018) during a psychedelic trip and that, from the perspective of predictive processing, the brain's higher-level priors ("beliefs") relax and allow for more uncertainty (Carhart-Harris and Friston 2019). We should be careful in making strong inferences from the results of neuroimaging studies to conclusions about what people experience and how their beliefs change. However, it does seem plausible that this evidence indicates that psychedelics help the mind to relax its usual overfitted patterns of thought, including those that would normally cause and reinforce a state of ignorance. In other words, by "freeing up" the mind, psychedelics may help people dissolve their ignorance and become aware of what they are truly uncertain of (among other things). From this perspective, it may be that overconfidence is a psychological disorder that results from overly rigid modes of cognition—much like depression, addiction, obsessive-compulsive disorder, etc.—that can be treated with psychedelics. A psychedelic trip, then, in the appropriate context and with careful measures in place, could be the magic wand that Kahneman would use to treat this most destructive of cognitive biases.

Next, let's turn to the connection between psychedelics and *phronēsis*. A lot of the enthusiasm about the psychedelic renaissance stems from the observation that people tend to make better decisions and live better lives as a result of their psychedelic sessions—particularly when psychedelics are used within in a psychotherapeutic context (there are, of course, plenty of exceptions outside of this context). The fact that psychedelics can promote well-being in a variety of ways suggests that people become more practically wise. The details of many of the anecdotal reports reinforce this point. For example, consider the following report from a psilocybin session:

> I remember thinking through, career wise, whether I should go do something more entrepreneurial and thinking that I really needed to do something like that in my life, and that I don't think I'd ever be fulfilled just doing what I did at that time. I've known I needed to make that change, but [my experience] helped to cement that a bit. And since then, it's been 8 or 9 months, but since then, I've moved in that direction and changed my career path. [...] I think [my

---

innate grasping of the self. If correct, this explanation would bolster the case for combining psychedelic methods (in this case, meditation) with analytic methods (in this case, studying doctrinal texts).

[43] Grube and Cooper 2002, p. 104.

experience] helped me to kind of push myself and force myself to make changes and make decisions that I was scared to, but that I knew would lead to happiness. Ultimately... it's kind of led me to lead a more fulfilling life down the road. I'm still kind of on that path, but I feel like I'm shifting in the right direction.

Zamaria 2016, p. 294

And here's another example, which we saw in Chapter 9, that highlights how the experience can facilitate access to knowledge of what is good for one:

I don't know if I really *learned*—it was more like letting back in stuff that I had blocked out?...I don't think I changed my values, just remembered more of them. Or just remembered to honour them more, or... *allow* them more.

Noorani et al. 2018, p. 759

In Chapter 9, I presented this example to demonstrate how psychedelics can enhance the memory aspect of one's mindfulness, and here we see how that contributes to *phronēsis* in a particular way—namely, awareness of what is good for one's self. This also lines up with Aristotle's explanation of *akrasia* (weakness of will) in Book VII of *Nicomachean Ethics*. Roughly speaking, Aristotle argued that it's not quite true that people do wrong things only out of ignorance (as Socrates thought), but rather it is because they lose the connection between their knowledge and their actions. Relatedly, there is reason to think that addiction can usefully be thought of as a form of *akrasia* (Heather 2020), which may speak to why psychedelics are so effective at treating it.

We've also already noted the evidence that psychedelics tend to promote increases in mindfulness.[44] Since mindfulness is an important part of *phronēsis*, it follows that psychedelics also tend to promote *phronēsis* (at least in this respect). The other component of *phronēsis* involves being experienced in life, and we've also already noted the evidence that psychedelics tend to promote increases in the core personality trait of openness to experience.[45] The natural thought, then, is that people will become more experienced than they otherwise would as they continue to move through life. Given the argument in Section 11.2 that *phronēsis* can be usefully approximated as mindfulness plus life experience, it seems quite plausible that psychedelics tend to promote *phronēsis* in these two respects. To be clear, the evidence in both cases involves the use of psychedelics in therapeutic—

[44] For example, see Thomas et al. 2013, Soler et al. 2016, 2018, Sampedro et al. 2017, Domínguez-Clavé et al. 2019, Smigielski et al. 2019, Uthaug et al. 2019, Mian et al. 2020, Uthaug et al. 2020, Davis et al. 2020, Madsen et al. 2020, Murphy-Beiner and Soar 2020, Oorsouw et al. 2022, and Søndergaard et al. 2022; and see Radakovic et al. 2022 for a meta-analysis.

[45] For example, see MacLean et al. 2011, Lebedev et al. 2016, Nour et al. 2017, Bouso et al. 2018, Erritzoe et al. 2018, Erritzoe et al. 2019, and Madsen et al. 2020. However, see also Griffiths et al. 2018, Schmid et al. 2018, Barrett et al. 2020, and Rocha et al. 2021 for less consistent findings.

or, at least, carefully controlled—contexts. So, there are surely situations in which psychedelics have the opposite effect. However, when used appropriately, there seems to be a positive relationship with *phronēsis*.

Let's now turn to the evidence concerning meditation, beginning again with aporetic wisdom.

The anecdotal evidence—or rather, the evidence from meditative traditions— also seems to indicate that the practice of meditation has a tendency to dissolve our ignorance by helping us see what we are uncertain of. Indeed, in the case of Zen, it is often said that a point of the practice is to bring forth doubt:

> In Zen practice, the essential point is to rouse doubt. What is this doubt? When you are born, for example, where do you come from? You cannot help but remain in doubt about this. When you die, where do you go? Again, you cannot help but remain in doubt. Since you cannot pierce this barrier of life and death, suddenly doubt will coalesce right before your eyes. Try to put it down, you cannot; try to push it away, you cannot. Eventually you will break through this doubt block and realize what a worthless notion life and death is—ha! As the old worthies said: 'Great doubt, great awakening; small doubt, small awakening; no doubt, no awakening'.
>
> Shore 2016, p. 10[46]

Again, this is similar to Socrates' point that a fear of death comes from the mistake of thinking one knows something when one does not.[47] It's worth noting that 'doubt' in this context may be better understood as *wonder* (Shore 2016), and so it is also worth noting Aristotle's famous comment about philosophy beginning in wonder and the philosophical value of myth:

> It is through wonder that men now begin and originally began to philosophize; wondering in the first place at obvious perplexities, and then by gradual progression raising questions about the greater matters too, e.g. about the changes of the moon and of the sun, about the stars and about the origin of the universe. Now he who wonders and is perplexed feels that he is ignorant (thus the myth-lover is in a sense a philosopher, since myths are composed of wonders) [...]
>
> Aristotle, *Metaphysics* 982b[48]

---

[46] Shore 2016.
[47] However, we should be careful not to focus too much on birth and death, as Shore writes: 'Once we open up, however, we realize that we don't really know **anything**—we don't even know where we really are right now. **Here** Great Doubt manifests. Otherwise you may be preoccupied only with the first and last moments of birth and death, or get lost in morbid notions of past or future lives, heaven and hell, and so on. Start where you actually are, with your present experience—not some concept or theory, or someone else's words or experience. Then you won't go astray'. (Emphasis in original).
[48] Tredennick 1989.

Doubt, or wonder, is also closely related to *shoshin*, or beginner's mind, which, roughly speaking, is the mindset that is open and clear of preconceptions about what is being perceived or contemplated by the mind (Suzuki 1970).

With respect to the scientific evidence, there is surprisingly little on the connection between meditation and aporetic wisdom. There is some evidence suggesting that meditation, similar to psychedelics, increases brain entropy (Vivot et al. 2020). This fits well with idea that various meditative practices aim to reduce our mental grasping and relax the grip of our hidden assumptions. Otherwise, the little evidence we have comes by way of mindfulness studies, which meditation is thought to promote. Lakey et al. 2007 found that mindfulness, as measured by MAAS, was negatively associated with overconfidence, as measured by individual calibration in a general knowledge task, among frequent gamblers. Kalafatoglu and Turgut 2017a found a negative relationship between mindfulness and *overplacement*, a particular form of overconfidence in which an individual overrates themselves as better than others in some respect (intelligence, driving ability, etc.). Kartelaia and Reb 2015 report an analysis of preliminary data indicating that mindfulness (as measured by MAAS) is negatively related to dispositional intolerance of uncertainty, which is likely a driver of overconfidence, and argue that mindfulness may help decision-makers become more aware of the uncertainty surrounding them. More generally, it has been proposed that intolerance of uncertainty underlies various psychological conditions, including major depressive, obsessive-compulsive, and generalized anxiety disorders (Boswell et al. 2013). This suggests that one way in which interventions involving meditation (and psychedelics) may help treat such conditions may involve the reduction of uncertainty intolerance. Indeed, some recent evidence indicates that mindfulness-based interventions can reduce the symptoms of such disorders and that these reductions are mediated by reductions of intolerance of uncertainty (Mathur et al. 2021 and Papenfuss et al. 2022).

Finally, let's consider the evidence concerning the connection between meditation and *phronēsis*.

Again, the anecdotal/traditional evidence is strong, since meditation is thought to cultivate mindfulness, which I've argued is an important component of *phronēsis*. There is also an even more direct argument here, which is that *phronēsis* concerns living well, and mindfulness is part of the Noble Eightfold Path (Chapter 9) for freeing one's self from *duhkha*—that is, suffering or dissatisfaction. In other words, mindfulness also concerns living well. There is also growing contemporary anecdotal evidence. For example:

> Many people only see the conscious mind and aren't aware of the benefits of connecting it to the subconscious. They believe that the way to accomplish more is to cram more into the conscious mind and make it work harder, but this is

often counterproductive. While it may seem counterintuitive, clearing your head can be the best way to make progress.

Knowing this, I now understand why creativity comes to me when I relax (like when I'm in the shower) and how meditation helps open this connection.

Dalio 2017, pp. 380–1

Indeed, as 'mindfulness' has entered the corporate world, there is increasing testimonial evidence of meditation helping people make better decisions.

There is also some scientific evidence in support of this. For example, we've noted the evidence that interventions involving meditation can enhance well-being in virtue of their psychotherapeutic effects (for reviews, see Wielgosz et al. 2019 and Heuschkel and Kuypers 2020). We've also seen the evidence that meditation improves various components of mindfulness, such as attention and awareness (Chapter 5) and memory recollection (Chapter 6), which are also components of *phronēsis*. Moreover, discussions of *phronēsis* often focus on its deliberative component, and so the evidence that meditation improves working memory (Chapter 6) suggests that it will also enhance this aspect of *phronēsis*. It should be noted, however, that we can't yet infer that meditation also enhances phronēsis by helping one develop life experience, since it isn't clear that meditation enhances openness (Section 11.2).

There are also now several studies that indicate that meditation and/or mindfulness are associated with better decision-making in a variety of ways. Kartelaia and Reb 2015 give a detailed review of the reasons why mindfulness is likely to lead to improved decision-making. Coming back to the study by Lakey et al. 2007, they explain their result that mindfulness correlated with reduced overconfidence (improved calibration) in a way that highlights the overlap between *phronēsis* and mindfulness:

[...] perhaps as a function of their heightened awareness and attention to present events and experiences, more mindful individuals displayed greater accuracy when answering general knowledge questions on the [Georgia Gambling Task]. Moreover, they exhibited better calibration between their confidence and accuracy (i.e., less overconfidence). [...] The fact that mindful individuals were more accurate suggests that mindfulness may inhibit distraction from intrusive thoughts, allowing for deeper processing of relevant stimuli. [...]

Lakey et al. 2007, p. 1707

Wenk-Sormaz 2005 found that 20 minutes of focused-attention meditation reduced habitual responding as measured by performance on the Stroop task and an atypical-word-production task. Chatzisarantis and Hagger 2007 found that dispositional mindfulness (MAAS) moderated the intention-behaviour gap in a leisure-time physical activity, such that more mindful individuals were more likely to align their behaviour with their intentions. Ruedy and Schweitzer 2010 found that mindfulness promotes ethical decision-making. Kiken and Shook 2011 found that 15 minutes of a mindfulness meditation intervention reduced the negative bias effect (the tendency to weigh negative information more heavily than positive information). Grégoire et al. 2012 found that mindfulness helps people set and fulfil self-concordant goals (see also Smyth et al. 2020), where self-concordance is the extent to which individuals' goals reflect their personal values and interests as opposed to internal or external pressures (Sheldon and Elliot 1999). In a study involving nuclear power plant operators, Zhang et al. 2013 found a positive effect of mindfulness on task performance that was moderated by task complexity. Hafenbrack et al. 2014 found that a mindfulness meditation intervention reduced the sunk cost bias, with Schmitzer-Torbert 2020 later finding a similar effect. Kalafatoğlu and Turgut 2017b found that mindfulness correlated with ethical behaviour. Raphiphatthana et al. 2018 found that mindfulness correlated with higher levels of grit (tenacity). And, finally, Battaglia et al. 2020 found that mindfulness correlates with the quality of legislative decision-making. As throughout the rest of this book, we should be cautious in drawing conclusions from this empirical work since the research is still nascent, but the evidence so far does seem to indicate that meditation and mindfulness are associated with good decision-making.

There is one final line of evidence that is particularly interesting. Libet et al. 1983 famously found evidence that we make decisions before we are aware of them. Although this result sparked controversy, especially in debates about free will (Dennett 1991, Mele 2014), the basic result has been replicated and extended several times (see Braun et al. 2021 for a recent meta-analysis). For example, Soon et al. 2008 found that predictive neural activity in the frontopolar cortex can exist up to 10 seconds before a decision appears in awareness. This also fits well with the fact that people are often unaware of what drives their decisions and are thus open to suboptimal influences on the decisions and even outright manipulation (Nisbett and Wilson 1977). However, Dreyfus 2011 (p. 53) argued that meditators should be more aware of their decisions and the processes that lead to them in comparison to non-meditators. Interestingly, Lush et al. 2016 found that meditators had an earlier awareness of their decision to act in comparison with non-meditators and especially with subjects that were highly hypnotizable. They also found that the degree to which subjects were hypnotizable correlated with delays in awareness. In fact, they found that, in some cases, highly hypnotizable subjects would report awareness of the decisions after they performed the *action* of the decision. Dienes et al. 2016 argue, based on these results and those of related studies, that mindfulness can be thought of as a form of *self-insight*, and hypnotizability as a form of *self-deception*. Their results support the idea that meditation improves self-knowledge or, at the very least, awareness of decisions and the early stages of decision processes. This doesn't entail that meditators therefore make better decisions. However, it does open up the possibility that meditators have greater opportunity to intervene on some of the suboptimal influences on their decision-making and therefore achieve a higher quality of deliberative capacity—thereby manifesting a core aspect of *phronēsis*.

11.7 Conclusion

At its core, philosophy is about how to live a good life, which is something that concerns us all. The activity of philosophy is directed at figuring out what makes for good thinking and decision-making and how we can best implement these practices in our lives. The ultimate goal is human flourishing across the full spectrum of human existence—and so philosophy, in its essence, concerns everything from the practical to the spiritual.

There are different approaches to doing philosophy. While this is an outdated way of speaking, science is essentially a form of philosophy and has historically been known as *natural philosophy*.[49] This book is mostly a project in *analytic philosophy*, but it has made extensive use of the outputs of science. It has also drawn inspiration from various other approaches to philosophy, especially Buddhist philosophy (and Zen). What makes these approaches distinct from one another is the different methods they tend to rely on and the aspects of wisdom they tend to focus on. Modern science focuses on knowledge about the natural world and relies heavily on statistical methods for generating that knowledge. Buddhist philosophy focuses on knowledge of the self (or non-self) and relies heavily on various methods of meditation. These two characterizations are broad brushstrokes and as such, they don't capture all of the details of these two approaches. However, they give us a good sense of the relevant differences. In this chapter, I've made the case for recognizing another kind of approach, with its own distinctive methods and aspects of focus, which I call *psychedelic philosophy*.

Although natural and analytic philosophy focus on different aspects of wisdom, both rely heavily on analytic methods. These are precise, language-based methods for sequential, conscious reasoning—methods such as logic, probability, decision theory, conceptual analysis, and so on. In contrast, psychedelic philosophy puts emphasis on methods that unlock the power of our unconscious thought processes. The defining characteristic of psychedelic methods is that they invoke mind-revealing experiences that help us become wiser. Whereas analytic methods help us with inferences, psychedelic methods help us have experiences that bring

---

[49] This construal of science may irk some readers but nothing of substance hangs on it. If one really wants to draw a distinction between the two, then instead of simply speaking of 'philosophy', we can speak of 'science and philosophy'.

our unconscious knowledge and processes into conscious awareness. These experiences can be powerful ways of achieving some of the same philosophical goals that we would normally rely on analytic methods for achieving. The difference is similar to that of using a CPU for a machine learning task versus using a GPU for the same task—both can do it, but the parallel processing of the GPU makes it superior for this kind of task.

However, although psychedelic methods are more powerful in this respect, they are not perfectly reliable, and need to be kept in check by our analytic methods. For example, insights that arise via the use of psychedelic methods can be false even though they may come attached with strong feelings of certainty. That means such insights need to be carefully examined for consistency and coherence with the rest of our knowledge (and perhaps especially our scientific knowledge). Moreover, as I argued, analytic methods can also be used to enhance the psychedelic ones. Therefore, the best overall approach to philosophy is one that integrates the methods of the various approaches.

12

Conclusion

A central thesis of this book is that we should disentangle our concept of a psychedelic experience from our methods for inducing such experiences, particularly those that involve the consumption of so-called psychedelic drugs. Following Osmond's 1957 introduction of the term 'psychedelic', I argued that we should understand a psychedelic experience as a *mind-revealing experience*. It is an experience in which one becomes aware of hidden parts or aspects of one's mind.

With this understanding in place, it is then an open question as to whether so-called psychedelic drugs tend to cause such experiences. It is also an open question as to whether these substances have other important effects on the mind, perhaps in addition to their psychedelic effects. This approach also allows us to consider whether there are other, and potentially better, ways of bringing about psychedelic experiences. In particular, I have argued that the practice of meditation is another reliable way of inducing psychedelic experiences. I have also discussed the typical similarities and differences between the psychedelic experiences induced by meditation and those induced by psychedelics, and their tendency to vary over time and with set and setting.

An important point of emphasis throughout the book is that these are contingent statements that could easily be false. For example, it is an empirical hypothesis that drugs such as psilocybin, mescaline, LSD, and DMT tend to cause mind-revealing experiences. As Carhart-Harris 2018 has pointed out, this hypothesis has never been systematically tested and it often remains a mere assumption in many discussions about psychedelic substances. One reason for this oversight is that the hypothesis is articulated in terms of the mind rather than in terms of behaviour or neurobiology, which are more amenable to empirical investigation. Another reason is that the hypothesis, as originally articulated by Osmond, is quite abstract. Left unpacked, it is not entirely clear how we can use the idea of a mind-revealing experience to understand the effects of psychedelics (or meditation) in any precise way.

One of the core goals of this book is to show that we can use the tools of analytic philosophy to make the hypothesis less abstract and connect it to other ideas that we have a better handle on—particularly those from cognitive science. The motivation behind this approach is that we need something like this to happen in order for us to develop a satisfactory understanding of the effects of psychedelics. At the moment, much of the basic research into psychedelics focuses on their neurocognitive effects and correlating them with subjective reports and ratings. Although some initial progress has been made that moves us beyond these correlations, this research is still in its early days. For example, the introduction of *entropy* to characterize the effects of psychedelics at the neurocognitive level has the potential to give us an explanatory bridge to the effects at the experiential level (Carhart-Harris et al. 2014). However, there is still much more work to be done along these lines. I have tried to help build the bridge by approaching the explanatory divide from the other direction: starting by analysing the effects at the experiential level, then thinking about how these can be explained at the neurocognitive level. In addition to bridging the divide from the experiential side, one advantage of this approach is that it has the potential to draw upon the wisdom of the mystical traditions and give us tools we can use to better navigate these experiences and integrate them effectively into our daily lives.

To demonstrate how we may connect the experiential level to the cognitive, I argued in Chapter 5 that we can use the cognitive faculty of *attention* to help bridge the explanatory divide. The outline of this argument went as follows. First, we have the hypothesis that psychedelics cause mind-revealing experiences, which are understood as certain kinds of *expansions of awareness*—that is, hidden parts or aspects of the unconscious are suddenly brought into the sphere of conscious experience. Second, we know that awareness and attention are intimately related with each other: attention helps bring things in and out of awareness, and it also affects our experience of them. Third, we have independent reason to think that meditation causes psychedelic experiences. Fourth, we know that the primary mechanism of action of meditation occurs via its effects on attention—briefly, meditation improves the allocation of our attentional resources. Putting all these ideas together, and completing the "triangle" (see Figure 12.1), it seems reasonable to infer, as a plausible hypothesis, that psychedelics must have some important effect on our attentional resources that we should try to understand.

While we do not yet have decisive empirical evidence on what that effect is, I proposed that it may be that psychedelics tend to release our attentional resources from their usual structures of automatic allocation, and thereby create a kind of *surplus* of attention. This surplus of attention is then shaped by one's set and setting, including one's ability to manage one's attention, and the general quality of a psychedelic trip will depend upon how one's attentional resources end up flowing. For example, attentional surplus could end up being yanked around chaotically and reactively, which appears to be typical of "bad" trips. However, it could also easily arrive at a more stable and non-reactive state, which appears to be characteristic of mystical experiences, with their equanimity and blissfulness. Where the attentional surplus lands determines the nature of the psychedelic experiences one may have during a psychedelic trip. For example, if it flows towards long-lost memories from childhood, then those memories may be sufficiently activated so that they appear in awareness. Similarly, if the surplus

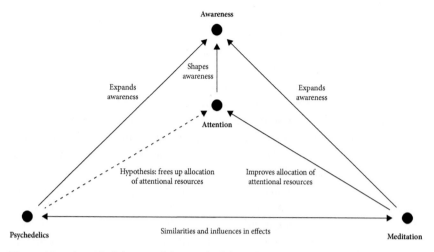

Figure 12.1 A unified theory of the psychedelic effects of psychedelics and meditation in terms of their impact on attentional resource allocation.

flows into the visual field, then visual sensations will appear more vividly—things will seem brighter and more colourful, for instance. I don't claim that all of the effects of psychedelics can be explained in these terms, but my proposal is that perhaps all of their *psychedelic* effects may be adequately explained in this way.

An important implication of this way of thinking is that some of the effects of psychedelics may not actually be psychedelic in nature (in the sense that they may not be mind-revealing). It may be the case that psychedelics increase the entropy of the brain, which is responsible for the freeing up of attentional resources— but *also* responsible for the various perceptual and cognitive distortions that psychedelics are known to cause, which may not involve the revelation of the mind. For example, the experience of synaesthesia may be the result of an increase in entropy—a kind of dissolving of the usual structures of experience—that is not psychedelic in any direct way.[1] This is just one potential example couched in terms of the entropic brain hypothesis. It is easy to imagine other examples that are just as plausible—for example, some effects that result from disrupted thalamic gating may be psychedelic, while others are not. However, I think it is plausible that many, if not all, of the mind-revealing effects of psychedelics come by way of the effects that these substances have on how our attentional resources are allocated.

How these effects on attention are accounted for at the neurocognitive level is a separate question, but there are plausible options on the table, including the

---

[1] It is possible that synaesthesia facilitates the experience of unconscious content that cannot easily be experienced by other means. However, even if this is the case, a synaesthetic experience itself may not be a psychedelic effect (unless we assume that there are synaesthetically fused representations stored deep in the mind).

relaxation of high-level priors (Carhart-Harris and Friston 2019) and disruptions to thalamic gating (Vollenweider and Geyer 2001, Preller et al. 2019) and attention-related networks such as the DMN, SN, and DAN (Stoliker et al. 2023). One challenge in investigating these hypotheses is that it is difficult to disentangle deteriorative effects on the *control* of attention from the effects that result from the release of attentional resources. Perhaps one way to make progress on this issue is to draw upon some of the research on attentional disorders. An intriguing line of thought in that literature that seems to be growing in popularity is that ADHD is not actually reflective of a deficit of attention but rather of an overabundance of attention that can potentially be managed and harnessed in productive, fulfilling ways (Hallowell and Ratey 2021). The deficit, then, in so far as there is one, is in the ability to *control* the overabundance of attentional resources. Perhaps not surprisingly, initial research indicates that mindfulness training programmes may be effective in treating ADHD (Xue et al. 2019, Cairncross and Miller 2020). Therefore, it is plausible that by better integrating the research on psychedelics, meditation, and ADHD, each will shed new light on the other.

Although the phenomenon of psychedelic experience is the primary focus of this book, another important idea of the book is that we can't properly understand the phenomenon until we also have a solid understanding of *mindfulness* and how the two phenomena relate to each other. Roughly speaking, a psychedelic experience is like suddenly finding your keys, and mindfulness is like not having lost them in the first place. Whereas a psychedelic experience involves the revelation of a hidden part of the mind, mindfulness involves that part of the mind not being hidden in the first place—it can be called into awareness at will. As I pointed out, there is more to mindfulness than this. Mindfulness also involves *retention*: being able to hold something in awareness indefinitely. Mindfulness also involves *clarity*: being able to see a part of the mind *as it is*, uncontaminated by our desires or conceptualizations. Finally, it can also be related to the here and now: your present thoughts and sensations, your present quality of consciousness, and even awareness itself.

I also proposed that the relationship between psychedelic experience and mindfulness can be put into sharper focus with the introduction of a third concept: that of a *psychecryptic state*. Whereas a psychedelic experience is a mind-revealing experience, a psychecryptic experience is a *mind-concealing* experience, and a psychedelic state is one in which some part or aspect of the mind is hidden from awareness. Just as some experiences are more psychedelic than others, because they reveal more of the mind, some states are more psychecryptic than others, because they conceal more of the mind. This gives us another way to characterize mindfulness: the more mindful one's default state is, the less psychecryptic it is.

Understanding this relationship can help us better understand the effects of psychedelic substances, which are commonly thought to bring about psychedelic experiences, and meditative practices, which are commonly thought to bring about improvements in mindfulness. Although it is common to think of the effects of psychedelics and meditation as neatly divided in this way, it turns out that there is a substantial overlap to them. As we have seen, there is growing evidence that psychedelics have a tendency to bring about long-lasting improvements in mindfulness. And there is also evidence that meditative practices regularly bring about psychedelic experiences, especially in the form of insights. For some readers, these points may come as a surprise: at first glance, it doesn't seem that the effects of psychedelics are anything like mindfulness, and the practice of meditation looks nothing like a psychedelic trip. However, when we understand the relationship between psychedelic experience and mindfulness, the overlap in effects becomes much less surprising. To use our analogy again: once you have finally found your keys (revelation), you know where they are, and it becomes easier for you to continue knowing where they are (mindfulness).

The conceptual framework of psychedelic space (which I introduced in Chapter 3) also makes it easier to understand the deep similarities and differences between the effects of psychedelics and meditation. As a "broad brushstroke" hypothesis, it seems that psychedelic substances tend to cause experiences that are very high in scope and novelty but low in clarity and duration. Conversely, it seems that meditative practices tend to cause experiences that are low in scope and novelty but high in clarity and duration. However, as I argued in Chapter 4, we need to be very careful with such hypotheses. As is well known, the qualities of a psychedelic experience depend heavily on its set and setting, irrespective of what intervention is used to bring it about. For example, the experiences during a psychedelic trip of someone who is very mindful and at peace with themselves are going to be quite different from the experiences of someone struggling with severe trauma at a silent meditation retreat. Also, in some cases, one can use mindfulness or surrogates for mindfulness to intervene on the experiences one has during a psychedelic trip to make them more psychedelic (e.g. by increasing their clarity and duration). However, in many cases, particularly high-dose psychedelic trips, this may be practically impossible since the release of attentional resources will outstrip one's ability to manage them. While such experiences may be experienced as difficult—and often referred to as "bad" trips—they can also be of incredible value to the individual in question, and clear the way for new levels of mindfulness and psychedelic experiences. Nevertheless, with these qualifications in mind, we can see how there may be some rough tendencies in the qualities of experiences brought about by different methods. The framework of psychedelic space gives us a set of useful, and easy-to-use, conceptual tools for thinking about these differences.

Another point of the book that highlights the importance of the connection between psychedelic experience and mindfulness concerns the reason why psychedelics can have such profound effects on well-being. In Chapter 9, I argued that one potential explanation for these benefits is that the psychedelic experiences that psychedelics typically induce have two features that involve improvements in mindfulness. The first feature is the one I mentioned earlier: there is growing evidence that psychedelic trips, when embedded in appropriate contexts, have a tendency to bring about long-lasting increases in mindfulness. The second feature is that psychedelic experiences themselves are approximations to temporary increases in mindfulness, and some of them can be very good approximations. Putting these two features together, we get the following explanation (and prediction): a psychedelic trip is conducive to well-being to the degree to which it results in long-lasting increases in mindfulness or involves experiences that approximate temporary increases in mindfulness.

This explanation obviously relies on there being a positive relationship between mindfulness and well-being. As discussed in Chapter 9, the evidence for such a relationship is accumulating—although more research needs to be done (and substantial methodological improvements need to be made). Also, there are good theoretical reasons to think there is this connection. From the perspective of Buddhism, mindfulness is an indispensable component of the Noble Eightfold Path, which leads one away from *dhukka* (suffering/unsatisfactoriness). Given my analysis of mindfulness, there is also a connection that we can explain in terms that are familiar to cognitive science: all else being equal, more mindfulness entails a variety of improvements to cognitive functioning that are good for well-being. For example, increased mindfulness should improve memory encoding and retrieval by improving awareness of the present moment and the ability to recollect events from the past. Learning and being able to apply what one has learned are obviously crucial skills for living a good life. Mindfulness should also improve performance related to working memory, by improving one's ability to hold parts or aspects of the mind in awareness indefinitely and engaging with their true form (unclouded by one's beliefs and desires, for instance). Working memory performance is crucial for good planning and decision-making, which are indispensable for living well. Although we should be wary of reducing the value of mindfulness exclusively to such practical benefits, they nonetheless exist, and can help us explain many of the observed benefits of psychedelics and meditation.

If we're willing to move away from purely psychological effects and more towards the psycho-spiritual end of the spectrum, we can also explain some of the more profound benefits of psychedelics and meditation. For example, although there is much debate as to whether anything such as a *self* exists, there is fairly widespread agreement that the practice of meditation and certain kinds of experiences with psychedelics can teach us something profoundly important about the self. Indeed, the literature on psychedelic-assisted psychotherapy appears to indicate that acquiring fresh insights about the self is of tremendous benefit to well-being. Whatever it is about the self that is revealed in these experiences, if we assume it involves some part or aspect of the mind, then it follows that developing mindfulness should help us experience this truth.

Although I think the connection between psychedelic experience and mindfulness is vital for understanding the benefits of psychedelics (and meditation), I am not committed to the view that all of the benefits can be explained in these terms. As before, other explanations are available that are plausible and complementary to this mindfulness-based explanation. Two such explanations involve the hypotheses that (i) psychedelics temporarily increase neuroplasticity, and (ii) psychedelics have long-term anti-inflammatory effects. I think there is potential for these explanations to be eventually unified under a common framework, but it is entirely possible that a piecemeal approach is warranted.

As I mentioned earlier, one of the central goals of this book has been to use the tools of analytic philosophy to help develop our understanding of psychedelic experience. Mystical experiences constitute the ultimate test for this sort of approach. As I argued in Chapter 10, mystical experience presents a kind of *singularity* for analytic philosophy. It is tempting to shoehorn mystical experience into the framework of analytic philosophy, by trying to argue for some sort of theory that best systematizes the various descriptions of the experience that mystics have given over the centuries. Given the importance of the *ineffability* that many mystics attribute to the experience, I argued that we shouldn't take this shoehorning approach. If we wish to truly understand mystical experience, we have to tackle it head on—that is, not as scholars of mysticism, but by engaging with it directly. Nevertheless, I think there is a way for us to use the tools of analytic philosophy to help us do this. We have well-developed theories of uncertainty (such as Bayesianism), and when we look closer at how they work in the extreme case of modelling maximal uncertainty, they manifest conceptual issues that are remarkably similar to those of mystical experiences. Although we need to be careful to not accidentally give a theory of mystical experience in the process, I think we can use this insight to point in the direction of the singularity. By engaging with ineffability and its deep uncertainty, and by contemplating these conceptual issues, I think there is a way for us to understand mystical experiences.

In Chapter 11, I flipped the central goal of the book around: I argued that we can use psychedelic experiences to help us do philosophy (including analytic philosophy). We can think of this as a transition from philosophy of psychedelics (and meditation) to what I called *psychedelic philosophy*. Certainly, a full and careful discussion of this idea requires the space of another book. However, I've hoped to put an initial brushstroke on this particular canvas. As discussed in that chapter, I take the ultimate goal of philosophy to be the pursuit of wisdom (even though this may not be apparent in much of the day-to-day activity of contemporary philosophy). I argued that we can use psychedelic experiences effectively to help us in that pursuit. Again, mindfulness played a key role in this argument. In short, it is best to be mindful, but this is difficult and takes time to develop. In contrast, psychedelic experiences can be easier to have, they can be good immediate approximations to mindfulness, and they can help us develop mindfulness in the long run. Because of this, I argued that our ability to do philosophy can be dramatically improved if we incorporate psychedelic methods into this discipline.

Chapter 11 focused on how we can use psychedelic experiences to pursue wisdom in ways that should be recognizable to any scientist, analytic philosopher, or, indeed, anyone with a naturalistic, "no nonsense" worldview. For example, psychedelic experiences can help us attain insights about important truths (theoretical wisdom), they can help release us from the bondage of our ignorance of our ignorance (aporetic wisdom), and they can help us make better decisions (practical wisdom). These forms of wisdom are certainly valuable and worth pursuing, but it was actually in Chapters 9 and 10 that we encountered the ultimate form of wisdom that psychedelic experiences can help us attain.

Although this form of wisdom is ineffable, we were able to circle around it a few times and get a sense of its character. It has something to do with the true nature of one's self, it is intimately related to our well-being, and it is something that can be revealed in a psychedelic experience but also be fully present in everyday life. Many authors have also attempted to say definitively what this wisdom is: an awareness of the oneness of everything, the realization that there is no self, the revelation of a true Self, a union or communion with God, and so on. There may be some truth in each of these statements, but I think the real wisdom is in not clinging to any of them—no matter how appealing they may seem. The trick is to let yourself not know.

Bibliography

Aday, J. S., J. R. Wood, E. K. Bloesch, and C. C. Davoli (2021). Psychedelic drugs and perception: a narrative review of the first era of research. *Reviews in the Neurosciences 32*(5), 559–71.

Agin-Liebes, G., T. F. Haas, R. Lancelotta, M. V. Uthaug, J. G. Ramaekers, and A. K. Davis (2021). Naturalistic use of mescaline is associated with self-reported psychiatric improvements and enduring positive life changes. *ACS Pharmacology & Translational Science 4*(2), 543–52.

Alais, D., J. J. v. Boxtel, A. Parker, and R. v. Ee (2010, 5). Attending to auditory signals slows visual alternations in binocular rivalry. *Vision Research 50*(10), 929–35.

Albahari, M. (2002). Against no-Ātman theories of Anattā. *Asian Philosophy 12*(1), 5–20.

Albahari, M. (2006). *Analytical Buddhism: The Two-Tiered Illusion of the Self.* New York: Palgrave Macmillan.

Albahari, M. (2019). The mystic and the metaphysician. *Journal of Consciousness Studies 26*(7–8), 12–36.

Alberts, H. J. E. M., H. Otgaar, and J. Kalagi (2017). Minding the source: the impact of mindfulness on source monitoring. *Legal and Criminological Psychology 22*(2), 302–13.

Ames, R. and D. Hall (2002). *Dao De Jing: A Philosophical Translation.* New York: Ballantine Books.

Anderson, B. (2011). There is no such thing as attention. *Frontiers in Psychology 2*, 246.

Anderson, J. R. (2007). *How Can the Human Mind Occur in the Physical Universe?* Oxford: Oxford University Press.

Andonovski, N. (2020). Memory as triage: facing up to the hard question of memory. *Review of Philosophy and Psychology 12*(2), 227–56.

Antinori, A., O. L. Carter, and L. D. Smillie (2017). Seeing it both ways: openness to experience and binocular rivalry suppression. *Journal of Research in Personality 68*, 15–22.

Anālayo, B. (2004). *Satipatthana: The Direct Path to Realization.* Cambridge: Windhorse Publications.

Anālayo, B. (2019). The insight knowledge of fear and adverse effects of mindfulness practices. *Mindfulness 10*(10), 2172–85.

Aqil, M. and L. Roseman (2023). More than meets the eye: the role of sensory dimensions in psychedelic brain dynamics, experience, and therapeutics. *Neuropharmacology, 223*.

Araujo, D. B. d., S. Ribeiro, G. A. Cecchi, F. M. Carvalho, T. A. Sanchez, J. P. Pinto, B. S. d. Martinis, J. A. Crippa, J. E. C. Hallak, and A. C. Santos (2012). Seeing with the eyes shut: neural basis of enhanced imagery following Ayahuasca ingestion. *Human Brain Mapping 33*(11), 2550–60.

Argento, E., R. Capler, G. Thomas, P. Lucas, and K. W. Tupper (2019). Exploring ayahuasca-assisted therapy for addiction: a qualitative analysis of preliminary findings among an Indigenous community in Canada. *Drug and Alcohol Review 38*(7), 781–9.

Audi, R. (2001). A Kantian intuitionism. *Mind 110*(439), 601–35.

Baars, B. J. (1993). *A Cognitive Theory of Consciousness.* Cambridge: Cambridge University Press.

Baas, M., B. Nevicka, and F. S. T. Velden (2014). Specific mindfulness skills differentially predict creative performance. *Personality and Social Psychology Bulletin 40*(9), 1092–106.

Badiner, A., A. Grey, and S. Batchelor (2015). *Zig Zag Zen: Buddhism and Psychedelics*. Santa Fe and London: Synergetic Press.

Baer, R., C. Crane, E. Miller, and W. Kuyken (2019). Doing no harm in mindfulness-based programs: conceptual issues and empirical findings. *Clinical Psychology Review 71*, 101–14.

Baer, R. A., G. T. Smith, and K. B. Allen (2004). Assessment of mindfulness by self-report. *Assessment 11*(3), 191–206.

Baggott, M. J. (2015). Psychedelics and creativity: a review of the quantitative literature. *PeerJ PrePrints 3*, e1202v1.

Baird, B., B. A. Riedner, M. Boly, R. J. Davidson, and G. Tononi (2019). Increased lucid dream frequency in long-term meditators but not following mindfulness-based stress reduction training. *Psychology of Consciousness: Theory, Research, and Practice 6*(1), 40–54.

Baker, T. I. and J. D. Cowan (2009). Spontaneous pattern formation and pinning in the primary visual cortex. *Journal of Physiology-Paris 103*(1–2), 52–68.

Ball, C. T. and J. C. Little (2006). A comparison of involuntary autobiographical memory retrievals. *Applied Cognitive Psychology 20*(9), 1167–79.

Baltes, P. (2004). *Wisdom as Orchestration of Mind and Virtue*. Unpublished book manuscript.

Banicki, K. (2009). The Berlin wisdom paradigm: a conceptual analysis of a psychological approach to wisdom. *History & Philosophy of Psychology 11*(2), 25–36.

Baranski, M. and C. A. Was (2017). Mindfulness meditation may not increase false-memory and may instead protect from false-memory susceptibility. *Mindfulness 8*(6), 1569–79.

Baranski, M. F. S. and C. A. Was (2018). A more rigorous examination of the effects of mindfulness meditation on working memory capacity. *Journal of Cognitive Enhancement 2*(3), 225–39.

Barner, C. P. and R. W. Barner (2011). Mindfulness, openness to experience, and transformational learning. In C. Hoare (ed.), *The Oxford Handbook of Reciprocal Adult Development and Learning*, pp. 347–62. New York: Oxford University Press.

Barrett, D. (1993). The 'committee of sleep': a study of dream incubation for problem solving. *Dreaming 3*(2), 115–22.

Barrett, D. (2001). *The Committee of Sleep: How Artists, Scientists, and Athletes Use Dreams for Creative Problem Solving—and How You Can Too*. New York: Crown/Random House.

Barrett, D. (2017). Dreams and creative problem-solving. *Annals of the New York Academy of Sciences 1406*(1), 64–7.

Barrett, F. S., M. K. Doss, N. D. Sepeda, J. J. Pekar, and R. R. Griffiths (2020). Emotions and brain function are altered up to one month after a single high dose of psilocybin. *Scientific Reports 10*(1), 2214.

Bartha, P. (2004). Countable additivity and the de Finetti lottery. *British Journal for the Philosophy of Science 55*(2), 301–21.

Barzykowski, K. and A. Niedźwieńska (2018). Involuntary autobiographical memories are relatively more often reported during high cognitive load tasks. *Acta Psychologica 182*, 119–28.

Barzykowski, K., A. Niedźwieńska, and G. Mazzoni (2019). How intention to retrieve a memory and expectation that a memory will come to mind influence the retrieval of autobiographical memories. *Consciousness and Cognition 72*, 31–48.

Barzykowski, K. and S. R. Staugaard (2016). Does retrieval intentionality really matter? Similarities and differences between involuntary memories and directly and generatively retrieved voluntary memories. *British Journal of Psychology 107*(3), 519–36.

Barzykowski, K. and S. R. Staugaard (2018). How intention and monitoring your thoughts influence characteristics of autobiographical memories. *British Journal of Psychology 109*(2), 321–40.

Basso, J. C., A. McHale, V. Ende, D. J. Oberlin, and W. A. Suzuki (2019). Brief, daily meditation enhances attention, memory, mood, and emotional regulation in non-experienced meditators. *Behavioural Brain Research 356*, 208–20.

Baston, R. and G. Vosgerau (2016). Implicit attitudes and implicit prejudices. *Philosophical Psychology 29*(6), 1–15.

Battaglia, A., D. Bilimoria, K. J. Lyytinen, E. Doherty-Sil, and K. Buse (2020). Does mindful decision-making matter? A study of legislators' decision-making. In *The Tenth International Conference on Engaged Management Scholarship*, SSRN Electronic Journal.

Baumgartner, G. (1960). Indirekte Größenbestimmung der rezeptiven Felder der Retina beim Menschen Mittels der Hermannschen Gittertauschung. *Pflugers Archiv für die gesamte Physiologie 272*, 21–2.

Beall, J. and G. Restall (2006). *Logical Pluralism*. Oxford: Clarendon Press.

Bellgrove, M. A., R. Hester, and H. Garavan (2004). The functional neuroanatomical correlates of response variability: evidence from a response inhibition task. *Neuropsychologia 42*(14), 1910–16.

Belser, A. B., G. Agin-Liebes, T. C. Swift, S. Terrana, N. Devenot, H. L. Friedman, J. Guss, A. Bossis, and S. Ross (2017). Patient experiences of psilocybin-assisted psychotherapy: an interpretative phenomenological analysis. *Journal of Humanistic Psychology 57*(4), 354–88.

Berens, S. C., B. A. Richards, and A. J. Horner (2020). Dissociating memory accessibility and precision in forgetting. *Nature Human Behaviour 4*(8), 866–77.

Berntsen, D. (1996). Involuntary autobiographical memories. *Applied Cognitive Psychology 10*, 435–54.

Berntsen, D. (1998). Voluntary and involuntary access to autobiographical memory. *Memory 6*(2), 113–41.

Berridge, K. and P. Winkielman (2003). What is an unconscious emotion? (The case for unconscious 'liking'). *Cognition & Emotion 17*(2), 181–211.

Billock, V. A. and B. H. Tsou (2012, 7). Elementary visual hallucinations and their relationships to neural pattern-forming mechanisms. *Psychological Bulletin 138*(4), 744.

Bird, C. M. and N. Burgess (2008). The hippocampus and memory: insights from spatial processing. *Nature Reviews Neuroscience 9*(3), 182–94.

Bisbee, C. C., P. Bisbee, E. Dyck, J. Sexton, and J. W. Spisak (2018). *Psychedelic Prophets: The Letters of Aldous Huxley and Humphry Osmond*. Montreal: McGill-Queen's University Press.

Block, N. (1995). On a confusion about a function of consciousness. *Behavioral and Brain Sciences 18*(2), 227–47.

Block, N. (2010). Attention and mental paint. *Philosophical Issues 20*(1), 23–63.

Blood, B. P. (1874). *The Anaesthetic Revelation and the Gist of Philosophy*. Amsterdam, NY

Boccia, M., L. Piccardi, and P. Guariglia (2015). The Meditative mind: a comprehensive meta-analysis of MRI studies. *BioMed Research International 2015*, 1–11.

Boden, M. A. (1990). *The Creative Mind: Myths and Mechanisms*. London: Psychology Press.

Bodhi, B. (2000). *Samyutta Nikāya*. Somerville, MA: Wisdom Publications.

Bodhi, B. (2011). What does mindfulness really mean? A canonical perspective. *Contemporary Buddhism 12*(1), 19–39.

Boer, J. d., J. Hale, and J. Chanton (2001). New evidence for the geological origins of the ancient Delphic oracle (Greece). *Geology 29*(8), 707–10.

Boswell, J. F., J. Thompson-Hollands, T. J. Farchione, and D. H. Barlow (2013). Intolerance of uncertainty: a common factor in the treatment of emotional disorders. *Journal of Clinical Psychology 69*(6), 630–45.

Bouso, J. C., R. G. d. Santos, M. A. Alcázar-Córcoles, and J. E. Hallak (2018). Serotonergic psychedelics and personality: a systematic review of contemporary research. *Neuroscience & Biobehavioral Reviews 87*, 118–32.

Bouyer, L. (1980). Mysticism: an essay on the history of the word. In R. Woods (ed.), *Understanding Mysticism*, pp. 42–56. Garden City, NJ: Image Books.

Bowden, E. M., M. Jung-Beeman, J. Fleck, and J. Kounios (2005). New approaches to demystifying insight. *Trends in Cognitive Sciences 9*(7), 322–8.

Bower, J. E. and M. R. Irwin (2015). Mind-body therapies and control of inflammatory biology: a descriptive review. *Brain, Behavior, and Immunity 51*, 1–11.

Bowers, J. S. and C. J. Davis (2012). Bayesian just-so stories in psychology and neuroscience. *Psychological Bulletin 138*(3), 389–414.

Bowers, K. S., G. Regehr, C. Balthazard, and K. Parker (1990). Intuition in the context of discovery. *Cognitive Psychology 22*(1), 72–110.

Boys-Stones, G., J. M. Dillon, and L. P. Gerson (2018). *Plotinus: The Enneads*. Cambridge: Cambridge University Press.

Braak, A. v. d. (2011). *Nietzsche and Zen: Self-Overcoming without a Self*. Plymouth: Lexington Books.

Braun, M. N., J. Wessler, and M. Friese (2021). A meta-analysis of Libet-style experiments. *Neuroscience and Biobehavioral Reviews 128*, 182–98.

Breeksema, J. J. and M. v. Elk (2021). Working with weirdness: a response to 'Moving Past Mysticism in Psychedelic Science'. *ACS Pharmacology & Translational Science 4*(4), 1471–4.

Breeksema, J. J., A. R. Niemeijer, E. Krediet, E. Vermetten, and R. A. Schoevers (2020). Psychedelic treatments for psychiatric disorders: a systematic review and thematic synthesis of patient experiences in qualitative studies. *CNS Drugs 34*(9), 925–46.

Bremmer, J. N. (1986). *Interpretations of Greek Mythology*. London: Routledge.

Bressloff, P. C., J. D. Cowan, M. Golubitsky, P. J. Thomas, and M. C. Wiener (2002). What geometric visual hallucinations tell us about the visual cortex. *Neural Computation 14*(3), 473–91.

Brewer, J. A., P. D. Worhunsky, J. R. Gray, Y.-Y. Tang, J. Weber, and H. Kober (2011). Meditation experience is associated with differences in default mode network activity and connectivity. *Proceedings of the National Academy of Sciences 108*(50), 20254–9.

Brigard, F. D. and J. Prinz (2010). Attention and consciousness. *Wiley Interdisciplinary Reviews: Cognitive Science 1*(1), 51–9.

Brown, K. W., R. J. Goodman, R. M. Ryan, and B. Anālayo (2016). Mindfulness enhances episodic memory performance: evidence from a multimethod investigation. *PLOS One 11*(4), e0153309.

Brown, K. W. and R. M. Ryan (2003). The benefits of being present: mindfulness and its role in psychological well-being. *Journal of Personality and Social Psychology 84*(4), 822–48.

Brown, R. and J. Kulik (1977). Flashbulb memories. *Cognition 5*(1), 73–99.

Bruya, B. and Y.-Y. Tang (2018). Is attention really effort? Revisiting Daniel Kahneman's influential 1973 book *Attention and Effort*. *Frontiers in Psychology 9*, 1133.

Buckner, C. and J. Garson (2018). Connectionism and post-connectionist models. In M. Sprevak and M. Colombo (eds.), *The Routledge Handbook of the Computational Mind*. London: Routledge.

Buddharakkhita, A. (1996). Maggavagga: The Path, *Dhammapada*, url: https://www.accesstoinsight.org/tipitaka/kn/dhp/dhp.20.budd.html

Buric, I., M. Farias, J. Jong, C. Mee, and I. A. Brazil (2017). What is the molecular signature of mind-body interventions? A systematic review of gene expression changes induced by meditation and related practices. *Frontiers in Immunology 8*, 670.

Burkert, W. (1985). *Greek Religion*. Cambridge, MA: Harvard University Press.

Busch, A. K. and W. C. Johnson (1950). L.S.D. 25 as an aid in psychotherapy: preliminary report of a new drug. *Diseases of the Nervous System 11*(8), 241–3.

Byrne, A. (2012). Hmm... Hill on the paradox of pain. *Philosophical Studies 161*(3), 489–96.

Cai, D. J., S. A. Mednick, E. M. Harrison, J. C. Kanady, and S. C. Mednick (2009). REM, not incubation, improves creativity by priming associative networks. *Proceedings of the National Academy of Sciences 106*(25), 10130–4.

Cairncross, M. and C. J. Miller (2020). The effectiveness of mindfulness-based therapies for ADHD: a meta-analytic review. *Journal of Attention Disorders 24*(5), 627–43.

Calvillo, D. P., A. N. Flores, and L. C. Gonzales (2018). A brief mindfulness induction after encoding decreases false recognition in the Deese-Roediger-McDermott paradigm. *Psychology of Consciousness: Theory, Research, and Practice 5*(2), 131–9.

Carbonaro, T. M., M. W. Johnson, E. Hurwitz, and R. R. Griffiths (2017). Double-blind comparison of the two hallucinogens psilocybin and dextromethorphan: similarities and differences in subjective experiences. *Psychopharmacology 235*(2), 521–34.

Carhart-Harris, R. (2007). Waves of the unconscious: the neurophysiology of dreamlike phenomena and its implications for the psychodynamic model of the mind. *Neuropsychoanalysis 9*(2), 183–211.

Carhart-Harris, R. and D. Nutt (2014). Was it a vision or a waking dream? *Frontiers in Psychology 5*, 255.

Carhart-Harris, R. L. (2018). The entropic brain—revisited. *Neuropharmacology 142*, 167–78.

Carhart-Harris, R. L. (2019). How do psychedelics work? *Current Opinion in Psychiatry 32*(1), 16–21.

Carhart-Harris, R. L., D. Erritzoe, E. Haijen, M. Kaelen, and R. Watts (2018). Psychedelics and connectedness. *Psychopharmacology 235*(2), 547–50.

Carhart-Harris, R. L., D. Erritzoe, T. Williams, J. M. Stone, L. J. Reed, A. Colasanti, R. J. Tyacke, R. Leech, A. L. Malizia, K. Murphy, P. Hobden, J. Evans, A. Feilding, R. G. Wise, and D. J. Nutt (2012). Neural correlates of the psychedelic state as determined by fMRI studies with psilocybin. *Proceedings of the National Academy of Sciences 109*(6), 2138–43.

Carhart-Harris, R. L. and K. J. Friston (2010). The default-mode, ego-functions and free-energy: a neurobiological account of Freudian ideas. *Brain 133*(4), 1265–83.

Carhart-Harris, R. L. and K. J. Friston (2019). REBUS and the anarchic brain: toward a unified model of the brain action of psychedelics. *Pharmacological Reviews 71*(3), 316–44.

Carhart-Harris, R. L., R. Leech, P. J. Hellyer, M. Shanahan, A. Feilding, E. Tagliazucchi, D. R. Chialvo, and D. Nutt (2014). The entropic brain: a theory of conscious states informed by neuroimaging research with psychedelic drugs. *Frontiers in Human Neuroscience 8*, 20.

Carhart-Harris, R. L., R. Leech, T. M. Williams, D. Erritzoe, N. Abbasi, T. Bargiotas, P. Hobden, D. J. Sharp, J. Evans, A. Feilding, R. G. Wise, and D. J. Nutt (2012). Implications for psychedelic-assisted psychotherapy: functional magnetic resonance imaging study with psilocybin. *British Journal of Psychiatry 200*(3), 238–44.

Carhart-Harris, R. L., S. Muthukumaraswamy, L. Roseman, M. Kaelen, W. Droog, K. Murphy, E. Tagliazucchi, E. E. Schenberg, T. Nest, C. Orban, R. Leech, L. T. Williams, T. M. Williams, M. Bolstridge, B. Sessa, J. McGonigle, M. I. Sereno, D. Nichols, P. J. Hellyer, P. Hobden, J. Evans, K. D. Singh, R. G. Wise, H. V. Curran, A. Feilding, and D. J. Nutt (2016). Neural correlates of the LSD experience revealed by multimodal neuroimaging. *Proceedings of the National Academy of Sciences of the United States of America 113*(17), 4853–8.

Carlson, V. R. (1958). Effect of lysergic acid diethylamide (LSD-25) on the absolute visual threshold. *Journal of Comparative and Physiological Psychology 51*(5), 528–31.

Carnap, R. (1951). *The Nature and Application of Inductive Logic: Consisting of Six Sections from Logical Foundations of Probability*. Chicago: University of Chicago Press.

Carrasco, M. and A. Barbot (2019). Spatial attention alters visual appearance. *Current Opinion in Psychology 29*, 56–64.

Carrasco, M., S. Ling, and S. Read (2004). Attention alters appearance. *Nature Neuroscience 7*(3), nn1194.

Carruthers, L., R. MacLean, and A. Willis (2018). The relationship between creativity and attention in adults. *Creativity Research Journal 30*(4), 370–9.

Carruthers, P. (2011). *The Opacity of Mind: An Integrative Theory of Self-Knowledge*. Oxford: Oxford University Press.

Carter, O., D. Presti, C. Callistemon, Y. Ungerer, G. Liu, and J. Pettigrew (2005). Meditation alters perceptual rivalry in Tibetan Buddhist monks. *Current Biology 15*(11), R412–R413.

Carter, O. L., D. C. Burr, J. D. Pettigrew, G. M. Wallis, F. Hasler, and F. X. Vollenweider (2005). Using psilocybin to investigate the relationship between attention, working memory, and the serotonin 1A and 2A receptors. *Journal of Cognitive Neuroscience 17*(10), 1497–1508.

Carter, O. L., F. Hasler, J. D. Pettigrew, G. M. Wallis, G. B. Liu, and F. X. Vollenweider (2007). Psilocybin links binocular rivalry switch rate to attention and subjective arousal levels in humans. *Psychopharmacology 195*(3), 415–24.

Carter, O. L., J. D. Pettigrew, D. C. Burr, D. Alais, F. Hasler, and F. X. Vollenweider (2004). Psilocybin impairs high-level but not low-level motion perception. *NeuroReport 15*(12), 1947–51.

Carter, O. L., J. D. Pettigrew, F. Hasler, G. M. Wallis, G. B. Liu, D. Hell, and F. X. Vollenweider (2005). Modulating the rate and rhythmicity of perceptual rivalry alternations with the mixed 5-HT2A and 5-HT1A agonist psilocybin. *Neuropsychopharmacology 30*(6), 1300621.

Cebolla, A., M. Demarzo, P. Martins, J. Soler, and J. Garcia-Campayo (2017). Unwanted effects: is there a negative side of meditation? A multicentre survey. *PLOS One 12*(9), e0183137.

Chalmers, D. (1996). *The Conscious Mind*. Oxford: Oxford University Press.

Chan, E. Y. and Y. Wang (2019). Mindfulness changes construal level: an experimental investigation. *Journal of Experimental Psychology: General 148*(9), 1656–64.

Chatzisarantis, N. L. D. and M. S. Hagger (2007). Mindfulness and the intention-behavior relationship within the theory of planned behavior. *Personality and Social Psychology Bulletin 33*(5), 663–76.

Cheng, J. T., C. Anderson, E. R. Tenney, S. Brion, D. A. Moore, and J. M. Logg (2020). The social transmission of overconfidence. *Journal of Experimental Psychology: General 150*(1), 157–86.

Christoff, K., A. M. Gordon, J. Smallwood, R. Smith, and J. W. Schooler (2009). Experience sampling during fMRI reveals default network and executive system contributions to mind wandering. *Proceedings of the National Academy of Sciences of the United States of America 106*(21), 8719–24.

Chun, M. M., J. D. Golomb, and N. B. Turk-Browne (2011). A taxonomy of external and internal attention. *Annual Review of Psychology 62*(1), 73–101.

Clancy, S. A., D. L. Schacter, R. J. McNally, and R. K. Pitman (2000). False recognition in women reporting recovered memories of sexual abuse. *Psychological Science 11*(1), 26–31.

Clark, A. (2015). *Surfing Uncertainty: Prediction, Action, and the Embodied Mind*. Oxford: Oxford University Press.

Clark, M. (2017). *The Tawny One: Soma, Haoma and Ayahuasca*. London: Muswell Hill Press.

Clark, M. (2019). Soma and haoma: ayahuasca analogues from the Late Bronze Age. *Journal of Psychedelic Studies 3*(2), 104–16.

Cleary, J. and T. F. Cleary (1994). *Zen Letters: Teachings of Yuanwu*. Boston: Shambhala Publications.

Cleary, T. (1986). *Shobogenzo: Zen Essay by Dogen*. Honolulu: University of Hawaii Press.

Cleary, T. F. (1995). *Minding Mind: A Course in Basic Meditation*. Boston: Shambhala Publications.

Cleary, T. F. (1998). *The Sutra of Hui-Neng, Grand Master of Zen: With Hui-Neng's Commentary on the Diamond Sutra*. Boston: Shambhala Publications.

Coe, D. K. (1983). Zen and sophia. *Philosophy Today 27*(2), 169–77.

Cohen, S. (1964). *The Beyond Within: The LSD Story*. New York: Atheneum.

Coleridge, S. T. (1816). *Christabel &c*. London: William Bulmer and Co.

Collobert, C., P. Destrée, and F. J. Gonzalez (2012). *Plato and Myth: Studies on the Use and Status of Platonic Myths*. Leiden and Boston: Brill.

Colzato, L. S., R. Sellaro, I. Samara, M. Baas, and B. Hommel (2015). Meditation-induced states predict attentional control over time. *Consciousness and Cognition 37*, 57–62.

Colzato, L. S., A. Szapora, D. Lippelt, and B. Hommel (2014). Prior meditation practice modulates performance and strategy use in convergent- and divergent-thinking problems. *Mindfulness 8*(1), 10–16.

Cooper, J. M. and D. Hutchinson (1997). *Plato: Complete Works*. Indianapolis, IN: Hackett Publishing.

Corlett, P. R., C. D. Frith, and P. C. Fletcher (2009). From drugs to deprivation: a Bayesian framework for understanding models of psychosis. *Psychopharmacology 206*(4), 515–30.

Corlett, P. R., G. Horga, P. C. Fletcher, B. Alderson-Day, K. Schmack, and A. R. Powers (2018). Hallucinations and strong priors. *Trends in Cognitive Sciences 23*, 114–27.

Cottingham, J. (1985). *The Philosophical Writings of Descartes*. Cambridge: Cambridge University Press.

Cowan, J. D. (2014). Geometric visual hallucinations and the structure of the visual cortex. In *The Neuroscience of Visual Hallucinations*, pp. 219–53. New York: John Wiley and Sons.

Coward, H. (1979). Mysticism in the analytical psychology of Carl Jung and the yoga psychology of Patanjali: a comparative study. *Philosophy East and West 29*(3), 323.

Cox, R. E. and A. J. Barnier (2015). A hypnotic analogue of clinical confabulation. *International Journal of Clinical and Experimental Hypnosis 63*(3), 249–73.

Crawley, R. (2015). Trait mindfulness and autobiographical memory specificity. *Cognitive Processing 16*(1), 79–86.

Crescentini, C., A. Matiz, M. Cimenti, E. Pascoli, R. Eleopra, and F. Fabbro (2018). The effect of mindfulness meditation on personality and psychological well-being in patients with multiple sclerosis. *International Journal of MS Care 20*(3), 101–8.

Creswell, J. D., A. A. Taren, E. K. Lindsay, C. M. Greco, P. J. Gianaros, A. Fairgrieve, A. L. Marsland, K. W. Brown, B. M. Way, R. K. Rosen, and J. L. Ferris (2016).

Alterations in resting-state functional connectivity link mindfulness meditation with reduced interleukin-6: a randomized controlled trial. *Biological Psychiatry 80*(1), 53–61.

Crisp, R. (2000). *Nicomachean Ethics*. Cambridge: Cambridge University Press.

Crowley and A. Shulgin (2019). *Secret Drugs of Buddhism: Psychedelic Sacraments and the Origins of the Vajrayana*. Santa Fe and London: Synergetic Press.

Curnow, T. (2011). Sophia and phronesis: past, present, and future. *Research in Human Development 8*(2), 95–108.

Cásedas, L., V. Pirruccio, M. A. Vadillo, and J. Lupiáñez (2020). Does mindfulness meditation training enhance executive control? A systematic review and meta-analysis of randomized controlled trials in adults. *Mindfulness 11*(2), 411–24.

Dalgleish, T., L. Navrady, E. Bird, E. Hill, B. D. Dunn, and A.-M. Golden (2013). Method-of-loci as a mnemonic device to facilitate access to self-affirming personal memories for individuals with depression. *Clinical Psychological Science 1*(2), 156–62.

Dalio, R. (2017). *Principles*. New York: Simon & Schuster.

Daly, C. (2010). *An Introduction to Philosophical Methods*. Peterborough, Ont.: Broadview Press.

Dam, N. T. V., M. K. v. Vugt, D. R. Vago, L. Schmalzl, C. D. Saron, A. Olendzki, T. Meissner, S. W. Lazar, J. Gorchov, K. C. R. Fox, B. A. Field, W. B. Britton, J. A. Brefczynski-Lewis, and D. E. Meyer (2018). Reiterated concerns and further challenges for mindfulness and meditation research: a reply to Davidson and Dahl. *Perspectives on Psychological Science 13*(1), 1745691617727529.

Dam, N. T. V., M. K. v. Vugt, D. R. Vago, L. Schmalzl, C. D. Saron, A. Olendzki, T. Meissner, S. W. Lazar, C. E. Kerr, J. Gorchov, K. C. R. Fox, B. A. Field, W. B. Britton, J. A. Brefczynski-Lewis, and D. E. Meyer (2018). Mind the hype: a critical evaluation and prescriptive agenda for research on mindfulness and meditation. *Perspectives on Psychological Science 13*(1), 36–61.

Davids, T. W. R. (1881). *Buddhist Suttas*. Oxford: Clarendon Press.

Davids, T. W. R. (1910). *Sacred Books of the Buddhists*. London: Oxford University Press.

Davidson, R. J. and C. J. Dahl (2018). Outstanding challenges in scientific research on mindfulness and Meditation. *Perspectives on Psychological Science 13*(1), 62–5.

Davies, O. (1994). *Meister Eckhart: Selected Writings*. London: Penguin Books.

Davis, A. K., F. S. Barrett, and R. R. Griffiths (2020). Psychological flexibility mediates the relations between acute psychedelic effects and subjective decreases in depression and anxiety. *Journal of Contextual Behavioral Science 15*, 39–45.

Davis, A. K., F. S. Barrett, S. So, N. Gukasyan, T. C. Swift, and R. R. Griffiths (2021). Development of the Psychological Insight Questionnaire among a sample of people who have consumed psilocybin or LSD. *Journal of Psychopharmacology 35*(4), 437–46.

Davis, A. K., Y. Xin, N. D. Sepeda, A. Garcia-Romeu, and M. T. Williams (2021). Increases in psychological flexibility mediate relationship between acute psychedelic effects and decreases in racial trauma symptoms among people of color. *Chronic Stress 5*, 247054702110356.

Daws, R. E., C. Timmermann, B. Giribaldi, J. D. Sexton, M. B. Wall, D. Erritzoe, L. Roseman, D. Nutt, and R. Carhart-Harris (2022). Increased global integration in the brain after psilocybin therapy for depression. *Nature Medicine 28*, 844–51.

Dennett, D. (1991). *Consciousness Explained*. Boston: Little, Brown and Co.

Dienes, Z., P. Lush, R. Semmens-Wheeler, J. Parkinson, R. Scott, and P. Naish (2016). Hypnosis as self-deception; meditation as self-insight. In A. Raz and M. Lifshitz (eds.), *Hypnosis and Meditation: Toward an Integrative Science of Conscious Planes*. Oxford: Oxford University Press.

Dieter, K. C., J. Brascamp, D. Tadin, and R. Blake (2016). Does visual attention drive the dynamics of bistable perception? *Attention, Perception, & Psychophysics 78*(7), 1861–73.

Dijksterhuis, A. and T. Meurs (2006). Where creativity resides: the generative power of unconscious thought. *Consciousness and Cognition 15*(1), 135–46.

Dijksterhuis, A. and L. F. Nordgren (2006). A theory of unconscious thought. *Perspectives on Psychological Science 1*(2), 95–109.

Dijksterhuis, A. and M. Strick (2016). A case for thinking without consciousness. *Perspectives on Psychological Science 11*(1), 117–32.

Diller, J. W. and K. A. Lattal (2008). Radical behaviorism and buddhism: complementarities and conflicts. *Behavior Analyst 31*(2), 163–77.

Doblin, R. and B. Burge (2014). Forward. In R. Doblin and B. Burge (eds.), *Manifesting Minds: A Review of Psychedelics in Science, Medicine, Sex, and Spirituality.* Berkeley, CA: Evolver Editions.

Doss, M. K., M. Považan, M. D. Rosenberg, N. D. Sepeda, A. K. Davis, P. H. Finan, G. S. Smith, J. J. Pekar, P. B. Barker, R. R. Griffiths, and F. S. Barrett (2021). Psilocybin therapy increases cognitive and neural flexibility in patients with major depressive disorder. *Translational Psychiatry 11*(1), 574.

Doss, M. K., J. Weafer, D. A. Gallo, and H. d. Wit (2018). MDMA impairs both the encoding and retrieval of emotional recollections. *Neuropsychopharmacology 43*(4), 791.

Downing, C. J. (1988). Expectancy and visual–spatial attention: effects on perceptual quality. *Journal of Experimental Psychology: Human Perception and Performance 14*(2), 188–202.

Dretske, F. (1997). *Naturalizing the Mind.* Cambridge, MA MIT Press.

Dreyfus, G. (2011). Is mindfulness present-centred and non-judgmental? A discussion of the cognitive dimensions of mindfulness. *Contemporary Buddhism 12*(1), 41–54.

Droit-Volet, S., M. Chaulet, and M. Dambrun (2018). Time and meditation: when does the perception of time change with mindfulness exercise? *Mindfulness 9*(5), 1557–70.

Droit-Volet, S., M. Fanget, and M. Dambrun (2015). Mindfulness meditation and relaxation training increases time sensitivity. *Consciousness and Cognition 31*, 86–97.

Droit-Volet, S. and J. Heros (2016). Time judgments as a function of mindfulness meditation, anxiety, and mindfulness awareness. *Mindfulness 8*(2), 266–75.

Dunning, D. (2011). Chapter five: the Dunning–Kruger Effect on being ignorant of one's own ignorance. *Advances in Experimental Social Psychology 44*, 247–96.

Eagleman and A. Brandt (2017). *The Runaway Species: How Human Creativity Remakes the World.* New York: Catapult.

Eagleman, D. (2011). *Incognito: The Secret Lives of the Brain.* New York: Pantheon.

Edwards, A. E. and S. Cohen (1961). Visual illusion, tactile sensibility and reaction time under LSD-25. *Psychopharmacologia 2*(5), 297–303.

Einstein, A. (1950). Letter to Robert S. Marcus.

Eisner, B. G. and S. Cohen (1959). Use of lysergic acid diethylamide in a psychotherapeutic setting. *Archives of Neurology and Psychiatry 81*(5), 615.

Ellenberger (1970). *The Discovery of the Unconscious: The History and Evolution of Dynamic Psychiatry*, Vol. 1. New York: Basic Books.

Ellenberger, H. F. (1966). The pathogenic secret and its therapeutics. *Journal of the History of the Behavioral Sciences 2*(1), 29–42.

Engelmann, M. L. (2018). Instructions for climbing the ladder (the minimalism of Wittgenstein's Tractatus). *Philosophical Investigations 41*(4), 446–70.

Eriksen, C. W. and J. D. S. James (1986). Visual attention within and around the field of focal attention: a zoom lens model. *Perception & Psychophysics 40*(4), 225–40.

Eriksen, C. W. and Y.-Y. Yeh (1985). Allocation of attention in the visual field. *Journal of Experimental Psychology: Human Perception and Performance 11*(5), 583–97.

Ermentrout, G. B. and J. D. Cowan (1979). A mathematical theory of visual hallucination patterns. *Biological Cybernetics 34*(3), 137–50.

Erritzoe, D., L. Roseman, M. M. Nour, K. MacLean, M. Kaelen, D. J. Nutt, and R. L. Carhart-Harris (2018). Effects of psilocybin therapy on personality structure. *Acta Psychiatrica Scandinavica 138*(5), 368–78.

Erritzoe, D., J. Smith, P. M. Fisher, R. Carhart-Harris, V. G. Frokjaer, and G. M. Knudsen (2019). Recreational use of psychedelics is associated with elevated personality trait openness: exploration of associations with brain serotonin markers. *Journal of Psychopharmacology 33*(9), 1068–75.

Fabbro, A., C. Crescentini, A. Matiz, A. Clarici, and F. Fabbro (2017). Effects of mindfulness meditation on conscious and non-conscious components of the mind. *Applied Sciences 7*(4), 349.

Fabio, R. A. and G. E. Towey (2018). Long-term meditation: the relationship between cognitive processes, thinking styles and mindfulness. *Cognitive Processing 19*(1), 73–85.

Family, N., D. Vinson, G. Vigliocco, M. Kaelen, M. Bolstridge, D. J. Nutt, and R. L. Carhart-Harris (2016). Semantic activation in LSD: evidence from picture naming. *Language, Cognition and Neuroscience 31*(10), 1–8.

Farb, N., A. Anderson, J. Irving, and Z. Segal (2014). Mindfulness interventions and emotion regulation. In J. J. Gross (ed.), *Handbook of Emotion Regulation*. Guilford Press.

Farias, M., E. Maraldi, K. C. Wallenkampf, and G. Lucchetti (2020). Adverse events in meditation practices and meditation-based therapies: a systematic review. *Acta Psychiatrica Scandinavica 142*(5), 374–93.

Fazekas, P. and B. Nanay (2021). Attention is amplification, not selection. *British Journal for the Philosophy of Science 72*(1), 299–324.

Feigenbaum, E. A. (1961). The simulation of verbal learning behavior. In *Papers presented at the May 9–11, 1961, western joint IRE-AIEE-ACM computer conference on IRE-AIEE-ACM '61 (Western)*, pp. 121–32.

Fernberger, S. W. (1923). Observations on taking peyote '(Anhalonium Lewinii)'. *American Journal of Psychology 34*(2), 267.

Feynman, R. (1974). Cargo cult science. *Engineering and Science 37*(7), 10–13.

Firestone, C. and B. J. Scholl (2015). Cognition does not affect perception: evaluating the evidence for 'top-down' effects. *Behavioral and Brain Sciences 39*, e229.

Fischer, E. (2011). *Philosophical Delusion and Its Therapy: Outline of a Philosophical Revolution*. New York: Routledge.

Fischer, R. and E. L. Mead (1966). Time contraction and psychomotor performance produced by 'psilocybin'. *Nature 209*(5021), 433–4.

Fischman, L. G. (1983). Dreams, hallucinogenic drug states, and schizophrenia: A psychological and biological comparison. *Schizophrenia Bulletin 9*(1), 73–94.

Flanagan, T. W. and C. D. Nichols (2018). Psychedelics as anti-inflammatory agents. *International Review of Psychiatry 30*(4), 363–75.

Fodor, J. (1975). *The Language of Thought*, Vol. 5. Cambridge, MA: Harvard University Press.

Fodor, J. (1983). *The Modularity of Mind*. Cambridge, MA: MIT Press.

Forman, R. K. C. (1999). *Mysticism, Mind, Consciousness*. New York: SUNY Press.

Forstmann, M., D. A. Yudkin, A. M. B. Prosser, S. M. Heller, and M. J. Crockett (2020). Transformative experience and social connectedness mediate the mood-enhancing effects of psychedelic use in naturalistic settings. *Proceedings of the National Academy of Sciences 117*(5), 2338–46.

Fortney, M. (2019). Conceptualizing intellectual attention. *Theory & Psychology 29*(6), 775–88.

Fox, K. C. and R. E. Beaty (2019). Mind-wandering as creative thinking: neural, psychological, and theoretical considerations. *Current Opinion in Behavioral Sciences 27*, 123–30.

Fox, C. R. and R. T. Clemen, (2005). Subjective probability assessment in decision analysis: partition dependence and bias toward the ignorance prior. *Management Science 51*(9), 1417–32.

Fox, K. C. R., M. Girn, C. C. Parro, and K. Christoff (2018). Functional neuroimaging of psychedelic experience: an overview of psychological and neural effects and their relevance to research on creativity, daydreaming, and dreaming. In R. E. Jung and O. Vartanian (eds.), *Cambridge Handbook of the Neuroscience of Creativity*, pp. 92–113. Cambridge: Cambridge University Press.

Fox, M. D., A. Z. Snyder, J. L. Vincent, M. Corbetta, D. C. V. Essen, and M. E. Raichle (2005). The human brain is intrinsically organized into dynamic, anticorrelated functional networks. *Proceedings of the National Academy of Sciences 102*(27), 9673–8.

Fox, K. C. R., P. Zakarauskas, M. Dixon, M. Ellamil, E. Thompson, and K. Christoff (2012). Meditation experience predicts introspective accuracy. *PLOS One 7*(9), e45370.

Fraassen, B. C. v. (1989). *Laws and Symmetry*. Oxford: Clarendon Press.

Frecska, E., K. D. White, and L. E. Luna (2003). Effects of the Amazonian psychoactive beverage ayahuasca on binocular rivalry: interhemispheric switching or interhemispheric fusion? *Journal of Psychoactive Drugs 35*(3), 367–74.

Frederking, W. (1955). Intoxicant drugs (mescaline and lysergic acid diethylamide) in psychotherapy. *Journal of Nervous and Mental Disease 121*(3), 262–6.

Freiberger, M. (2009). Uncoiling the spiral: maths and hallucinations, url: https://plus.maths.org/content/uncoiling-spiral-maths-and-hallucinations

Friston, K. (2002). Functional integration and inference in the brain. *Progress in Neurobiology 68*(2), 113–43.

Fromm, E. (1959). Psychoanalysis and Zen Buddhism. *Psychologia 2*(2), 79–99.

Fujino, M., Y. Ueda, H. Mizuhara, J. Saiki, and M. Nomura (2018). Open monitoring meditation reduces the involvement of brain regions related to memory function. *Scientific Reports 8*(1), 9968.

Fuller, S. and M. Carrasco (2006). Exogenous attention and color perception: performance and appearance of saturation and hue. *Vision Research 46*(23), 4032–47.

Gallimore, A. R. (2015). Restructuring consciousness—the psychedelic state in light of integrated information theory. *Frontiers in Human Neuroscience 9*, 346.

Gallimore, A. R. and R. J. Strassman (2016). A model for the application of target-controlled intravenous infusion for a prolonged immersive DMT psychedelic experience. *Frontiers in Pharmacology 7*, 211.

Galvão-Coelho, N. L., A. C. d. M. Galvão, R. N. d. Almeida, F. Palhano-Fontes, I. C. Braga, B. L. Soares, J. P. Maia-de Oliveira, D. Perkins, J. Sarris, and D. B. d. Araujo (2020). Changes in inflammatory biomarkers are related to the antidepressant effects of ayahuasca. *Journal of Psychopharmacology 34*(10), 1125–33.

Garcia-Romeu, A., A. K. Davis, F. Erowid, E. Erowid, R. R. Griffiths, and M. W. Johnson (2019). Cessation and reduction in alcohol consumption and misuse after psychedelic use. *Journal of Psychopharmacology 33*(9), 1088–1101.

Garrison, K. A., T. A. Zeffiro, D. Scheinost, R. T. Constable, and J. A. Brewer (2015). Meditation leads to reduced default mode network activity beyond an active task. *Cognitive, Affective & Behavioral Neuroscience 15*(3), 712–20.

Gassendi, P. (1641). Fifth set of objections and replies. In Cottingham et al. (eds.), The Philosophical Writings of Descartes Vol. 2, pp. 179–277. Cambridge: Cambridge University Press.

Gaut, B. (2003). Creativity and imagination. In The Creation of Art. New Essays in Philosophical Aesthetics, pp. 148–73. Cambridge: Cambridge University Press.

Geraerts, E., E. Smeets, M. Jelicic, J. v. Heerden, and H. Merckelbach (2005). Fantasy proneness, but not self-reported trauma is related to DRM performance of women reporting recovered memories of childhood sexual abuse. Consciousness and Cognition 14(3), 602–12.

Gethin, R. (2011). On some definitions of mindfulness. Contemporary Buddhism 12(1), 263–79.

Gilbert, D. T. (1999). What the mind's not. In S. Chaiken and Y. Trope (eds.), Dual Process Theories in Social Psychology, pp. 3–11. New York: Guilford Press.

Giluk, T. L. (2009). Mindfulness, Big Five personality, and affect: a meta-analysis. Personality and Individual Differences 47(8), 805–11.

Girn, M., C. Mills, L. Roseman, R. L. Carhart-Harris, and K. Christoff (2020). Updating the dynamic framework of thought: creativity and psychedelics. NeuroImage 213, 116726.

Gligorov, N. (2008). Unconscious pain. The American Journal of Bioethics 8(9), 27–8.

Goldberg, J. A., U. Rokni, and H. Sompolinsky (2004). Patterns of ongoing activity and the functional architecture of the primary visual cortex. Neuron 42(3), 489–500.

Goldpaugh, D. D. (2022). Finding the divine within: exploring the role of the sacred in psychedelic integration therapy for sexual trauma and dysfunction. Sexual and Relationship Therapy 37(3), 314–23.

Goodman, N. (1955). Fact, Fiction, and Forecast. Cambridge, MA: Harvard University Press.

Gouzoulis-Mayfrank, E., M. Schreckenberger, O. Sabri, C. Arning, B. Thelen, M. Spitzer, K.-A. Kovar, L. Hermle, U. Büll, and H. Sass (1999). Neurometabolic effects of psilocybin, 3, 4-methylenedioxyethylamphetamine (MDE) and d-methamphetamine in healthy volunteers: a double-blind, placebo-controlled PET study with [18F]FDG. Neuropsychopharmacology 20(6), 565–81.

Gouzoulis-Mayfrank, E., B. Thelen, S. Maier, K. Heekeren, K.-A. Kovar, H. Sass, and M. Spitzer (2002). Effects of the hallucinogen psilocybin on covert orienting of visual attention in humans. Neuropsychobiology 45(4), 205–12.

Green, R. P. H. (2008). On Christian Teaching. Oxford: Oxford University Press.

Greenberg, J., K. Reiner, and N. Meiran (2012, 5). 'Mind the trap': mindfulness practice reduces cognitive rigidity. PLOS One 7(5), e36206.

Greenwald, A. G. and M. R. Banaji (1995). Implicit social cognition: attitudes, self-esteem, and stereotypes. Psychological Review 102(1), 4–27.

Gregorio, D. D., J. Popic, J. P. Enns, A. Inserra, A. Skalecka, A. Markopoulos, L. Posa, M. Lopez-Canul, H. Qianzi, C. K. Lafferty, J. P. Britt, S. Comai, A. Aguilar-Valles, N. Sonenberg, and G. Gobbi (2021). Lysergic acid diethylamide (LSD) promotes social behavior through mTORC1 in the excitatory neurotransmission. Proceedings of the National Academy of Sciences 118(5), e2020705118.

Griffiths, R., W. Richards, M. Johnson, U. McCann, and R. Jesse (2008). Mystical-type experiences occasioned by psilocybin mediate the attribution of personal meaning and spiritual significance 14 months later. Journal of Psychopharmacology 22(6), 621–32.

Griffiths, R. R., M. W. Johnson, M. A. Carducci, A. Umbricht, W. A. Richards, B. D. Richards, M. P. Cosimano, and M. A. Klinedinst (2016). Psilocybin produces substantial and sustained decreases in depression and anxiety in patients with life-threatening cancer: a randomized double-blind trial. Journal of Psychopharmacology 30(12), 1181–97.

Griffiths, R. R., M. W. Johnson, W. A. Richards, B. D. Richards, R. Jesse, K. A. MacLean, F. S. Barrett, M. P. Cosimano, and M. A. Klinedinst (2018). Psilocybin-occasioned mystical-type experience in combination with meditation and other spiritual practices produces enduring positive changes in psychological functioning and in trait measures of prosocial attitudes and behaviors. *Journal of Psychopharmacology 32*(1), 49–69.

Griffiths, R. R., M. W. Johnson, W. A. Richards, B. D. Richards, U. McCann, and R. Jesse (2011). Psilocybin occasioned mystical-type experiences: immediate and persisting dose-related effects. *Psychopharmacology 218*(4), 649–65.

Griffiths, R. R., W. A. Richards, U. McCann, and R. Jesse (2006). Psilocybin can occasion mystical-type experiences having substantial and sustained personal meaning and spiritual significance. *Psychopharmacology 187*(3), 268–83.

Griffiths, T. L., C. Kemp, and J. B. Tenenbaum (2008). Bayesian models of cognition. In R. Sun (ed.), *Cambridge Handbook of Computational Cognitive Modeling*, pp. 59–100. Cambridge, MA: Cambridge University Press.

Grof, S. (1975). *Realms of the Human Unconscious: Observations from LSD Research*. New York: Viking Press.

Grof, S. (1980). *LSD Psychotherapy*. Nashville, TN: Hunter House.

Grof, S. (2009). *LSD: Doorway to the Numinous: The Groundbreaking Psychedelic Research into Realms of the Human Unconscious*. Rochester, VT: Park Street Press.

Grube, G. M. A. and J. M. Cooper (2002). *Five Dialogues*. Indianapolis, IN: Hackett Publishing.

Grégoire, S., T. Bouffar, and C. Vezeau (2012). Personal goal setting as a mediator of the relationship between mindfulness and wellbeing. *International Journal of Wellbeing 2*(3), 236–50.

Haase, J., P. H. P. Hanel, and N. Gronau (2022). Creativity enhancement methods for adults: a meta-analysis. *Psychology of Aesthetics, Creativity, and the Arts*. (In Press)

Habib, R. and L. Nyberg (2008). Neural correlates of availability and accessibility in memory. *Cerebral Cortex 18*(7), 1720–26.

Hafenbrack, A. C., Z. Kinias, and S. G. Barsade (2014). Debiasing the mind through meditation. *Psychological Science 25*(2), 369–76.

Hájek, A. (2014). Philosophical heuristics and philosophical creativity. In E. Paul and S. B. Kaufman (eds.), *The Philosophy of Creativity*, pp. 288–317. Oxford: Oxford University Press.

Hájek, A. (2016). Philosophical heuristics and philosophical methodology. In *The Oxford Handbook of Philosophical Methodology*, pp. 348–73. Oxford: Oxford University Press.

Hájek, A. (2018). Creating heuristics for philosophy creativity. In Berys Gaut and Matthew Kieran (eds.), *Creativity and Philosophy*, pp. 293–312. New York: Routledge.

Haliwa, I., J. M. Wilson, S. K. Spears, J. Strough, and N. J. Shook (2020). Exploring facets of the mindful personality: dispositional mindfulness and the Big Five. *Personality and Individual Differences 171*, 110469.

Hallowell, E. and J. J. Ratey (2021). *ADHD 2.0*. New York: Random House.

Hamilton, E. and H. Cairns (1980). *The Collected Works of Plato*. Princeton, NJ: Princeton University Press.

Hammond, L., G. F. Wagstaff, and J. Cole (2006). Facilitating eyewitness memory in adults and children with context reinstatement and focused meditation. *Journal of Investigative Psychology and Offender Profiling 3*(2), 117–30.

Happold, F. C. (1963). *Mysticism: A Study and an Anthology*. Harmondsworth, England: Penguin Books.

Hargus, E., C. Crane, T. Barnhofer, and J. M. G. Williams (2010). Effects of mindfulness on meta-awareness and specificity of describing prodromal symptoms in suicidal depression. *Emotion 10*(1), 34.

Harman, W. W. (1963). The issue of the consciousness-expanding drugs. *Main Currents in Modern Thought 20*(1), 5–14.

Harman, W. W., R. H. McKim, R. E. Mogar, J. Fadiman, and M. J. Stolaroff (1966). Psychedelic agents in creative problem-solving: a pilot study. *Psychological Reports 19*(1), 211–27.

Hartman, A. M. and L. E. Hollister (1963). Effect of mescaline, lysergic acid diethylamide and psilocybin on color perception. *Psychopharmacologia 4*(6), 441–51.

Hartogsohn, I. (2016). Set and setting, psychedelics and the placebo response: an extra-pharmacological perspective on psychopharmacology. *Journal of Psychopharmacology 30*(12), 1259–67.

Hartogsohn, I. (2018). The meaning-enhancing properties of psychedelics and their mediator role in psychedelic therapy, spirituality, and creativity. *Frontiers in Neuroscience 12*, 129.

Hasler, F., U. Grimberg, M. A. Benz, T. Huber, and F. X. Vollenweider (2004). Acute psychological and physiological effects of psilocybin in healthy humans: a double-blind, placebo-controlled dose?effect study. *Psychopharmacology 172*(2), 145–56.

Hassin, R. R. (2013). Yes it can. *Perspectives on Psychological Science 8*(2), 195–207.

Hassin, R. R., J. A. Bargh, A. D. Engell, and K. C. McCulloch (2009). Implicit working memory. *Consciousness and Cognition 18*(3), 665–78.

Haxton, B. (2001). *Fragments: The Collected Wisdom of Heraclitus*. New York: Penguin Classics.

Healy, C. J. (2021). The acute effects of classic psychedelics on memory in humans. *Psychopharmacology 238*(3), 639–53.

Heather, N. (2020). The concept of akrasia as the foundation for a dual systems theory of addiction. *Behavioural Brain Research 390*, 112666.

Heeren, A., N. V. Broeck, and P. Philippot (2009). The effects of mindfulness on executive processes and autobiographical memory specificity. *Behaviour Research and Therapy 47*(5), 403–9.

Hermans, D., K. V. d. Broeck, G. Belis, F. Raes, G. Pieters, and P. Eelen (2004). Trauma and autobiographical memory specificity in depressed inpatients. *Behaviour Research and Therapy 42*(7), 775–89.

Heron, W., B. K. Doane, and T. H. Scott (1956). Visual disturbances after prolonged perceptual isolation. *Canadian Journal of Psychology/Revue Canadienne de Psychologie 10*(1), 13–18.

Heuschkel, K. and K. P. Kuypers (2020). Depression, mindfulness, and psilocybin: possible complementary effects of mindfulness meditation and psilocybin in the treatment of depression. a review. *Frontiers in Psychiatry 11*, 224.

Hill, C. L. M. and J. A. Updegraff (2012). Mindfulness and its relationship to emotional regulation. *Emotion 12*(1), 81–90.

Hill, C. S. (2006). Ow! The paradox of pain. In *Pain: New Essays on Its Nature and the Methodology of Its Study*. Cambridge, MA: MIT Press.

Hillman, D. (2008). *The Chemical Muse: Drug Use and the Roots of Western Civilization*. Macmillan.

Hodgins, H. S. and K. C. Adair (2010). Attentional processes and meditation. *Consciousness and Cognition 19*(4), 872–8.

Hofmann, W. and T. D. Wilson (2010). Consciousness, introspection, and the adaptive unconscious. In B. Gawronski and B. Payne (eds.), *Handbook of Implicit Social Cognition: Measurement, Theory, and Applications*. Guilford Press.

Hohwy, J. (2013). *The Predictive Mind*. Oxford University Press.

Hommel, B. (2012). Convergent and divergent operations in cognitive search. In P. Todd, T. Hills, and T. Robbins (eds.), *Cognitive Search: Evolution, Algorithms, and the Brain*, Strüngmann Forum Reports, pp. 221–35. Cambridge, MA: MIT Press.

Hommel, B., C. S. Chapman, P. Cisek, H. F. Neyedli, J.-H. Song, and T. N. Welsh (2019). No one knows what attention is. *Attention, Perception, & Psychophysics 81*(7), 2288–303.

Hood, R. W. (1975). The Construction and preliminary validation of a measure of reported mystical experience. *Journal for the Scientific Study of Religion 14*(1), 29.

Hood, R. W., N. Ghorbani, P. J. Watson, A. F. Ghramaleki, M. N. Bing, H. K. Davison, R. J. Morris, and W. P. Williamson (2001). Dimensions of the mysticism scale: confirming the three-factor structure in the United States and Iran. *Journal for the Scientific Study of Religion 40*(4), 691–705.

Horan, R. (2009). The Neuropsychological connection between creativity and meditation. *Creativity Research Journal 21*(2-3), 199–222.

Horowitz, M. (1975). A cognitive model of hallucinations. *American Journal of Psychiatry 132*(8), 789–95.

Howatson, M. and F. C. C. Sheffield (2008). *Symposium*. Cambridge: Cambridge University Press.

Huemer, M. (2005). *Ethical Intuitionism*. Houndmills, Basingstoke, Hampshire, England: Palgrave Macmillan.

Hurk, P. A. M. v. d., T. Wingens, F. Giommi, H. P. Barendregt, A. E. M. Speckens, and H. T. v. Schie (2011). On the relationship between the practice of mindfulness meditation and personality—an exploratory analysis of the mediating role of mindfulness skills. *Mindfulness 2*(3), 194–200.

Huxley, A. (1945). *The Perennial Philosophy*. New York: Harper & Brothers.

Huxley, A. (1954). *The Doors of Perception*. New York: Harper & Row.

Huxley, A. (1956). *Heaven and Hell*. New York: Harper & Brothers.

Huxley, A., C. Palmer, and M. Horowitz (1977). *Moksha: Classic Writings on Psychedelics and the Visionary Experience*. New York: Stonehill Publishing Company.

Isaacson, W. (2011). *Steve Jobs*. New York: Simon & Schuster.

Iszáj, F., M. D. Griffiths, and Z. Demetrovics (2016). Creativity and psychoactive substance use: a systematic review. *International Journal of Mental Health and Addiction 15*(5), 1135–49.

Jacobs, B. L. (1978). Dreams and hallucinations: a common neurochemical mechanism mediating their phenomenological similarities. *Neuroscience & Biobehavioral Reviews 2*(1), 59–69.

James, W. (1882). On some Hegelisms. *Mind 7*(26), 186–208.

James, W. (1890). *The Principles of Psychology*. New York: Henry Holt and Company.

James, W. (1902). *The Varieties of Religious Experience: A Study in Human Nature*. London: Longmans, Green and Co.

James, W. (1910). A suggestion about mysticism. *Journal of Philosophy, Psychology and Scientific Methods 7*(4), 85.

Jamison, S. W. and J. P. Brereton (2014). *The Rigveda: The Earliest Religious Poetry of India*. South Asia Research.

Jarvik, M. E., H. A. Abramson, and M. W. Hirsch (1955). Lysergic acid diethylamide (LSD-25): VI. Effect upon recall and recognition of various stimuli. *The Journal of Psychology 39*(2), 443–54.

Jaspers, K. (1950). *Origin and Goal of History*. New Haven: Yale University Press.

Jaynes, E. T. (1973). The well-posed problem. *Foundations of Physics 3*(4), 477–92.

Jha, A. (2021). *Peak Mind: Find Your Focus, Own Your Attention, Invest 12 Minutes a Day*. London: Piatkus.

Jha, A., J. Krompinger, and M. Baime (2007). Mindfulness training modifies subsystems of attention. *Cognitive, Affective, & Behavioral Neuroscience 7*(2), 109–19.

Jha, A. P., E. Denkova, A. P. Zanesco, J. E. Witkin, J. Rooks, and S. L. Rogers (2019). Does mindfulness training help working memory 'work' better? *Current Opinion in Psychology 28*, 273–8.

Johnson-Laird, P. N. (2002). How jazz musicians improvise. *Music Perception 19*(3), 415–42.

Johnston, K. and B. Timney (2013). Alcohol and lateral inhibitory interactions in human vision. *Perception 42*(12), 1301–10.

Jonas, S. (2016). *Ineffability and its Metaphysics: The Unspeakable in Art, Religion, and Philosophy*. New York: Palgrave MacMillan.

Josipovic, Z., I. Dinstein, J. Weber, and D. J. Heeger (2012). Influence of meditation on anti-correlated networks in the brain. *Frontiers in Human Neuroscience 5*, 183.

Joyce, J. M. (2010). A defence of imprecise credences in inference and decision making. *Philosophical Perspectives 24*(1), 281–323.

Jung, C. (1949). Foreword. In *Introduction to Zen Buddhism*. New York: Philosophical Library.

Jung, C. (1953). *Collected Works (Volume 9, Part II)*. London: Routledge.

Jung, C. (1954). To Father Victor White. In *C.G. Jung Letters, Volume 2*. Princeton: Princeton University Press.

Jung, C. (1959). *The Archetypes and the Collective Unconscious*. Princeton: Princeton University Press.

Jung-Beeman, M., E. M. Bowden, J. Haberman, J. L. Frymiare, S. Arambel-Liu, R. Greenblatt, P. J. Reber, and J. Kounios (2004). Neural activity when people solve verbal problems with insight. *PLOS Biology 2*(4), e97.

Kabat-Zinn, J. (1990). *Full Catastrophe Living*. New York: Random House.

Kabat-Zinn, J. (1994). *Wherever You Go, There You Are*. West Port, CT: Hyperion.

Kabat-Zinn, J. (2005). *Coming to Our Senses*. West Port, CT: Hyperion.

Kabat-Zinn, J. (2011). Some reflections on the origins of MBSR, skillful means, and the trouble with maps. *Contemporary Buddhism 12*(1), 281–306.

Kahneman, D. (1978). *Attention and Effort*. Englewood Cliffs, NJ: Prentice-Hall.

Kahneman, D. and S. Frederick (2002). Representativeness revisited: attribute substitution in intuitive judgment. In T. Gilovich, D. Griffin, and D. Kahneman (eds.), *Heuristics and Biases: The Psychology of Intuitive Judgment*, pp. 49–81. New York: Cambridge University Press.

Kalafatoglu, Y. and T. Turgut (2017a). The effects of mindfulness on overconfidence. *Journal of Administrative Sciences 15*(29), 175–91.

Kalafatoğlu, Y. and T. Turgut (2017b). Another benefit of mindfulness: ethical behaviour. *International Journal of Social Sciences and Education Research 3*(3), 772–82.

Kapleau, R. P. (1965). *The Three Pillars of Zen*. New York: Anchor Books.

Kartelaia, N. and J. Reb (2015). Improving decision making through mindfulness. In J. Reb and P. Atkins (eds.), *Mindfulness in Organizations: Foundations, Research, and Applications*, pp. 163–89. Cambridge: Cambridge University Press.

Kashdan, T. B. and J. Rottenberg (2010). Psychological flexibility as a fundamental aspect of health. *Clinical Psychology Review 30*(7), 865–78.

Katyal, S. and P. Goldin (2021). Neural correlates of nonjudgmental perception induced through meditation. *Annals of the New York Academy of Sciences 1499*(1), 70–81.

Katz, S. T. (1978). Language, epistemology, and mysticism. In *Mysticism and Philosophical Analysis*, pp. 22–74. London: Sheldon Press.

Katz, S. T. (1983). *Mysticism and Religious Traditions*. New York: Oxford University Press.

Kaufman, S. B. (2020). *Transcend: The New Science of Self-Actualization*. New York: TarcherPerigee.

Keefe, J. M. and V. S. Störmer (2021). Lateralized alpha activity and slow potential shifts over visual cortex track the time course of both endogenous and exogenous orienting of attention. *NeuroImage 225*, 117495.

Kekes, J. (1983). Wisdom. *American Philosophical Quarterly 20*(3), 277–86.

Kelly, A. M. C., L. Q. Uddin, B. B. Biswal, F. X. Castellanos, and M. P. Milham (2008). Competition between functional brain networks mediates behavioral variability. *NeuroImage 39*(1), 527–37.

Kenet, T., D. Bibitchkov, M. Tsodyks, A. Grinvald, and A. Arieli (2003). Spontaneously emerging cortical representations of visual attributes. *Nature 425*(6961), 954–6.

Kenna, J. C. and G. Sedman (1964). The subjective experience of time during lysergic acid diethylamide (LSD-25) intoxication. *Psychopharmacologia 5*(4), 280–8.

Kentridge, R. (2013). Visual attention: bringing the unseen past into view. *Current Biology 23*(2), R69–R71.

Kiken, L. G., E. L. Garland, K. Bluth, O. S. Palsson, and S. A. Gaylord (2015). From a state to a trait: trajectories of state mindfulness in meditation during intervention predict changes in trait mindfulness. *Personality and Individual Differences 81*, 41–6.

Kiken, L. G. and N. J. Shook (2011). Looking up. *Social Psychological and Personality Science 2*(4), 425–31.

Kiraga, M. K., N. L. Mason, M. V. Uthaug, K. I. v. Oorsouw, S. W. Toennes, J. G. Ramaekers, and K. P. C. Kuypers (2021). Persisting effects of ayahuasca on empathy, creative thinking, decentering, personality, and well-being. *Frontiers in Pharmacology 12*, 721537.

Kirchhoff, M. D. (2018). Predictive processing, perceiving and imagining: is to perceive to imagine, or something close to it? *Philosophical Studies 175*(3), 751–67.

Klüver, H. (1928). *Mescal: The Divine Plant and Its Psychological Effects*. London: Kegan Paul, Trench, Trubner & Co.

Klüver, H. (1942). Mechanisms of hallucinations. In Terman and Merrill (eds.), *Studies in Personality*, pp. 175–207. New York: Mc-Graw-Hill.

Knafo, D. (2002). Revisiting Ernst Kris's concept of regression in the service of the ego in art. *Psychoanalytic Psychology 19*(1), 24–49.

Knauer, A. and W. J. M. A. Maloney (1913). A preliminary note on the psychic action of mescaline, with special reference to the mechanism of visual hallucinations. *Journal of Nervous and Mental Disease 40*(7), 425–36.

Kobori, N. (1957). A discussion between one and zero. *The Eastern Buddhist 8*, 43–9.

Koestler, A. (1954). *The Invisible Writing: The Second Volume of an Autobiography, 1932–40*. London: Collins, with H. Hamilton.

Koestler, A. (1964). *The Act of Creation*. New York: Macmillan.

Kometer, M., B. R. Cahn, D. Andel, O. L. Carter, and F. X. Vollenweider (2011). The 5-HT2A/1A agonist psilocybin disrupts modal object completion associated with visual hallucinations. *Biological Psychiatry 69*(5), 399–406.

Kometer, M. and F. X. Vollenweider (2018). Serotonergic hallucinogen-induced visual perceptual alterations. In A. Halberstadt, F. Vollenweider, and D. Nichols (eds.), *Behavioral Neurobiology of Psychedelic drugs*, Volume 36 of *Current Topics in Behavioral Neurosciences*, pp. 257–82. Berlin and Heidelberg: Springer.

Konjedi, S. and R. Maleeh (2020). Sleep and mindfulness meditation as they relate to false memory. *Psychological Research 84*(4), 1084–1111.

Kopec, M. and M. G. Titelbaum (2016). The uniqueness thesis. *Philosophy Compass 11*(4), 189–200.

Kotchoubey, B. (2018). Human consciousness: where is it from and what is it for. *Frontiers in Psychology 9*, 567.

Kouider, S., V. d. Gardelle, J. Sackur, and E. Dupoux (2010). How rich is consciousness? The partial awareness hypothesis. *Trends in Cognitive Sciences 14*(7), 301–7.

Kounios, J. and M. Beeman (2015). *The Eureka Factor: Aha Moments, Creative Insight, and the Brain*. New York: Random House.

Kounios, J., J. I. Fleck, D. L. Green, L. Payne, J. L. Stevenson, E. M. Bowden, and M. Jung-Beeman (2008). The origins of insight in resting-state brain activity. *Neuropsychologia 46*(1), 281–91.

Kozhevnikov, M., O. Louchakova, Z. Josipovic, and M. A. Motes (2009). The enhancement of visuospatial processing efficiency through buddhist deity meditation. *Psychological Science 20*(5), 645–53.

Kraehenmann, R. (2017). Dreams and psychedelics: neurophenomenological comparison and therapeutic implications. *Current Neuropharmacology 15*(7), 1032–42.

Kraehenmann, R., D. Pokorny, H. Aicher, K. H. Preller, T. Pokorny, O. G. Bosch, E. Seifritz, and F. X. Vollenweider (2017). LSD increases primary process thinking via serotonin 2A receptor activation. *Frontiers in Pharmacology 8*, 814.

Kraehenmann, R., D. Pokorny, L. Vollenweider, K. H. Preller, T. Pokorny, E. Seifritz, and F. X. Vollenweider (2017). Dreamlike effects of LSD on waking imagery in humans depend on serotonin 2A receptor activation. *Psychopharmacology 234*(13), 2031–46.

Kral, T. R., B. S. Schuyler, J. A. Mumford, M. A. Rosenkranz, A. Lutz, and R. J. Davidson (2018). Impact of short- and long-term mindfulness meditation training on amygdala reactivity to emotional stimuli. *NeuroImage 181*, 301–13.

Kramer, R. S. S., U. W. Weger, and D. Sharma (2013). The effect of mindfulness meditation on time perception. *Consciousness and Cognition 22*(3), 846–52.

Kranczioch, C. and J. D. Thorne (2013). Simultaneous and preceding sounds enhance rapid visual targets: evidence from the attentional blink. *Advances in Cognitive Psychology / University of Finance and Management in Warsaw 9*(3), 130–42.

Kreitz, C., G. Pugnaghi, and D. Memmert (2020). Guessing right: preconscious processing in inattentional blindness. *Quarterly Journal of Experimental Psychology 73*(7), 1055–65.

Kreitz, C., R. Schnuerch, H. Gibbons, and D. Memmert (2015). Some see it, some don't: exploring the relation between inattentional blindness and personality factors. *PLOS One 10*(5), e0128158.

Krippner, S. (1968). The hypnotic trance, the psychedelic experience, and the creative act. *Journal of Humanistic Psychology 8*(49), 40–67.

Kris, E. (1936). The psychology of caricature. *International Journal of Psychoanalysis 17*, 285–303.

Kuypers, K. P. C., J. Riba, M. d. l. F. Revenga, S. Barker, E. L. Theunissen, and J. G. Ramaekers (2016). Ayahuasca enhances creative divergent thinking while decreasing conventional convergent thinking. *Psychopharmacology 233*(18), 3395–403.

Kvavilashvili, L. and G. Mandler (2004). Out of one's mind: a study of involuntary semantic memories. *Cognitive Psychology 48*(1), 47–94.

LaBerge, D. and V. Brown (1989). Theory of attentional operations in shape identification. *Psychological Review 96*(1), 101–24.

Lachaud, L., B. Jacquet, and J. Baratgin (2022). Reducing choice-blindness? An experimental study comparing experienced meditators to non-meditators. *European Journal of Investigation in Health, Psychology and Education 12*(11), 1607–20.

Lakey, C. E., W. K. Campbell, K. W. Brown, and A. S. Goodie (2007). Dispositional mindfulness as a predictor of the severity of gambling outcomes. *Personality and Individual Differences 43*(7), 1698–1710.

Langs, R. J. (1967). Stability of earliest memories under LSD-25 and placebo. *Journal of Nervous and Mental Disease 144*(3), 171–84.

Lara-Carrasco, J., T. A. Nielsen, E. Solomonova, K. Levrier, and A. Popova (2009). Overnight emotional adaptation to negative stimuli is altered by REM sleep deprivation and is correlated with intervening dream emotions. *Journal of Sleep Research 18*(2), 178–87.

Laukkonen, R. E., B. T. Kaveladze, J. M. Tangen, and J. W. Schooler (2020). The dark side of eureka: artificially induced aha moments make facts feel true. *Cognition 196*, 104122.

Lebedev, A. V., M. Kaelen, M. Lövdén, J. Nilsson, A. Feilding, D. J. Nutt, and R. L. Carhart-Harris (2016). LSD-induced entropic brain activity predicts subsequent personality change: LSD-induced entropic brain activity. *Human Brain Mapping 37*(9), 3203–13.

Lebedev, A. V., M. Lövdén, G. Rosenthal, A. Feilding, D. J. Nutt, and R. L. Carhart-Harris (2015). Finding the self by losing the self: neural correlates of ego-dissolution under psilocybin. *Human Brain Mapping 36*(8), 3137–53.

Lebuda, I., D. L. Zabelina, and M. Karwowski (2016). Mind full of ideas: a meta-analysis of the mindfulness–creativity link. *Personality and Individual Differences 93*, 22–6.

Lee, C.-H. and F. Giuliani (2019). The role of inflammation in depression and fatigue. *Frontiers in Immunology 10*, 1696.

Lee, Y.-H., Y.-J. Shiah, S. C.-J. Chen, S.-F. Wang, M.-S. Young, and C.-L. Lin (2015). Improved emotional stability in experienced meditators with concentrative meditation based on electroencephalography and heart rate variability. *Journal of Alternative and Complementary Medicine 21*(1), 31–9.

Leeuwen, S. v., N. G. Müller, and L. Melloni (2009). Age effects on attentional blink performance in meditation. *Consciousness and Cognition 18*(3), 593–9.

Leeuwen, S. v., W. Singer, and L. Melloni (2012). Meditation increases the depth of information processing and improves the allocation of attention in space. *Frontiers in Human Neuroscience 6*, 133.

Lehrer, J. (2007). *Proust Was a Neuroscientist*. New York: Houghton Mifflin Company.

Leighton, T. D. and S. Okumura (2010). *Dogen's Extensive Record: A Translation of the Eihei Kōroku*. Somerville, MA: Wisdom Publications.

Leloup, J.-Y. and J. Rowe (2005). *The Gospel of Thomas: The Gnostic Wisdom of Jesus*. Rochester, VT: Inner Traditions.

Lennie, P. (2003). The cost of cortical computation. *Current Biology 13*(6), 493–7.

Letheby, C. (2021). *Philosophy of Psychedelics*. Oxford: Oxford University Press.

Letheby, C. and P. Gerrans (2017). Self unbound: ego dissolution in psychedelic experience. *Neuroscience of Consciousness 2017*(1), nix016.

Levi, U. and E. Rosenstreich (2019). Mindfulness and memory: a review of findings and a potential model. *Journal of Cognitive Enhancement 3*(3), 302–14.

Levinson, J. (2016). *Aesthetic Pursuits: Essays in Philosophy of Art*. Oxford: Oxford University Press.

Levman, B. (2017). Putting smrti back into sati (putting remembrance back into mindfulness). *Journal of the Oxford Centre for Buddhist Studies 13*, 121–49.

Levy, N. (2003). Analytic and continental philosophy: explaining the differences. *Metaphilosophy 34*(3), 284–304.

Lewis, C. R., K. H. Preller, R. Kraehenmann, L. Michels, P. Staempfli, and F. X. Vollenweider (2017). Two dose investigation of the 5-HT-agonist psilocybin on relative and global cerebral blood flow. *NeuroImage 159*, 70–8.

Lewis, D. (1976). The paradoxes of time travel. *American Philosophical Quarterly 13*(2), 145–52.

Lewis, D. (1980). Veridical hallucination and prosthetic vision. *Australasian Journal of Philosophy 58*(3), 239–49.

Lewis, P. A., G. Knoblich, and G. Poe (2018). How memory replay in sleep boosts creative problem-solving. *Trends in Cognitive Sciences 22*(6), 491–503.

Lichtenberg, G. (1971). *Schriften und Briefe, Vol. ii*. Munich: Carl Hanser Verlag.

Lichtenstein, S., B. Fischhoff, and L. Phillips (1982). Calibration of probabilities: the state of the art to 1980. In D. Kahneman, P. Slovic, and A. Tversky (eds.), *Judgment under Uncertainty: Heuristics and Biases*, pp. 306–44. Cambridge: Cambridge University Press.

Lifshitz, M., E. Sheiner, and L. J. Kirmayer (2018). Cultural neurophenomenology of psychedelic thought: guiding the 'unconstrained' mind through ritual context. In K. Christoff and K. C. Fox (eds.), *The Oxford Handbook of Spontaneous Thought: Mind-Wandering, Creativity, and Dreaming*, pp. 573–94. New York: Oxford University Press.

Lindahl, J. R., N. E. Fisher, D. J. Cooper, R. K. Rosen, and W. B. Britton (2017). The varieties of contemplative experience: a mixed-methods study of meditation-related challenges in Western Buddhists. *PLOS One 12*(5), e0176239.

Lindahl, J. R., C. T. Kaplan, E. M. Winget, and W. B. Britton (2014). A phenomenology of meditation-induced light experiences: traditional buddhist and neurobiological perspectives. *Frontiers in Psychology 4*, 973.

Lloyd, M., A. Szani, K. Rubenstein, C. Colgary, and L. Pereira-Pasarin (2016). A brief mindfulness exercise before retrieval reduces recognition memory false alarms. *Mindfulness 7*(3), 606–13.

Loftus, E. F. (1993). The reality of repressed memories. *American Psychologist 48*(5), 518–37.

Lollo, V. D. (2018). Attention is a sterile concept: iterative reentry is a fertile substitute. *Consciousness and Cognition 64*, 45–9.

Lopez, A. (2022). Vicarious attention, degrees of enhancement, and the contents of consciousness. *Philosophy and the Mind Sciences 3*, 1–42.

Lugg, A. (2014). Wittgenstein on showing what cannot be said. *Philosophical Investigations 37*(3), 246–57.

Luke, D. (2018). Reply to 'Ayahuasca turned on my mind's eye': a case of acquired versus congenital aphantasia, as evidenced with DMT use? *Journal of Psychedelic Studies 2*(2), 97–8.

Luria, A. (1968). *The Mind of a Mnemonist: A Little Book about a Vast Memory*. Cambridge, MA: Harvard University Press.

Lush, P., P. Naish, and Z. Dienes (2016). Metacognition of intentions in mindfulness and hypnosis. *Neuroscience of Consciousness 2016*(1), niw007.

Lycan, W. (1987). *Consciousness*. Cambridge, MA: MIT Press.

Lykins, E. L. B., R. A. Baer, and L. R. Gottlob (2012). Performance-based tests of attention and memory in long-term mindfulness meditators and demographically matched nonmeditators. *Cognitive Therapy and Research 36*(1), 103–14.

Lynch, D. (2007). *Catching the Big Fish: Meditation, Consciousness, and Creativity*. New York: Penguin Random House.

Lyon, A. (2016). Kolmogorov's axiomatisation and its discontents. In A. Hájek and C. Hitchcock (eds.), *The Oxford Handbook of Probability and Philosophy*. Oxford: Oxford University Press.

Lyon, A. and A. Farennikova (2022). Through the psychedelic looking-glass: the importance of phenomenal transparency in psychedelic transformation. *Philosophy and the Mind Sciences 3*(10).

Lyons, T. and R. L. Carhart-Harris (2018). More realistic forecasting of future life events after psilocybin for treatment-resistant depression. *Frontiers in Psychology 9*, 1721.

MacDonald, H. Z. and A. Olsen (2020). The role of attentional control in the relationship between mindfulness and anxiety. *Psychological Reports 123*(3), 33294119835756.

Mack, A. and I. Rock (1998). *Inattentional Blindness*. Cambridge, MA: MIT Press.

MacKenna, S. (1952). *Plotinus: The Enneads*. Erie, PA: Larson Publications.

MacLean, K. A., M. W. Johnson, and R. R. Griffiths (2011). Mystical experiences occasioned by the hallucinogen psilocybin lead to increases in the personality domain of openness. *Journal of Psychopharmacology (Oxford, England) 25*(11), 1453–61.

MacLean, M. H. and K. M. Arnell (2010). Personality predicts temporal attention costs in the attentional blink paradigm. *Psychonomic Bulletin & Review 17*(4), 556–62.

Macpherson, F. (2013). The philosophy and psychology of hallucination: an introduction. In F. Macpherson and D. Platchais (eds.), *Hallucination: Philosophy and Psychology*. Cambridge, MA: MIT Press.

Macpherson, F. and C. Batty (2016). Redefining illusion and hallucination in light of new cases. *Philosophical Issues 26*(1), 263–96.

Madsen, M. K., P. M. Fisher, D. S. Stenbæk, S. Kristiansen, D. Burmester, S. Lehel, T. Páleníček, M. Kuchař, C. Svarer, B. Ozenne, and G. M. Knudsen (2020). A single psilocybin dose is associated with long-term increased mindfulness, preceded by a proportional change in neocortical 5-HT2A receptor binding. *European Neuropsychopharmacology: Journal of the European College of Neuropsychopharmacology 33*, 71–80.

Madsen, M. K., D. S. Stenbæk, A. Arvidsson, S. Armand, M. R. Marstrand-Joergensen, S. S. Johansen, K. Linnet, B. Ozenne, G. M. Knudsen, and P. M. Fisher (2021). Psilocybin-induced changes in brain network integrity and segregation correlate with plasma psilocin level and psychedelic experience. *European Neuropsychopharmacology 50*, 121–32.

Maier, N. R. F. (1931). Reasoning in humans. II. The solution of a problem and its appearance in consciousness. *Journal of Comparative Psychology 12*(2), 181–94.

Maillart-Garg, M. and M. Winkelman (2019). The 'Kamasutra' temples of India: a case for the encoding of psychedelically induced spirituality. *Journal of Psychedelic Studies 3*(2), 81–103.

Malhotra, A. K. (2006). *Wisdom of the Tao Te Ching: The Code of a Spiritual Warrior*. State University of New York, Oneonta.

Malone, T. C., S. E. Mennenga, J. Guss, S. K. Podrebarac, L. T. Owens, A. P. Bossis, A. B. Belser, G. Agin-Liebes, M. P. Bogenschutz, and S. Ross (2018). Individual experiences in four cancer patients following psilocybin-assisted psychotherapy. *Frontiers in Pharmacology 9*, 256.

Mashour, G. A. (2022). Ketamine analgesia and psychedelia: can we dissociate dissociation? *Anesthesiology 136*(5), 675–77.

Maslow, A. H. (1963). *The Fartherest Reaches of Human Nature*. New York: McGraw-Hill Book Company.

Mason, M. F., M. I. Norton, J. D. V. Horn, D. M. Wegner, S. T. Grafton, and C. N. Macrae (2007). Wandering minds: the default network and stimulus-independent thought. *Science 315*(5810), 393–5.

Mason, N. L., K. P. C. Kuypers, F. Müller, J. Reckweg, D. H. Y. Tse, S. W. Toennes, N. R. P. W. Hutten, J. F. A. Jansen, P. Stiers, A. Feilding, and J. G. Ramaekers (2020). Me, myself, bye: regional alterations in glutamate and the experience of ego dissolution with psilocybin. *Neuropsychopharmacology 45*(12), 2003–11.

Mason, N., K. Kuypers, J. Reckweg, F. Muller, and J. Ramaekers (2021). P.214 (Sub)acute effects of psilocybin on creative cognition: a double-blind, placebo-controlled experimental study. *European Neuropsychopharmacology 44*, S25–S26.

Mason, N. L., K. P. C. Kuypers, J. T. Reckweg, F. Müller, D. H. Y. Tse, B. D. Rios, S. W. Toennes, P. Stiers, A. Feilding, and J. G. Ramaekers (2021). Spontaneous and deliberate creative cognition during and after psilocybin exposure. *Translational Psychiatry 11*(1), 209.

Mason, N. L., E. Mischler, M. V. Uthaug, and K. P. C. Kuypers (2019). Sub-acute effects of psilocybin on empathy, creative thinking, and subjective well-being. *Journal of Psychoactive Drugs 51*(2), 123–34.

Mason, O. J. and F. Brady (2009). The psychotomimetic effects of short-term sensory deprivation. *Journal of Nervous and Mental Disease 197*(10), 783–5.

Mathur, S., M. P. Sharma, S. Balachander, T. Kandavel, and Y. J. Reddy (2021). A randomized controlled trial of mindfulness-based cognitive therapy vs stress management training for obsessive-compulsive disorder. *Journal of Affective Disorders 282*, 58–68.

McEvilley, T. (2002). *The Shape of Ancient Thought: Comparative Studies in Greek and Indian Philosophies*. New York: Allworth Press.

McGlothlin, W., S. Cohen, and M. S. McGlothlin (1967). Long lasting effects of LSD on normals. *Archives of General Psychiatry 17*(5), 521.

McGuinness, B. F. (1966). The mysticism of the Tractatus. *Philosophical Review 75*(3), 305.

Mele, A. R. (2014). *Free: Why Science Hasn't Disproved Free Will*. Oxford: Oxford University Press.

Merabet, L. B., D. Maguire, A. Warde, K. Alterescu, R. Stickgold, and A. Pascual-Leone (2004). Visual hallucinations during prolonged blindfolding in sighted subjects. *Journal of Neuro-Ophthalmology 24*(2), 109–13.

Merikle, P. M., D, Smilek, and J. D. Eastwood (2001). Perception without awareness: perspectives from cognitive psychology. *Cognition, 79*(1–2), 115–34.

Metzinger, T. (2003). *Being No One: The Self-Model Theory of Subjectivity*. Cambridge, MA: MIT Press.

Metzner, R. and T. Leary (1967). On programming psychedelic experiences. *Psychedelic Review 9*, 5–19.

Mian, M. N., B. R. Altman, and M. Earleywine (2020). Ayahuasca's antidepressant effects covary with behavioral activation as well as mindfulness. *Journal of Psychoactive Drugs 52*(2), 1–8.

Miller, J. J. (1983). The unveiling of traumatic memories and emotions through mindfulness and concentration meditation. *Journal of Transpersonal Psychology 25*(2), 169–80.

Miller, R. F. (1981). *Dostoevsky and The Idiot*. Cambridge, MA and London: Harvard University Press.

Millière, R., R. L. Carhart-Harris, L. Roseman, F.-M. Trautwein, and A. Berkovich-Ohana (2018, 9). Psychedelics, meditation, and self-consciousness. *Frontiers in Psychology 9*, 1475.

Mirams, L., E. Poliakoff, R. J. Brown, and D. M. Lloyd (2013). Brief body-scan meditation practice improves somatosensory perceptual decision making. *Consciousness and Cognition 22*(1), 348–59.

Mitchell, S. (1988). *Tao Te Ching: A New English Version*. Harper Perennial Modern Classics.

Mohs, F. and W. Haidinger (1825). *Treatise on Mineralogy, or, The Natural History of the Mineral Kingdom by Frederick Mohs; Translated from the German, with Considerable Additions, by William Haidinger*. Edinburgh and London: Printed for Archibald Constable and Co.; and Hurst, Robinson, and Co.

Moll, A. (1890). *Hypnotism*. London: Walter Scott.

Moore, C. (2015). *Socrates and Self-Knowledge*. Cambridge: Cambridge University Press.

Moore, C. (2019). *Calling Philosophers Names: On the Origin of a Discipline*. Princeton: Princeton University Press.

Moore, C. M. and H. Egeth (1997). Perception without attention: evidence of grouping under conditions of inattention. *Journal of Experimental Psychology: Human Perception and Performance 23*(2), 339–52.

Mordvintsev, A., C. Olah, and M. Tyka (2015). Inceptionism: going deeper into neural networks, url: https://ai.googleblog.com/2015/06/inceptionism-going-deeper-into-neural.html

Moreton, S. G., L. Szalla, R. E. Menzies, and A. F. Arena (2020). Embedding existential psychology within psychedelic science: reduced death anxiety as a mediator of the therapeutic effects of psychedelics. *Psychopharmacology 237*(1), 21–32.

Morris, M. and J. Dodd (2007). Mysticism and nonsense in the Tractatus. *European Journal of Philosophy 17*(2), 247–76.

Mouly, A.-M. and R. Sullivan (2010). The neurobiology of olfaction. *Frontiers in Neuroscience 20092457*, 367–94.

Muraresku, B. C. (2020). *The Immortality Key: The Secret History of the Religion with No Name*. New York: St. Martin's Press.

Murphy, J. J. (1996). Meister Eckhart and the via negativa: epistemology and mystical language. *New Blackfriars 77*(908), 458–72.

Murphy-Beiner, A. and K. Soar (2020). Ayahuasca's 'afterglow': improved mindfulness and cognitive flexibility in ayahuasca drinkers. *Psychopharmacology 237*(4), 1161–9.

Murray, J. D. (2003). *Mathematical Biology: I. An Introduction.*, Vol. 17. New York: Springer Science & Business Media.

Müller, F., P. C. Dolder, A. Schmidt, M. E. Liechti, and S. Borgwardt (2018). Altered network hub connectivity after acute LSD administration. *NeuroImage: Clinical 18*, 694–701.

Müller, B. C. N., A. Gerasimova, and S. M. Ritter (2016). Concentrative meditation influences creativity by increasing cognitive flexibility. *Psychology of Aesthetics, Creativity, and the Arts 10*(3), 278–86.

Nagele, P., B. J. Palanca, B. Gott, F. Brown, L. Barnes, T. Nguyen, W. Xiong, N. C. Salloum, G. D. Espejo, C. N. Lessov-Schlaggar, N. Jain, W. W. L. Cheng, H. Komen, B. Yee, J. D. Bolzenius, A. Janski, R. Gibbons, C. F. Zorumski, and C. R. Conway (2021). A phase 2 trial of inhaled nitrous oxide for treatment-resistant major depression. *Science Translational Medicine 13*(597), eabe1376.

Namgyal, L. T. (2011). Introduction. In K. T. Rinpoche and L. T. Namgyal (eds.), *The Ninth Karmapa's Ocean of Definitive Meaning*, pp. 1–19. Boulder, CO: Snow Lion Publications.

Nanamoli, B. and B. Bodhi (1995). *The Middle Length Discourses of the Buddha: A Translation of the Majjhima Nikaya*. Somerville, MA: Wisdom Publications.

Nanay, B. (2014). An experiential account of creativity. In E. S. Paul and S. B. Kaufman (eds.), *The Philosophy of Creativity: New Essays*, pp. 17–35. Oxford: Oxford University Press.

Nanay, B. (2016a). *Aesthetics as Philosophy of Perception*. Oxford: Oxford University Press.

Nanay, B. (2016b). Hallucination as mental imagery. *Journal of Consciousness Studies*.

Nanay, B. (2021). Unconscious mental imagery. *Philosophical Transactions of the Royal Society B 376*(1817), 20190689.

Narby, J. (2001). Shamans and scientists. In J. Narby and F. Huxley (eds.), *Shamans through Time*. New York: Tarcher/Putnam.

Nau, F., B. Yu, D. Martin, and C. D. Nichols (2013). Serotonin 5-HT2A receptor activation blocks TNF-alpha mediated inflammation in vivo. *PLOS One 8*(10), e75426.

Neisser, U. and R. Becklen (1975). Selective looking: attending to visually specified events. *Cognitive Psychology 7*(4), 480–94.

Newen, A., S. Gallagher, and L. D. Bruin (2018). 4E cognition: historical roots, key concepts, and central issues. In A. Newen, L. D. Bruin, and S. Gallagher (eds.), *The Oxford Handbook of 4E Cognition*, pp. 2–16. Oxford: Oxford University Press.

Nichols, D., M. Johnson, and C. Nichols (2017). Psychedelics as medicines: an emerging new paradigm. *Clinical Pharmacology & Therapeutics 101*(2), 209–19.

Nichols, D. E. (1986). Differences between the mechanism of action of MDMA, MBDB, and the classic hallucinogens. Identification of a new therapeutic class: entactogens. *Journal of Psychoactive Drugs 18*(4), 305–13.

Nichols, S., N. Strohminger, A. Rai, and J. Garfield (2018). Death and the self. *Cognitive Science 42*, 314–32.

Nida-Rümelin, M. (2017). Self-awareness. *Review of Philosophy and Psychology 8*(1), 55–82.

Nieli, R. (1987). *Wittgenstein: From Mysticism to Ordinary Language*. New York: SUNY Press.

Nielsen, C. J. (2001). Effect of scenario and experience on interpretation of mach bands. *Journal of Endodontics 27*(11), 687–91.

Nielsen, L. and A. W. Kaszniak (2006). Awareness of subtle emotional feelings: a comparison of long-term meditators and nonmeditators. *Emotion 6*(3), 392–405.

Nisbett, R. E. and T. D. Wilson (1977). Telling more than we can know: verbal reports on mental processes. *Psychological Review 84*(3), 231–59.

Nobre, A. d. P., G. M. d. Melo, G. Gauer, and J. Wagemans (2020). Implicit processing during inattentional blindness: a systematic review and meta-analysis. *Neuroscience & Biobehavioral Reviews 119*, 355–75.

Noorani, T., A. Garcia-Romeu, T. C. Swift, R. R. Griffiths, and M. W. Johnson (2018). Psychedelic therapy for smoking cessation: qualitative analysis of participant accounts. *Journal of Psychopharmacology (Oxford, England) 32*(7), 269881118780612.

Norton, J. D. (2020). How NOT to build an infinite lottery machine. *Studies in History and Philosophy of Science Part A 82*, 1–8.

Nour, M. M., L. Evans, and R. L. Carhart-Harris (2017). Psychedelics, personality and political perspectives. *Journal of Psychoactive Drugs 49*(3), 1–10.

Nozick, R. (1989). *The Examined Life*. New York: Simon & Schuster.

Nutt, D. and R. Carhart-Harris (2020). The current status of psychedelics in psychiatry. *JAMA Psychiatry 78*(2), 121–2.

Nutt, D. J., L. A. King, and D. E. Nichols (2013). Effects of schedule I drug laws on neuroscience research and treatment innovation. *Nature Reviews Neuroscience 14*(8), 577–85.

Nyhus, E., W. A. Engel, T. D. Pitfield, and I. M. W. Vakkur (2019). Increases in theta oscillatory activity during episodic memory retrieval following mindfulness meditation training. *Frontiers in Human Neuroscience 13*, 311.

Nyhus, E., W. A. Engel, T. D. Pitfield, and I. M. W. Vakkur (2020, 5). Combining behavior and EEG to study the effects of mindfulness meditation on episodic memory. *Journal of Visualized Experiments : JoVE* (159).

O'Brien, G. and J. Jureidini (2002a). Dispensing with the dynamic unconscious. *Philosophy, Psychiatry, & Psychology 9*(2), 141–53.

O'Brien, G. and J. Jureidini (2002b). The last rites of the dynamic unconscious. *Philosophy, Psychiatry, & Psychology 9*(2), 161–6.

Ogren, B. (2016). Mysticism historicized: historical figures and movements. In A. D. DeConick (ed.), *Secret Religion*, pp. 315–29. Farmington Hills, MI: Gale, Cengage Learning: MacMillan Reference.

Oizumi, M., L. Albantakis, and G. Tononi (2014). From the phenomenology to the mechanisms of consciousness: integrated information theory 3.0. *PLOS Computational Biology 10*(5), e1003588.

Olivelle, P. (1998). *The Early Upanisads: An Annotated Text and Translation*. New York: Oxford University Press.

Oorsouw, K. v., S. W. Toennes, and J. G. Ramaekers (2022). Therapeutic effect of an ayahuasca analogue in clinically depressed patients: a longitudinal observational study. *Psychopharmacology 239*(6), 1–14.

Oroc, J. (2011). Psychedelics and extreme sports. *Multidisciplinary Association for Psychedelic Studies Bulletin 21*(1), 25–9.

Osmond, H. (1957). A review of the clinical effects of psychotomimetic agents. *Annals of the New York Academy of Sciences 66*(3), 418–34.

Ost, J., H. Blank, J. Davies, G. Jones, K. Lambert, and K. Salmon (2013). False memory [is not equal to] false memory: DRM errors are unrelated to the misinformation effect. *PLOS One 8*(4), e57939.

Ostafin, B. D. and K. T. Kassman (2012). Stepping out of history: mindfulness improves insight problem solving. *Consciousness and Cognition 21*(2), 1031–6.

Oster, G. (1966). Moiré patterns and visual hallucinations. *Psychedelic Review 7*, 33–40.

Otto, R. (1932). *Mysticism East and West: A Comparative Analysis of the Nature of Mysticism*. London: Macmillan & Co.

Outler, A. C. (2006). *Augustine: Confessions and Enchiridion*. Philadelphia: Westminster John Knox Press.

Paffen, C. L., D. Alais, and F. A. Verstraten (2006). Attention speeds binocular rivalry. *Psychological Science 17*(9), 752–6.

Pahnke, W. N. (1969). Psychedelic drugs and mystical experience. *International Psychiatry Clinics 5*(4), 149–62.

Pahnke, W. N. and W. A. Richards (1966). Implications of LSD and experimental mysticism. *Journal of Religion and Health 5*(3), 175–208.

Palhano-Fontes, F., K. C. Andrade, L. F. Tofoli, A. C. Santos, J. A. S. Crippa, J. E. C. Hallak, S. Ribeiro, and D. B. de. Araujo (2015). The psychedelic state induced by ayahuasca modulates the activity and connectivity of the default mode network. *PLOS One 10*(2), e0118143.

Pandit, A. S., M. de Gouveia, H. L. Horsfall, A. Reka, and H. J. Marcus (2022). Efficacy of a mindfulness-based intervention in ameliorating inattentional blindness amongst young neurosurgeons: a prospective, controlled pilot study. *Frontiers in Surgery 9*, 916228.

Papenfuss, I., M. J. J. Lommen, M. Huisman, and B. D. Ostafin (2022). Aversive response to uncertainty as a mediator for the effect of a mindfulness intervention on symptoms of anxiety. *International Journal of Psychophysiology 179*, 30–42.

Pasquini, L., F. Palhano-Fontes, and Araujo, D. B. (2020). Subacute effects of the psychedelic ayahuasca on the salience and default mode networks. *Journal of Psychopharmacology 34*(6), 623–35.

Patihis, L., S. J. Frenda, and E. F. Loftus (2018). False memory tasks do not reliably predict other false memories. *Psychology of Consciousness: Theory, Research, and Practice 5*(2), 140–60.

Payne, J. E., R. Chambers, and P. Liknaitzky (2021). Combining psychedelic and mindfulness interventions: synergies to inform clinical practice. *ACS Pharmacology & Translational Science 4*(2), 416–23.

Peacocke, C. (2012). I—Descartes defended. *Aristotelian Society Supplementary Volume 86*(1), 109–25.

Peelen, M. V., D. J. Heslenfeld, and J. Theeuwes (2004). Endogenous and exogenous attention shifts are mediated by the same large-scale neural network. *NeuroImage 22*(2), 822–30.

Peill, J. M., K. E. Trinci, H. Kettner, L. J. Mertens, L. Roseman, C. Timmermann, F. E. Rosas, T. Lyons, and R. L. Carhart-Harris (2022). Validation of the psychological insight scale: a new scale to assess psychological insight following a psychedelic experience. *Journal of Psychopharmacology 36*(1), 31–45.

Poincaré, H. (1910). Mathematical creation. *The Monist 20*(3), 321–35.

Pokorski, M. and A. Suchorzynska (2018). Psychobehavioral effects of meditation. *Advances in Experimental Medicine and Biology 1023*, 85–91.

Polanyi, M. (1966). *The Tacit Dimension*. Garden City, NY: Doubleday.

Pollan, M. (2018). *How to Change Your Mind: What the New Science of Psychedelics Teaches Us about Consciousness, Dying, Addiction, Depression, and Transcendence*. Penguin Books.

Polosmak, N. V. (2010). We drank soma, we became immortal... *Science First Hand 26*(2), 63–71.

Posner, M. I., C. R. Snyder, and B. J. Davidson (1980). Attention and the detection of signals. *Journal of Experimental Psychology: General 109*(2), 160–74.

Prado, C. G. (2003). *A House Divided: Comparing Analytic and Continental Philosophy*. San Jose, CA: Humanity Books.

Prasad, S. and R. K. Mishra (2019). The nature of unconscious attention to subliminal cues. *Vision 3*(3), 38.

Preller, K. H., A. Razi, P. Zeidman, P. Stämpfli, K. J. Friston, and F. X. Vollenweider (2019). Effective connectivity changes in LSD-induced altered states of consciousness in humans. *Proceedings of the National Academy of Sciences of the United States of America 116*(7), 2743–8 [LSD (analysis of original: Preller et al. 2018)].

Price, C. J., E. A. Thompson, S. Crowell, and K. Pike (2019). Longitudinal effects of interoceptive awareness training through mindful awareness in body-oriented therapy (MABT) as an adjunct to women's substance use disorder treatment: a randomized controlled trial. *Drug and Alcohol Dependence 198*, 140–9.

Prinz, J. (2012). Whose consciousness? The illusory self. In *The Conscious Brain: How Attention Engenders Experience*, pp. 213–40. Oxford: Oxford University Press.

Prochazkova, L. and B. Hommel (2020). Altered states of consciousness and creativity. In D. D. Preiss, D. Cosmelli, and J. C. Kaufman (eds.), *Creativity and the Wandering Mind: Spontaneous and Controlled Cognition*, pp. 121–58. London: Academic Press.

Proust M. (1913–27). 1982. Remembrance of Things Past. Volume 1: Swann's Way: Within a Budding Grove. The definitive French Pleiade edition translated by C.K. Scott Moncrieff and Terence Kilmartin. New York: Vintage. pp. 48–51.

Proverbio, A. M. and A. Zani (2002). Electrophysiological indexes of illusory contours perception in humans. *Neuropsychologia 40*(5), 479–91.

Purser, R. E. and J. Milillo (2015). Mindfulness revisited. *Journal of Management Inquiry 24*(1), 3–24.

Puxty, D. J., J. G. Ramaekers, R. d. l. Torre, M. Farré, N. Pizarro, M. Pujadas, and K. P. C. Kuypers (2017). MDMA-induced dissociative state not mediated by the 5-HT2A receptor. *Frontiers in Pharmacology 8*, 455.

Pylyshyn, Z. W. (1980). Computation and cognition: issues in the foundations of cognitive science. *Behavioral and Brain Sciences 3*(1), 111–32.

Quach, D., K. E. J. Mano, and K. Alexander (2016). A randomized controlled trial examining the effect of mindfulness meditation on working memory capacity in adolescents. *Journal of Adolescent Health 58*(5), 489–96.

Quednow, B. B., M. Kometer, M. A. Geyer, and F. X. Vollenweider (2012). Psilocybin-induced deficits in automatic and controlled inhibition are attenuated by ketanserin in healthy human volunteers. *Neuropsychopharmacology 37*(3), npp2011228.

Quincey, D. (1821). *Confessions of the Opium Eater*. London: New York: London Magazine.

Quine, W. V. O. (1960). *Word and Object*. New York: John Wiley.

Raffone, A., L. Marzetti, C. D. Gratta, M. G. Perrucci, G. L. Romani, and V. Pizzella (2019). Toward a brain theory of meditation. *Progress in Brain Research 244*, 207–32.

Ransom, M. and S. Fazelpour (2020). The many faces of attention: why precision optimization is not attention. In D. Mendonça, J. M. R. Curado, and S. Gouveia (eds.), *The Philosophy and Science of Predictive Processing*, pp. 119–39. London: Bloomsbury Academic.

Raphiphatthana, B., P. Jose, and K. Salmon (2018). Does dispositional mindfulness predict the development of grit? *Journal of Individual Differences 39*(2), 76–87.

Rawls, J. (1971). *A Theory of Justice*. Cambridge, MA: Harvard University Press.

Rayo, A. (2011). A puzzle about ineffable propositions. *Australasian Journal of Philosophy 89*(2), 289–95.

Reber, A. S. (1989). Implicit learning and tacit knowledge. *Journal of Experimental Psychology: General 118*(3), 219–35.

Reeve, C. (2012). *A Plato Reader*. Indianapolis, IN: Hackett Publishing.

Ren, J., Z. Huang, J. Luo, G. Wei, X. Ying, Z. Ding, Y. Wu, and F. Luo (2011). Meditation promotes insightful problem-solving by keeping people in a mindful and alert conscious state. *Science China Life Sciences 54*(10), 961–5.

Reveal (2020). *Cambridge English Dictionary*. Available at: https://dictionary.cambridge.org/dictionary/english/reveal (Accessed 20 April, 2020).

Rice, F., A. Rawal, L. Riglin, G. Lewis, G. Lewis, and S. Dunsmuir (2015). Examining reward-seeking, negative self-beliefs and over-general autobiographical memory as mechanisms of change in classroom prevention programs for adolescent depression. *Journal of Affective Disorders 186*, 320–7.

Rich, A. N. and J. B. Mattingley (2013). The role of attention in synesthesia. In J. Simner and E. Hubbard (eds.), *Oxford Handbook of Synesthesia*. Oxford: Oxford University Press.

Richards, W. (1975). Counseling, peak experiences and the human encounter with death: an empirical study of the efficacy of DPT-assisted counseling in enhancing the quality of life of persons with terminal cancer and their closest family members. Ph.D. thesis.

Richards, W. A. (2015). *Sacred Knowledge: Psychedelics and Religious Experiences*. New York: Columbia University Press.

Rieser, N. M., M. Herdener, and K. H. Preller (2021). Psychedelic-assisted therapy for substance use disorders and potential Mechanisms of action. *Current Topics in Behavioral Neurosciences*, 1–25.

Ringach, D. L. (2009). Spontaneous and driven cortical activity: implications for computation. *Current Opinion in Neurobiology 19*(4), 439–44.

Rinpoche, K. T. (2011). *The Ninth Karmapa's Ocean of Definitive Meaning*. Ithaca: Snow Lion.

Rios, M. D. d. and O. Janiger (2003). *LSD, Spirituality and the Creative Process*. Rochester: Park Street Press.

Ritchie, T. D., J. J. Skowronski, W. R. Walker, and S. E. Wood (2006). Comparing two perceived characteristics of autobiographical memory: memory detail and accessibility. *Memory 14*(4), 471–85.

Roca, P. and C. Vazquez (2020). Brief meditation trainings improve performance in the emotional attentional blink. *Mindfulness 11*(7), 1613–22.

Rocha, J. M., G. N. Rossi, F. L. Osório, J. C. B. Saiz, G. D. O. Silveira, M. Yonamine, E. J. Crevelin, M. E., Queiroz, J. E. C. Hallak, and R. G. D. Santos (2021). Effects of ayahuasca on personality: results of two randomized, placebo-controlled trials in healthy volunteers. *Frontiers in Psychiatry 12*, 688439.

Roediger, H. L. and K. B. McDermott (1995). Creating false memories: remembering words not presented in lists. *Journal of Experimental Psychology: Learning, Memory, and Cognition 21*(4), 803–14.

Rorty, R. (1967). *The Linguistic Turn*. Chicago: Chicago University Press.

Roseman, L., E. Haijen, K. Idialu-Ikato, M. Kaelen, R. Watts, and R. Carhart-Harris (2019). Emotional breakthrough and psychedelics: validation of the emotional breakthrough inventory. *Journal of Psychopharmacology 33*(9), 1076–87.

Roseman, L., D. J. Nutt, and R. L. Carhart-Harris (2018). Quality of acute psychedelic experience predicts therapeutic efficacy of psilocybin for treatment-resistant depression. *Frontiers in Pharmacology 8*, 974.

Rosenkranz, M. A., R. J. Davidson, D. G. Maccoon, J. F. Sheridan, N. H. Kalin, and A. Lutz (2013). A comparison of mindfulness-based stress reduction and an active control in modulation of neurogenic inflammation. *Brain, Behavior, and Immunity 27*(1), 174–84.

Rosenstreich, E. (2016). Mindfulness and false-memories: the impact of mindfulness practice on the DRM paradigm. *Journal of Psychology 150*(1), 58–71.

Rosenstreich, E. and L. Ruderman (2017). A dual-process perspective on mindfulness, memory, and consciousness. *Mindfulness 8*(2), 505–16.

Ross, S., A. Bossis, J. Guss, G. Agin-Liebes, T. Malone, B. Cohen, S. E. Mennenga, A. Belser, K. Kalliontzi, J. Babb, Z. Su, P. Corby, and B. L. Schmidt (2016). Rapid and sustained symptom reduction following psilocybin treatment for anxiety and depression in patients with life-threatening cancer: a randomized controlled trial. *Journal of Psychopharmacology 30*(12), 1165–80.

Ruedy, N. E. and M. E. Schweitzer (2010). In the moment: the effect of mindfulness on ethical decision making. *Journal of Business Ethics 95*(Suppl 1), 73–87.

Rumelhart, D. E., J. L. McClelland, and P. R. Group (1986). *Parallel Distributed Processing*, Vols. 1–2. Cambridge, MA: MIT Press.

Runco, M. A. and G. J. Jaeger (2012). The standard definition of creativity. *Creativity Research Journal 24*(1), 92–6.

Russell, B. (1910a). Knowledge by acquaintance and knowledge by description. *Proceedings of the Aristotelian Society 11*(1), 108–28.

Russell, B. (1910b). *Mysticism and Logic and Other Essays*. London: George Allen & Unwin Ltd.

Russell, B. (1912). *The Problems of Philosophy*. New York: H. Holt and Co.

Russell, B. (1945). *A History of Western Philosophy and Its Connection with Political and Social Circumstances from the Earliest Times to the Present Day*. New York: Simon and Schuster.

Russell, B. (1950). Philosophy for laymen. In *Unpopular Essays*, pp. 38–49. New York: Simon & Schuster.

Russell, B. (1951). *New Hopes for a Changing World*. New York: Simon & Schuster.

Ryan, S. (2020). Wisdom. In Edward N. Zalta (ed.), *The Stanford Encyclopedia of Philosophy* (Spring 2020 edition), url: https://plato.stanford.edu/archives/spr2020/entries/wisdom/

Ryff, C. D. (1989). Happiness is everything, or is it? Explorations on the meaning of psychological well-being. *Journal of Personality and Social Psychology 57*(6), 1069–81.

Safron, A. (2020). On the varieties of conscious experiences: altered beliefs under psychedelics (ALBUS). *PsyArXiv Preprints*.

Sahn, S. (2012). *The Compass of Zen*. Boston: Shambala.

Sampedro, F., M. d. l. F. Revenga, M. Valle, N. Roberto, E. Domínguez-Clavé, M. Elices, L. E. Luna, J. A. S. Crippa, J. E. C. Hallak, D. B. d. Araujo, P. Friedlander, S. A. Barker, E. Álvarez, J. Soler, J. C. Pascual, A. Feilding, and J. Riba (2017). Assessing the psychedelic 'after-glow' in ayahuasca users: post-acute neurometabolic and functional connectivity changes are associated with enhanced mindfulness capacities. *International Journal of Neuropsychopharmacology 20*(9), pyx036–.

Sanders, J. W. and J. Zijlmans (2021). Moving past mysticism in psychedelic science. *ACS Pharmacology & Translational Science 4*(3), 1253–55.

Sandison, Spencer, and Whitelaw (1954). The therapeutic value of lysergic acid diethylamide in mental illness. *Journal of Mental Science 100*(419), 491–507.

Sandison, R. A. (1959). The role of psychotropic drugs in individual therapy. *Bulletin of the World Health Organisation 21*, 495–503.

Sandison, R. A. (1963). Certainty and uncertainty in the LSD treatment of psychoneurosis. In R. Crockett, R. Sanderson, and A. Wolk (eds.), *Hallucinogenic Drugs and Their Psychotherapeutic Use*. Springfield, IL: Charles C. Thomas.

Santos, R. G. d., S. Enyart, J. C. Bouso, O. Pares, and J. E. C. Hallak (2018). AAA. *Journal of Psychedelic Studies 2*(2), 74–7.

Sanz, C., F. Zamberlan, E. Erowid, F. Erowid, and E. Tagliazucchi (2018). The experience elicited by hallucinogens presents the highest similarity to dreaming within a large database of psychoactive substance reports. *Frontiers in Neuroscience 12*, 7.

Sasaki, K. J. (1974). *Buddha Is the Center of Gravity*. San Cristobal, NM: Lama Foundation.

Sasaki, R. F. (2009). *The Record of Linji*. Honolulu: University of Hawaii Press.

Sastri, A. M. (1921). *Amritabindu and Kaivalya Upanishads*. Madras: V. Ramaswami Sastrulu & Sons.

Savage, C. (1952). Lysergic acid diethylamide (LSD-25). *American Journal of Psychiatry 108*(12), 896–900.

Scarpelli, S., C. Bartolacci, A. D'Atri, M. Gorgoni, and L. D. Gennaro (2019). The functional role of dreaming in emotional processes. *Frontiers in Psychology 10*, 459.

Scheibner, H. J., C. Bogler, T. Gleich, J.-D. Haynes, and F. Bermpohl (2017). Internal and external attention and the default mode network. *NeuroImage 148*, 381–9.

Schiff, N. D., S. A. Shah, A. E. Hudson, T. Nauvel, S. F. Kalik, and K. P. Purpura (2013). Gating of attentional effort through the central thalamus. *Journal of Neurophysiology, 109*(4), 1152–63.

Schiffman, R. (2016). Psilocybin: a journey beyond the fear of death? *Scientific American*, url: https:// www.scientificamerican.com/article/psilocybin-a-journey-beyond-the-fear-of-death/

Schiller, P. H. and C. E. Carvey (2005). The Hermann grid illusion revisited. *Perception 34*(11), 1375–97.

Schlosser, M., T. Sparby, S. Vörös, R. Jones, and N. L. Marchant (2019). Unpleasant meditation-related experiences in regular meditators: prevalence, predictors, and conceptual considerations. *PLOS One 14*(5), e0216643.

Schmid, Y. and M. E. Liechti (2018). Long-lasting subjective effects of LSD in normal subjects. *Psychopharmacology 235*(2), 535–45.

Schmitzer-Torbert, N. (2020). Mindfulness and decision making: sunk costs or escalation of commitment? *Cognitive Processing 21*(3), 391–402.

Schofield, T. P., J. D. Creswell, and T. F. Denson (2015). Brief mindfulness induction reduces inattentional blindness. *Consciousness and Cognition 37*, 63–70.

Schultes, R. E., A. Hofmann, and C. Ratsch (2001). *Plants of the Gods: Their Sacred, Healing, and Hallucinogenic Powers*. Rochester, VT: Healing Arts Press.

Schwitzgebel, E. (2002). How well do we know our own conscious experience? The case of visual imagery. *Journal of Consciousness Studies 9*(5–6), 35–53.

Seligman, M. E. P. (2011). *Flourish: A Visionary New Understanding of Happiness and Well-Being*. New York: Free Press.

Sergent, C., V. Wyart, M. Babo-Rebelo, L. Cohen, L. Naccache, and C. Tallon-Baudry (2013). Cueing attention after the stimulus is gone can retrospectively trigger conscious perception. *Current Biology : CB 23*(2), 150–5.

Sessa, B. (2008). Is it time to revisit the role of psychedelic drugs in enhancing human creativity? *Journal of Psychopharmacology 22*(8), 821–7.

Shah, D. and L. M. Knott (2018). The role of attention at retrieval on the false recognition of negative emotional DRM lists. *Memory 26*(2), 1–8.

Shanon, B. (2002). *The Antipodes of the Mind: Charting the Phenomenology of the Ayahuasca Experience*. Oxford: Oxford University Press on Demand.

Sharf, R. (1995). Buddhist modernism and the rhetoric of meditative experience. *Numen 42*(3), 228–83.

Sharf, R. (2000). The rhetoric of experience and the study of religion. *Journal of Consciousness Studies 7*(11–12), 267–87.

Shariatmadari, D. (2015). Daniel Kahneman: 'What would I eliminate if I had a magic wand? Overconfidence', url: https://www.theguardian.com/books/2015/jul/18/daniel-kahneman-books-interview.

Sheldon, K. M. and A. J. Elliot (1999). Goal striving, need satisfaction, and longitudinal well-being: the self-concordance model. *Journal of Personality and Social Psychology 76*(3), 482–97.

Sherman, S. M. and J. A. Grange (2020). Exploring the impact of mindfulness on false-memory susceptibility. *Psychological Science 31*(8), 968–77.

Shields, G. S., A. C. Skwara, B. G. King, A. P. Zanesco, F. S. Dhabhar, and C. D. Saron (2020). Deconstructing the effects of concentration meditation practice on interference control: the roles of controlled attention and inflammatory activity. *Brain, Behavior, and Immunity 89*, 256–67.

Shore, J. (2016). *Great Doubt: Practicing Zen in the World*. Somerville, MA Wisdom Publications.

Short, E. B., S. Kose, Q. Mu, J. Borckardt, A. Newberg, M. S. George, and F. A. Kozel (2010). Regional brain activation during meditation shows time and practice effects: an exploratory FMRI study. *Evidence-Based Complementary and Alternative Medicine 7*(1), 121–7.

Shrader, D. W. (2008). Seven characteristics of mystical experiences. *Proceedings of the 6th Annual Hawaii International Conference on Arts and Humanities*.

Shulman, E. (2010). Mindful wisdom: the Sati-pahāna-sutta on mindfulness, memory, and liberation. *History of Religions 49*(4), 393–420.

Siderits, M., E. Thompson, and D. Zahavi (2011). Self, no self?: Perspectives from analytical, phenomenological, and Indian traditions. In *Perspectives from Analytical, Phenomenological, and Indian Traditions*. Oxford: Oxford Scholarship Online.

Siegler, R. S. (2000). Unconscious insights. *Current Directions in Psychological Science 9*(3), 79–83.

Silverman, J. (1971). Research with psychedelics. *Archives of General Psychiatry 25*(6), 498.

Silvia, P. J., E. C. Nusbaum, C. Berg, C. Martin, and A. O'Connor (2009). Openness to experience, plasticity, and creativity: exploring lower-order, high-order, and interactive effects. *Journal of Research in Personality 43*(6), 1087–90.

Simmons, A. (2012). Cartesian consciousness reconsidered. *Philosophers Imprint 12*(2), 1–21.

Simons, D. J. and C. F. Chabris (1999). Gorillas in our midst: sustained inattentional blindness for dynamic events. *Perception 28*(9), 1059–74.

Simonsson, O. and S. B. Goldberg (2022). Linkages between psychedelics and meditation in a population-based sample in the United States. *Journal of Psychoactive Drugs*, 1–8.

Simonton, D. K. (2013). What is a creative idea? Little-c versus big-C creativity. In K. Thomas and J. Chan (eds.), *Handbook of Research on Creativity*, pp. 69–83. London: Edward Elgar Publishing.

Singh, A. and N. Srinivasan (2019). Concentrative (Sahaj Samadhi) meditation expands subjective time. *PsyCh Journal 8*(1), 28–35.

Sjöstedt-Hughes, P. (2022). The white sun of substance: Spinozism and the psychedelic amor dei intellectualis. In C. Hauskeller and P. Sjöstedt-Hughes (eds.), *Philosophy and Psychedelics: Frameworks for Exceptional Experience*. London: Bloomsbury Academic.

Slagter, H. A., A. Lutz, L. L. Greischar, A. D. Francis, S. Nieuwenhuis, J. M. Davis, and R. J. Davidson (2007). Mental training affects distribution of limited brain resources. *PLOS Biology 5*(6), e138.

Sloane, B. and J. W. L. Doust (1954). Psychophysiological investigations in experimental psychoses: results of the exhibition of D-lysergic acid diethylamide to psychiatric patients. *Journal of Mental Science 100*(418), 129–44.

Smigielski, L., M. Kometer, M. Scheidegger, R. Krähenmann, T. Huber, and F. X. Vollenweider (2019). Characterization and prediction of acute and sustained response to psychedelic psilocybin in a mindfulness group retreat. *Scientific Reports 9*(1), 14914.

Smith, A. (1776). *The Wealth of Nations*. London: W. Strahan and T. Cadell.

Smith, H. (1964). Do drugs have religious import? *Journal of Philosophy 61*(18), 517–30.

Smith, H., C. Grob, R. Jesse, G. Bravo, A. Agar, and R. Walsh (2004). Do drugs have religious import? A 40-year retrospective. *Journal of Humanistic Psychology 44*(2), 120–40.

Smith, M. F. (2014). Lucid dreaming as a problem-solving method. Ph.D. thesis.

Smyth, A., K. M. Werner, M. Milyavskaya, A. Holding, and R. Koestner (2020). Do mindful people set better goals? Investigating the relation between trait mindfulness, self-concordance, and goal progress. *Journal of Research in Personality 88*, 104015.

Smythies, J. R. (1960). The stroboscopic patterns: III. Further experiments and discussion. *British Journal of Psychology 51*(3), 247–55.

Soler, J., M. Elices, E. Dominguez-Clavé, J. C. Pascual, A. Feilding, M. Navarro-Gil, J. García-Campayo, and J. Riba (2018). Four weekly ayahuasca sessions lead to increases in 'acceptance' capacities: a comparison study with a standard 8-week mindfulness training program. *Frontiers in Pharmacology 9*, 224.

Soler, J., M. Elices, A. Franquesa, S. Barker, P. Friedlander, A. Feilding, J. C. Pascual, and J. Riba (2016). Exploring the therapeutic potential of ayahuasca: acute intake increases mindfulness-related capacities. *Psychopharmacology 233*(5), 823–9.

Sollberger, M. (2013). Rethinking synesthesia. *Philosophical Psychology 26*(2), 171–87.

Soon, C. S., M. Brass, H.-J. Heinze, and J.-D. Haynes (2008). Unconscious determinants of free decisions in the human brain. *Nature Neuroscience 11*(5), 543–5.

Spilka, B., R. Hood, B. Hunsberger, and R. Gorsuch (2005). *The Psychology of Religion: An Empirical Approach*. New York: Guilford Press.

Spiller, H. A., J. R. Hale, and J. Z. D. Boer (2002). The Delphic oracle: a multidisciplinary defense of the gaseous vent theory. *Journal of Toxicology: Clinical Toxicology 40*(2), 189–96.

Spitzer, M., M. Thimm, L. Hermle, P. Holzmann, K.-A. Kovar, H. Heimann, E. Gouzoulis-Mayfrank, U. Kischka, and F. Schneider (1996). Increased activation of indirect semantic associations under psilocybin. *Biological Psychiatry 39*(12), 1055–7.

Srinivasan, N. and A. Singh (2017). Concentrative meditation influences visual awareness: a study with color afterimages. *Mindfulness 8*(1), 17–26.

Srinivasan, N., S. Tripathi, and I. Singhal (2020). Meditators exercise better endogenous and exogenous control of visual awareness. *Mindfulness 11*(12), 2705–14.

Stace, W. T. (1960). *Mysticism and Philosophy*. New York: Palgrave Macmillan.

Steinhart, E. (2017). *More Precisely: The Math You Need to Do Philosophy*. Peterborough, Ont.: Broadview Press.

Stern, P. (1997). The rule of wisdom and the rule of law in Plato's statesman. *American Political Science Review 91*(2), 264–76.

Stoliker, D., L. Novelli, F. X. Vollenweider, G. F. Egan, K. H. Preller, and Razi, A. (2023). Effective connectivity of functionally anticorrelated networks under lysergic acid diethylamide. *Biological Psychiatry 93*(3), 224–32.

Strawson, G. (2009). *Selves: An Essay in Revisionary Metaphysics*. Oxford: Oxford University Press.

Strick, M., T. H. v. Noorden, R. R. Ritskes, J. R. d. Ruiter, and A. Dijksterhuis (2012, 4). Zen meditation and access to information in the unconscious. *Consciousness and Cognition 21*(3), 1476–81.

Studerus, E., A. Gamma, M. Kometer, and F. X. Vollenweider (2012). Prediction of psilocybin response in healthy volunteers. *PLOS One 7*(2), e30800.

Studerus, E., A. Gamma, and F. X. Vollenweider (2010). Psychometric evaluation of the altered states of consciousness rating scale (OAV). *PLOS One 5*(8), e12412.

Stumbrys, T. and M. Daniels (2010). An exploratory study of creative problem solving in lucid dreams: preliminary findings and methodological considerations. *International Journal of Dream Research 3*(2), 121–9.

Stuss, D. T., K. J. Murphy, M. A. Binns, and M. P. Alexander (2003). Staying on the job: the frontal lobes control individual performance variability. *Brain 126*(11), 2363–80.

Sumantry, D. and K. E. Stewart (2021). Meditation, mindfulness, and attention: a meta-analysis. *Mindfulness 12*(6), 1332–49.

Suzuki, D. T. (1957). *Mysticism: Christian and Buddhist*. New York: Harper and Row.

Suzuki, D. T. (1964). An Introduction to Zen Buddhism. New York: Grove Press.

Suzuki, D. T. (1971). Religion and drugs. *The Eastern Buddhist 4*(2), 128–33.

Suzuki, D. T. (2014). On Satori—the revelation of a new truth in Zen Buddhism. In R. M. Jaffe (ed.), *Selected Works of D.T. Suzuki, Volume I*, pp. 14–38.

Suzuki, S. (1970). *Zen Mind, Beginner's Mind: Informal Talks on Zen Meditation and Practice*. New York: Walker/Weatherhill.

Swanson, L. R. (2018). Unifying theories of psychedelic drug effects. *Frontiers in Pharmacology 9*, 172.

Sweat, N. W., L. W. Bates, and P. S. Hendricks (2016). The associations of naturalistic classic psychedelic use, mystical experience, and creative problem solving. *Journal of Psychoactive Drugs 48*(5), 344–50.

Swift, T. C., A. B. Belser, G. Agin-Liebes, N. Devenot, S. Terrana, H. L. Friedman, J. Guss, A. P. Bossis, and S. Ross (2017). Cancer at the dinner table: experiences of psilocybin-assisted psychotherapy for the treatment of cancer-related distress. *Journal of Humanistic Psychology 57*(5), 488–519.

Swift, V., K. E. Wilson, and J. B. Peterson (2020). Zooming in on the attentional foundations of the Big Five. *Personality and Individual Differences 164*, 110000.

Sytsma, J. and J. Livengood (2015). *The Theory and Practice of Experimental Philosophy.* Peterborough, Ont.: Broadview Press.

Szabo, A. (2015). Psychedelics and immunomodulation: novel approaches and therapeutic opportunities. *Frontiers in Immunology 6*, 358.

Szabo, A. (2019). Effects of psychedelics on inflammation and immunity. In M. Winkelman and B. Sessa (eds.), *Advances in Psychedelic Medicine: State-of-the-Art Therapeutic Applications.* Goleta, CA: Praeger.

Szabo, A. and E. Frecska (2016). Dimethyltryptamine (DMT): a biochemical Swiss Army knife in neuroinflammation and neuroprotection? *Neural Regeneration Research 11*(3), 396–7.

Tagliazucchi, E., R. Carhart-Harris, R. Leech, D. Nutt, and D. R. Chialvo (2014). Enhanced repertoire of brain dynamical states during the psychedelic experience. *arXiv 35*(11), 5442–56.

Tass, P. (1995). Cortical pattern formation during visual hallucinations. *Journal of Biological Physics 21*(3), 177–210.

Taves, A. (2020). Mystical and other alterations in sense of self: an expanded framework for studying nonordinary experiences. *Perspectives on Psychological Science 15*(3), 669–90.

Teasdale, J. D., Z. Segal, and J. G. Williams (1995). How does cognitive therapy prevent depressive relapse and why should attentional control (mindfulness) training help? *Behaviour Research and Therapy 33*(1), 25–39.

Teper, R., Z. V. Segal, and M. Inzlicht (2013). Inside the mindful mind. *Current Directions in Psychological Science 22*(6), 449–54.

Thanissaro, B. (2014). There is no self, url: https://tricycle.org/magazine/there-no-self/.

Thibault, L., R. v. d. Berg, P. Cavanagh, and C. Sergent (2016). Retrospective attention gates discrete conscious access to past sensory stimuli. *PLOS One 11*(2), e0148504.

Thompson, B. L. and J. Waltz (2007). Everyday mindfulness and mindfulness meditation: overlapping constructs or not? *Personality and Individual Differences 43*(7), 1875–85.

Thompson, C. and A. Szabo (2020). Psychedelics as a novel approach to treating autoimmune conditions. *Immunology Letters 228*, 45–54.

Thompson, E. (2020). *Why I Am Not a Buddhist.* New Haven: Yale University Press.

Thānissaro, B. (2012). *Right Mindfulness.* Valley Center, CA: self published.

Titelbaum, M. G. (2011). Symmetry and evidential support. *Symmetry 3*(3), 680–98.

Tomasi, D., G.-J. Wang, and N. D. Volkow (2013). Energetic cost of brain functional connectivity. *Proceedings of the National Academy of Sciences 110*(33), 13642–7.

Tomasino, B., S. Fregona, M. Skrap, and F. Fabbro (2013). Meditation-related activations are modulated by the practices needed to obtain it and by the expertise: an ALE meta-analysis study. *Frontiers in Human Neuroscience 6*, 346.

Tononi, G. (2004). An information integration theory of consciousness. *BMC Neuroscience 5*(1), 42.

Tredennick, H. (1989). *Aristotle in 23 Volumes.* Cambridge, MA: Cambridge University Press.

Treves, I. N., L. Y. Tello, R. J. Davidson, and S. B. Goldberg (2019). The relationship between mindfulness and objective measures of body awareness: a meta-analysis. *Scientific Reports 9*(1), 17386.

Tse, P. U. (2005). Voluntary attention modulates the brightness of overlapping transparent surfaces. *Vision Research 45*(9), 1095–8.

Tulving, E. and Z. Pearlstone (1966). Availability versus accessibility of information in memory for words. *Journal of Verbal Learning and Verbal Behavior 5*(4), 381–91.

Turing, A. M. (1952). The chemical basis of morphogenesis. *Philosophical Transactions of the Royal Society of London. Series B, Biological Sciences 237*(641), 37–72.

Uthaug, M. V., R. Lancelotta, K. v. Oorsouw, K. P. C. Kuypers, N. Mason, J. Rak, A. Šuláková, R. Jurok, M. Maryška, M. Kuchař, T. Páleníček, J. Riba, and J. G. Ramaekers (2019). A single inhalation of vapor from dried toad secretion containing 5-methoxy-N,N-dimethyltryptamine (5-MeO-DMT) in a naturalistic setting is related to sustained enhancement of satisfaction with life, mindfulness-related capacities, and a decrement of psychopathological symptoms. *Psychopharmacology 236*(9), 2653–66.

Uthaug, M. V., R. Lancelotta, A. Szabo, A. K. Davis, J. Riba, and J. G. Ramaekers (2020). Prospective examination of synthetic 5-methoxy-N,N-dimethyltryptamine inhalation: effects on salivary IL-6, cortisol levels, affect, and non-judgment. *Psychopharmacology 237*(3), 773–85.

Uthaug, M. V., K. v. Oorsouw, K. P. C. Kuypers, M. v. Boxtel, N. J. Broers, N. L. Mason, S. W. Toennes, J. Riba, and J. G. Ramaekers (2018). Sub-acute and long-term effects of ayahuasca on affect and cognitive thinking style and their association with ego dissolution. *Psychopharmacology 235*(10), 2979–89.

VandenBos, G. (2015). *APA Dictionary of Psychology* (2nd ed.). Washington, DC: American Psychological Association.

Vannucci, M., C. Pelagatti, M. Hanczakowski, and C. Chiorri (2019). Visual attentional load affects the frequency of involuntary autobiographical memories and their level of meta-awareness. *Memory & Cognition 47*(1), 117–29.

Vervaeke, J. and L. Ferraro (2016). Reformulating the mindfulness construct: the cognitive processes at work in mindfulness, hypnosis, and mystical states. In A. Raz and M. Lifshitz (eds.), *Hypnosis and Meditation: Towards an Integrative Science of Conscious Planes*, pp. 241–68. Oxford: Oxford University Press.

Visser, T., P. Merikle, and V. D. Lollo (2005). Priming in the attentional blink: perception without awareness? *Visual Cognition 12*(7), 1362–72.

Vivot, R. M., C. Pallavicini, F. Zamberlan, D. Vigo, and E. Tagliazucchi (2020). Meditation increases the entropy of brain oscillatory activity. *Neuroscience 431*, 40–51.

Vollenweider, F. (1998). Advances and pathophysiological models of hallucinogenic drug actions in humans: a preamble to schizophrenia research. *Pharmacopsychiatry 31*(S 2), 92–103.

Vollenweider, F. X., P. A. Csomor, B. Knappe, M. A. Geyer, and B. B. Quednow (2007). The effects of the preferential 5-HT2A agonist psilocybin on prepulse inhibition of startle in healthy human volunteers depend on interstimulus interval. *Neuropsychopharmacology 32*(9), 1876–87.

Vollenweider, F. X. and M. A. Geyer (2001). A systems model of altered consciousness: integrating natural and drug-induced psychoses. *Brain Research Bulletin 56*, 495–507.

Vollenweider, F., K. Leenders, C. Scharfetter, P. Maguire, O. Stadelmann, and J. Angst (1997). Positron emission tomography and fluorodeoxyglucose studies of metabolic hyperfrontality and psychopathology in the psilocybin model of psychosis. *Neuropsychopharmacology 16*(5), 357–72.

Vugt, M. K. v., P. Hitchcock, B. Shahar, and W. Britton (2012). The effects of mindfulness-based cognitive therapy on affective memory recall dynamics in depression: a mechanistic model of rumination. *Frontiers in Human Neuroscience 6*, 257.

Vugt, M. K. v. and H. A. Slagter (2014). Control over experience? Magnitude of the attentional blink depends on meditative state. *Consciousness and Cognition 23*, 32–9.

Wackermann, J., M. Wittmann, F. Hasler, and F. X. Vollenweider (2008). Effects of varied doses of psilocybin on time interval reproduction in human subjects. *Neuroscience Letters 435*(1), 51–5.

Wagstaff, G., J. Brunas-Wagstaff, J. Cole, and J. Wheatcroft (2004). New directions in forensic hypnosis: facilitating memory with a focused meditation technique. *Contemporary Hypnosis 21*(1), 14–27.

Wagstaff, G. F., J. Brunas-Wagstaff, J. Cole, L. Knapton, J. Winterbottom, V. Crean, and J. Wheatcroft (2004). Facilitating memory with hypnosis, focused meditation, and eye closure. *International Journal of Clinical and Experimental Hypnosis 52*(4), 434–55.

Wagstaff, G. F., J. M. Wheatcroft, C. L. Burt, H. J. Pilkington, K. Wilkinson, and J. D. Hoyle (2011). Enhancing witness memory with focused meditation and eye-closure: assessing the effects of misinformation. *Journal of Police and Criminal Psychology 26*(2), 152–61.

Wahn, B. and P. König (2017). Is attentional resource allocation across sensory modalities task-dependent? *Advances in Cognitive Psychology 13*(1), 83–96.

Walbridge, J. and H. Ziai (1999). *The Philosophy of Illumination*. Provo, UT: Brigham Young University Press.

Wallace, A. (1998). *Bridge of Quiescence: Experiencing Tibetan Buddhist Meditation*. Chicago: Open Court.

Wallace, B. A. (2006). *The Attention Revolution: Unlocking the Power of the Focused Mind*. Somerville, MA: Wisdom Publications.

Walley, S. M. (2012). Historical origins of indentation hardness testing. *Materials Science and Technology 28*(9–10), 1028–44.

Walshe, M. O. (2010). *The Complete Mystical Works of Meister Eckhart*. New York: Crossroads.

Wamsley, E. J. and R. Stickgold (2019). Dreaming of a learning task is associated with enhanced memory consolidation: replication in an overnight sleep study. *Journal of Sleep Research 28*(1), e12749.

Wamsley, E. J., M. Tucker, J. D. Payne, J. A. Benavides, and R. Stickgold (2010). Dreaming of a learning task is associated with enhanced sleep-dependent memory consolidation. *Current Biology 20*(9), 850–5.

Wang, Y., L. Xiao, W. Gong, Y. Chen, X. Lin, Y. Sun, N. Wang, J. Wang, and F. Luo (2022). Mindful non-reactivity is associated with improved accuracy in attentional blink testing: a randomized controlled trial. *Current Psychology 41*(12), 1–13.

Ward, L. M. (2013). The thalamus: gateway to the mind. *Wiley Interdisciplinary Reviews: Cognitive Science 4*(6), 609–22.

Watts, R., C. Day, J. Krzanowski, D. Nutt, and R. Carhart-Harris (2017). Patients' accounts of increased 'connectedness' and 'acceptance' after psilocybin for treatment-resistant depression. *Journal of Humanistic Psychology 57*(5), 520–64.

Watzl, S. (2017). *Structuring Mind: The Nature of Attention and How It Shapes Consciousness*. Oxford: Oxford University Press.

Weisberg, R. W. (1993). *Creativity: Beyond the Myth of Genius*. New York: Freeman.

Weiss, M. N. (2017). Philosophical mindfulness. An essay about the art of philosophizing. *Haser 8*, 91–138.

Wells, B. (1974). *Psychedelic Drugs*. New York: Jason Aronson.

Wendt, B. A., H. B. Bell, O. G. Buroker, and A. C. G. Hall (2021). Using a false memory paradigm to understand the cognitive effects of meditation. *Mindfulness 12*(4), 1022–33.

Wenk-Sormaz, H. (2005). Meditation can reduce habitual responding. *Alternative Therapies in Health and Medicine 11*(2), 42–58.

Werner-Seidler, A. and T. Dalgleish (2016). The method of loci improves longer-term retention of self-affirming memories and facilitates access to mood-repairing memories in recurrent depression. *Clinical Psychological Science 4*(6), 1065–72.

Wheatstone, C. (1838). XVIII. Contributions to the physiology of vision.—Part the first. On some remarkable, and hitherto unobserved, phenomena of binocular vision. *Philosophical Transactions of the Royal Society of London 128*(128), 371–94.

Whitehead, A. N. (1938). *Modes of Thought*. New York: Macmillan Company.

Whitfield, H. J. (2021). A spectrum of selves reinforced in multilevel coherence: a contextual behavioural response to the challenges of psychedelic-assisted therapy development. *Frontiers in Psychiatry 12*, 727572.

Wielgosz, J., S. B. Goldberg, T. R. A. Kral, J. D. Dunne, and R. J. Davidson (2019). Mindfulness meditation and psychopathology. *Annual Review of Clinical Psychology 15*(1), 285–316.

Williams, J. M. G., J. D. Teasdale, Z. V. Segal, and J. Soulsby (2000). Mindfulness-based cognitive therapy reduces overgeneral autobiographical memory in formerly depressed patients. *Journal of Abnormal Psychology 109*(1), 150.

Wilson, B. M., L. Mickes, S. Stolarz-Fantino, M. Evrard, and E. Fantino (2015). Increased false-memory susceptibility after mindfulness meditation. *Psychological Science 26*(10), 1567–73.

Wilson, T. D. (2002). *Strangers to Ourselves: Discovering the Adaptive Unconscious*. Cambridge, MA: Belknarp Press.

Wilson, T. D. (2009). Know thyself. *Perspectives on Psychological Science 4*(4), 384–9.

Wilson, T. D. and E. W. Dunn (2004). Self-knowledge: its limits, value, and potential for improvement. *Annual Review of Psychology 55*(1), 493–518.

Wilson, T. R. (1974). *Review of Psychedelic Drugs: Psychological, Medical and Social Issues*. By Brian Wells. London: Penguin Books. 1973. *British Journal of Psychiatry 124*(580), 309.

Winkelman, M. J. (2017). The mechanisms of psychedelic visionary experiences: hypotheses from evolutionary psychology. *Frontiers in Neuroscience 11*, 539.

Wittgenstein, L. (1999). *Tractatus Logico-Philosophicus*. Mineola, NY: Dover Publications.

Wittmann, M., O. Carter, F. Hasler, B. R. Cahn, U. Grimberg, P. Spring, D. Hell, H. Flohr, and F. X. Vollenweider (2007). Effects of psilocybin on time perception and temporal control of behaviour in humans. *Journal of Psychopharmacology 21*(1), 50–64.

Wood, K. and D. J. Simons (2019). Processing without noticing in inattentional blindness: a replication of Moore and Egeth (1997) and Mack and Rock (1998). *Attention, Perception, & Psychophysics 81*(1), 1–11.

Wright, R. (2017). *Why Buddhism Is True*. New York: Simon & Schuster.

Wronska, M. K., A. Kolańczyk, and B. A. Nijstad (2018). Engaging in creativity broadens attentional scope. *Frontiers in Psychology 9*, 1–14.

Xu, J., A. Vik, I. R. Groote, J. Lagopoulos, A. Holen, O. Ellingsen, A. K. Håberg, and S. Davanger (2014). Nondirective meditation activates default mode network and areas associated with memory retrieval and emotional processing. *Frontiers in Human Neuroscience 8*, 86.

Xue, J., Y. Zhang, and Y. Huang (2019). A meta-analytic investigation of the impact of mindfulness-based interventions on ADHD symptoms. *Medicine 98*(23), e15957.

Yaden, D. B., J. C. Eichstaedt, H. A. Schwartz, M. L. Kern, K. D. L. Nguyen, N. A. Wintering, R. W. H. Jr., and A. B. Newberg (2015). The language of ineffability: linguistic analysis of mystical experiences. *Psychology of Religion and Spirituality 8*(3), 244.

Yaden, D. B., J. Iwry, K. J. Slack, J. C. Eiechstaedt, Y. Zhao, G. E. Vaillant, and A. B. Newberg (2016). The overview effect: awe and self-transcendent experience in space flight. *Psychology of Consciousness: Theory, Research, and Practice 3*(1), 1–11.

Yaden, D. B., K. D. L. Nguyen, M. L. Kern, A. B. Belser, J. C. Eichstaedt, J. Iwry, M. E. Smith, N. A. Wintering, R. W. Hood, and A. B. Newberg (2017). Of roots and fruits:

a comparison of psychedelic and nonpsychedelic mystical experiences. *Journal of Humanistic Psychology 57*(4), 338–53.

Yanakieva, S., N. Polychroni, N. Family, L. T. J. Williams, D. P. Luke, and D. B. Terhune (2018). The effects of microdose LSD on time perception: a randomised, double-blind, placebo-controlled trial. *Psychopharmacology 236*(4), 1159–70.

Young, M. S. and N. A. Stanton (2002). Malleable attentional resources theory: a new explanation for the effects of mental underload on performance. *Human Factors: Journal of Human Factors and Ergonomics Society 44*(3), 365–75.

Zabelina, D. L. (2018). Creativity and attention. In R. E. Jung and O. Vartanian (eds.), *The Cambridge Handbook of the Neuroscience of Creativity*, pp. 161–79. Cambridge: Cambridge University Press.

Zaehner, R. C. (1957). *Mysticism, Sacred and Profane: An Inquiry into Some Varieties of Praeternatural Experience*. Oxford: Oxford University Press.

Zaehner, R. C. (1972). *Drugs, Mysticism and Make-Believe*. London: William Collins.

Zahavi, D. and U. Kriegel (2016). For-me-ness: what it is and what it is not. In D. Dahistrom, L. Elpidorou, and W. Hopp (eds.), *Philosophy of Mind and Phenomenology: Conceptual and Empirical Approaches*, pp. 36–53. London: Routledge.

Zakay, D. and R. A. Block (1995). An attentional gate model of prospective time estimation. In V. D. Keyser, G. d'Ydewalle, and A. Vandierendonck (eds.), *Time and the Dynamic Control of Behavior*, pp. 167–78. Liege, Belgium: Universite de Liege.

Zamaria, J. A. (2016). A Phenomenological Examination of Psilocybin and its Positive and Persisting Aftereffects. *NeuroQuantology, 14*(2). https://doi.org/10.14704/nq. 2016.14.2.943

Zanesco, A. P., B. G. King, C. Powers, R. D. Meo, K. Wineberg, K. A. MacLean, and C. D. Saron (2019). Modulation of event-related potentials of visual discrimination by meditation training and sustained attention. *Journal of Cognitive Neuroscience 31*(8), 1184–204.

Zegans, L. S., J. C. Pollard, and D. Brown (1967). The effects of LSD-25 on creativity and tolerance to regression. *Archives of General Psychiatry 16*(6), 740.

Zeidan, F., S. K. Johnson, B. J. Diamond, Z. David, and P. Goolkasian (2010). Mindfulness meditation improves cognition: evidence of brief mental training. *Consciousness and Cognition 19*(2), 597–605.

Zhang, J., W. Ding, Y. Li, and C. Wu (2013). Task complexity matters: the influence of trait mindfulness on task and safety performance of nuclear power plant operators. *Personality and Individual Differences 55*(4), 433–9.

Zhang, P., S. Engel, C. Rios, B. He, and S. He (2010). Binocular rivalry requires visual attention: evidence from EEG. *Journal of Vision 9*(8), 291, url: https://jov.arvojournals. org/article.aspx?articleid=2135693.

Zhang, R., S. A. Engel, and K. Kay (2017). Binocular rivalry: a window into cortical competition and suppression. *Journal of the Indian Institute of Science 97*(4), 477–85.

Zhong, C.-B., A. Dijksterhuis, and A. D. Galinsky (2008, 3). The merits of unconscious thought in creativity. *Psychological Science 19*(9), 912–18.

Zivony, A., S. Shanny, and D. Lamy (2018). Perceptual processing is not spared during the attentional blink. *Journal of Cognition 1*(1), 18.

Index